DSM-IV
TRAINING GUIDE

DSM-IV
TRAINING GUIDE

WILLIAM H. REID, M.D., M.P.H.

Medical Director
Texas Department of Mental Health and Retardation

Professor of Psychiatry
Liaison for Mental Health and Mental Retardation Affairs
The University of Texas System

Adjunct Professor of Psychiatry
Texas A & M College of Medicine

MICHAEL G. WISE, M.D.

Clinical Professor of Psychiatry
Louisiana State University School of Medicine
Tulane School of Medicine
Uniformed Services University of the Health Sciences,
F. Edward Hebert School of Medicine

BRUNNER/MAZEL *PUBLISHERS* • NEW YORK

Note: "DSM-III-R," "DSM-IV," and the contents of the American Psychiatric
Association's *Diagnostic and Statistical Manuals of Mental Disorders* are copyrighted by the
American Psychiatric Association.

Library of Congress Cataloging-in-Publication Data

Reid, William H.
    DSM-IV training guide
  fourth edition / William H. Reid and Michael G. Wise.
      p. cm.
    Includes bibliographical references and index.
    ISBN 0-87630-763-2 (pbk.).—ISBN 0-87630-768-3 (cloth)
    1. Mental illness—Classification. 2. Mental illness—Diagnosis.
  3. Diagnostic and statistical manual of mental disorders. I. Wise,
  Michael G. II. Diagnostic and statistical manual of
  mental disorders. III. Title.
    [DNLM: 1. Mental Disorders—classification. 2. Mental Disorders—
  diagnosis. WM 15 R359d 1995]
  RC455.2.C4R45 1995
  616.89′075—dc20
  DNLM/DLC
  for Library of Congress   95-9947
                                          CIP

Published by Brunner/Mazel, Inc.
19 Union Square West
New York, New York 10003

Designed by Susan Phillips

Manufactured in the United States of America

10 9 8 7 6 5 4 3 2

To our patients, and to those who help them receive proper diagnosis and treatment

CONTENTS*

*See list of DSM-IV and corresponding ICD-10 classifications for a chapter-by-chapter breakdown of every disorder discussed in this book.

LIST OF *DSM-IV* AND CORRESPONDING *ICD-10* CLASSIFICATIONS

Disorders Usually First Diagnosed in Infancy, Childhood, or Adolescence (Chapter 10)

MENTAL RETARDATION

317	Mild Mental Retardation	F70.9
318.0	Moderate Mental Retardation	F71.9
318.1	Severe Mental Retardation	F72.9
318.2	Profound Mental Retardation	F73.9
319	Mental Retardation, Severity Unspecified	F79.9

LEARNING DISORDERS

315.00	Reading Disorder	F81.0
315.1	Mathematics Disorder	F81.2
315.2	Disorder of Written Expression	F81.8
315.9	Learning Disorder NOS	F81.9

MOTOR SKILLS DISORDER

315.4	Developmental Coordination Disorder	F82

COMMUNICATION DISORDERS

315.31	Expressive Language Disorder	F80.1
315.31	Mixed Receptive-Expressive Language Disorder	F80.2
315.39	Phonological Disorder	F80.0
307.0	Stuttering	F98.5
307.9	Communication Disorder NOS	F80.9

Pervasive Developmental Disorders

299.00	Autistic Disorder	F84.0
299.80	Rett's Disorder	F84.2
299.10	Childhood Disintegrative Disorder	F84.3
299.80	Asperger's Disorder	F84.5
299.80	Pervasive Developmental Disorder NOS	F84.9

Attention-Deficit and Disruptive Behavior Disorders

314.xx	Attention-Deficit/Hyperactivity Disorder	
.01	Combined Type	F90.0
.00	Predominantly Inattentive Type	F98.8
.01	Predominantly Hyperactive-Impulsive Type	F90.0
314.9	Attention-Deficit/Hyperactivity Disorder NOS	F90.9
312.8	Conduct Disorder	F91.8
313.81	Oppositional Defiant Disorder	F91.3
312.9	Disruptive Behavior Disorder NOS	F91.9

Feeding and Eating Disorders of Infancy or Early Childhood

307.52	Pica	F98.3
307.53	Rumination Disorder	F98.2
307.59	Feeding Disorder of Infancy or Early Childhood	F98.2

Tic Disorders

307.23	Tourette's Disorder	F95.2
307.22	Chronic Motor or Vocal Tic Disorder	F95.1
307.21	Transient Tic Disorder	F95.0
307.20	Tic Disorder NOS	F95.9

Elimination Disorders

	Encopresis	
787.6	With Constipation and Overflow Incontinence	R15
307.7	Without Constipation and Overflow Incontinence	F98.1
307.6	Enuresis (Not Due to a General Medical Condition)	F98.0

Other Disorders of Infancy, Childhood, or Adolescence

309.21	Separation Anxiety Disorder	F93.0
313.23	Selective Mutism	F94.0

Amphetamine (or Amphetamine-Like)–Related Disorders

AMPHETAMINE USE DISORDERS

304.40	Amphetamine Dependence	F15.2x
305.70	Amphetamine Abuse	F15.1

AMPHETAMINE-INDUCED DISORDERS

292.89	Amphetamine Intoxication	F15.00
	With Perceptual Disturbances	F15.04
292.0	Amphetamine Withdrawal	F15.3
292.81	Amphetamine Intoxication Delirium	F15.03
292.xx	Amphetamine-Induced Psychotic Disorder	F15.xx
.11	With Delusions	.51
.12	With Hallucinations	.52
292.84	Amphetamine-Induced Mood Disorder	F15.8
292.89	Amphetamine-Induced Anxiety Disorder	F15.8
292.89	Amphetamine-Induced Sexual Dysfunction	F15.8
292.89	Amphetamine-Induced Sleep Disorder	F15.8
292.9	Amphetamine-Related Disorder NOS	F15.9

Caffeine-Related Disorders

CAFFEINE-INDUCED DISORDERS

305.90	Caffeine Intoxication	F15.00
292.89	Caffeine-Induced Anxiety Disorder	F15.8
292.89	Caffeine-Induced Sleep Disorder	F15.8
292.9	Caffeine-Related Disorder NOS	F15.9

Cannabis-Related Disorders

CANNABIS USE DISORDERS

304.30	Cannabis Dependence	F12.2x
305.20	Cannabis Abuse	F12.1

CANNABIS-INDUCED DISORDERS

292.89	Cannabis Intoxication	F12.00
	With Perceptual Disturbances	F12.04
292.81	Cannabis Intoxication Delirium	F12.03
292.xx	Cannabis-Induced Psychotic Disorder	F12.xx
.11	With Delusions	.51
.12	With Hallucinations	.52

292.89 Cannabis-Induced Anxiety Disorder   F12.8
292.9   Cannabis-Related Disorder NOS   F12.9

Cocaine-Related Disorders

COCAINE USE DISORDERS

304.20 Cocaine Dependence   F14.2x
305.60 Cocaine Abuse   F14.1

COCAINE-INDUCED DISORDERS

292.89 Cocaine Intoxication   F14.00
            With Perceptual Disturbances   F14.04
292.0   Cocaine Withdrawal   F14.3
292.81 Cocaine Intoxication Delirium   F14.03
292.xx Cocaine-Induced Psychotic Disorder
    .11   With Delusions   F14.51
    .12   With Hallucinations   F14.52
292.84 Cocaine-Induced Mood Disorder   F14.8
292.89 Cocaine-Induced Anxiety Disorder   F14.8
292.89 Cocaine-Induced Sexual Dysfunction   F14.8
292.89 Cocaine-Induced Sleep Disorder   F14.8
292.9   Cocaine-Related Disorder NOS   F14.9

Hallucinogen-Related Disorders

HALLUCINOGEN USE DISORDERS

304.50 Hallucinogen Dependence   F16.2x
305.30 Hallucinogen Abuse   F16.1

HALLUCINOGEN-INDUCED DISORDERS

292.89 Hallucinogen Intoxication   F16.00
292.89 Hallucinogen Persisting Perception Disorder   F16.70
            (Flashbacks)
292.81 Hallucinogen Intoxication Delirium   F16.03
292.xx Hallucinogen-Induced Psychotic Disorder   F16.xx
    .11   With Delusions   .51
    .12   With Hallucinations   .52
292.84 Hallucinogen-Induced Mood Disorder   F16.8
292.89 Hallucinogen-Induced Anxiety Disorder   F16.8
292.9   Hallucinogen-Related Disorder NOS   F16.9

Inhalant-Related Disorders

INHALANT USE DISORDERS

304.60	Inhalant Dependence	F18.2x
305.90	Inhalant Abuse	F18.1

INHALANT-INDUCED DISORDERS

292.89	Inhalant Intoxication	F18.00
292.81	Inhalant Intoxication Delirium	F18.03
292.82	Inhalant-Induced Persisting Dementia	F18.73
292.xx	Inhalant-Induced Psychotic Disorder	F18.xx
.11	With Delusions	.51
.12	With Hallucinations	.52
292.84	Inhalant-Induced Mood Disorder	F18.8
292.89	Inhalant-Induced Anxiety Disorder	F18.8
292.9	Inhalant-Related Disorder NOS	F18.9

Nicotine-Related Disorders

NICOTINE USE DISORDER

305.10	Nicotine Dependence	F17.2x

NICOTINE-INDUCED DISORDER

292.0	Nicotine Withdrawal	F17.3
292.9	Nicotine-Related Disorder NOS	F17.9

Opioid-Related Disorders

OPIOID USE DISORDERS

304.00	Opioid Dependence	F11.2x
305.50	Opioid Abuse	F11.1

OPIOID-INDUCED DISORDERS

292.89	Opioid Intoxication	F11.00
	With Perceptual Disturbances	F11.04
292.0	Opioid Withdrawal	F11.3
292.81	Opioid Intoxication Delirium	F11.03
292.xx	Opioid-Induced Psychotic Disorder	F11.xx
.11	With Delusions	.51
.12	With Hallucinations	.52
292.84	Opioid-Induced Mood Disorder	F11.8

292.84	Sedative-, Hypnotic-, or Anxiolytic-Induced Mood Disorder	F13.8
292.89	Sedative-, Hypnotic-, or Anxiolytic-Induced Anxiety Disorder	F13.8
292.89	Sedative-, Hypnotic-, or Anxiolytic-Induced Sexual Dysfunction	F13.8
292.89	Sedative-, Hypnotic-, or Anxiolytic-Induced Sleep Disorder	F13.8
292.9	Sedative-, Hypnotic-, or Anxiolytic-Related Disorder NOS	F13.9

Polysubstance-Related Disorders

| 304.80 | Polysubstance Dependence | F19.2x |

Other (or Unknown) Substance-Related Disorders

OTHER (OR UNKNOWN) SUBSTANCE USE DISORDERS

| 304.90 | Other (or Unknown) Substance Dependence | F19.2x |
| 305.90 | Other (or Unknown) Substance Abuse | F19.1 |

OTHER (OR UNKNOWN) SUBSTANCE-INDUCED DISORDERS

292.89	Other (or Unknown) Substance Intoxication	F19.00
	With Perceptual Disturbances	F19.04
292.0	Other (or Unknown) Substance Withdrawal	F19.3
292.81	Other (or Unknown) Substance-Induced Delirium	F19.03
292.82	Other (or Unknown) Substance-Induced Persisting Dementia	F19.73
292.83	Other (or Unknown) Substance-Induced Persisting Amnestic Disorder	F19.6
292.xx	Other (or Unknown) Substance-Induced Psychotic Disorder	F19.xx
.11	With Delusions	.51
.12	With Hallucinations	.52
292.84	Other (or Unknown) Substance-Induced Mood Disorder	F19.8
292.89	Other (or Unknown) Substance-Induced Anxiety Disorder	F19.8
292.89	Other (or Unknown) Substance-Induced Sexual Dysfunction	F19.8
292.89	Other (or Unknown) Substance-Induced Sleep Disorder	F19.8
292.9	Other (or Unknown) Substance-Related Disorder NOS	F19.9

Schizophrenia and Other Psychotic Disorders (Chapter 14)

295.xx	Schizophrenia	F20.xx
.30	Paranoid Type	.0x
.10	Disorganized Type	.1x
.20	Catatonic Type	.2x
.90	Undifferentiated Type	.3x
.60	Residual Type	.5x
295.40	Schizophreniform Disorder	F20.8
295.70	Schizoaffective Disorder	F25.x
	Bipolar Type	.0
	Depressive Type	.1
297.1	Delusional Disorder	F22.0
298.8	Brief Psychotic Disorder	F23.xx
	With Marked Stressor(s)	.81
	Without Marked Stressor(s)	.80
297.3	Shared Psychotic Disorder	F24
293.xx	Psychotic Disorder Due to . . . [Indicate the General Medical Condition]	F06.x
.81	With Delusions	.2
.82	With Hallucinations	.0
	Substance-Induced Psychotic Disorder	
298.9	Psychotic Disorder NOS	F29

Mood Disorders (Chapter 15)

DEPRESSIVE DISORDERS

296.2x	Major Depressive Disorder, Single Episode	F32.x
296.3x	Major Depressive Disorder, Recurrent	F33.x
300.4	Dysthymic Disorder	F34.1
311	Depressive Disorder NOS	F32.9

BIPOLAR DISORDERS

296.xx	Bipolar I Disorder	
.0x	Single Manic Episode	F30.x
.40	Most Recent Episode Hypomanic	F31.0
.4x	Most Recent Episode Manic	F31.x
.6x	Most Recent Episode Mixed	F31.6
.5x	Most Recent Episode Depressed	F31.x
.7	Most Recent Episode Unspecified	F31.9
296.89	Bipolar II Disorder	F31.8
301.13	Cyclothymic Disorder	F34.0
296.80	Bipolar Disorder NOS	F31.9

Anxiety Disorders (Chapter 16)

Somatoform Disorders (Chapter 17)

Factitious Disorders (Chapter 18)

Dissociative Disorders (Chapter 19)

Sexual and Gender Identity Disorders (Chapter 20)

Sexual Dysfunctions

SEXUAL DESIRE DISORDERS

SEXUAL AROUSAL DISORDERS

ORGASMIC DISORDERS

SEXUAL PAIN DISORDERS

Sexual Dysfunction Due to a Medical Condition

625.8	Female Hypoactive Sexual Desire Disorder Due to . . . [Indicate the General Medical Condition]	N94.8
608.89	Male Hypoactive Sexual Desire Disorder Due to . . . [Indicate the General Medical Condition]	N50.8
607.84	Male Erectile Disorder Due to . . . [Indicate the General Medical Condition]	N48.4
625.0	Female Dyspareunia Due to . . . [Indicate the General Medical Condition]	N94.1
608.89	Male Dyspareunia Due to . . . [Indicate the General Medical Condition]	N50.8
625.8	Other Female Sexual Dysfunction Due to . . . [Indicate the General Medical Condition]	N94.8
608.89	Other Male Sexual Dysfunction Due to . . . [Indicate the General Medical Condition] Substance-Induced Sexual Dysfunction	N50.8
302.70	Sexual Dysfunction NOS	F52.9

Paraphilias

302.4	Exhibitionism	F65.2
302.81	Fetishism	F65.0
302.89	Frotteurism	F65.8
302.2	Pedophilia	F65.4
302.83	Sexual Masochism	F65.5
302.84	Sexual Sadism	F65.5
302.3	Transvestic Fetishism	F65.1
302.82	Voyeurism	F65.3
302.9	Paraphilia NOS	F65.9

Gender Identity Disorders

302.xx	Gender Identity Disorder	F64.x
.6	In Children	.2
.85	In Adolescents or Adults	.0
302.6	Gender Identity Disorder NOS	F64.9
302.9	Sexual Disorder NOS	F52.9

Eating Disorders (Chapter 21)

307.1	Anorexia Nervosa	F50.0
307.51	Bulimia Nervosa	F50.2
307.50	Eating Disorder NOS	F50.9

Sleep Disorders (Chapter 22)

Primary Sleep Disorders

DYSSOMNIAS

307.42	Primary Insomnia	F51.0
307.44	Primary Hypersomnia	F51.1
347	Narcolepsy	G47.4
780.59	Breathing-Related Sleep Disorder	G47.3
307.45	Circadian Rhythm Sleep Disorder	F51.2
307.47	Dyssomnia NOS	F51.9

PARASOMNIAS

307.47	Nightmare Disorder	F51.5
307.46	Sleep Terror Disorder	F51.4
307.46	Sleepwalking Disorder	F51.3
307.47	Parasomnia NOS	F51.8

SLEEP DISORDERS RELATED TO ANOTHER MENTAL DISORDER

307.42	Insomnia Related to . . . [Indicate the Axis I or Axis II Disorder]	F51.0
307.44	Hypersomnia Related to . . . [Indicate the Axis I or Axis II Disorder]	F51.1

OTHER SLEEP DISORDERS

780.xx	Sleep Disorder Due to . . . [Indicate the General Medical Condition]	G47.x
.52	Insomnia Type	.0
.54	Hypersomnia Type	.1
.59	Parasomnia Type	.8
.59	Mixed Type	.8
	Substance-Induced Sleep Disorder	

Impulse Control Disorders Not Elsewhere Classified (Chapter 23)

312.34	Intermittent Explosive Disorder	F63.8
312.32	Kleptomania	F63.2
312.33	Pyromania	F63.1
312.31	Pathological Gambling	F63.0
312.39	Trichotillomania	F63.3
312.30	Impulse Control Disorder NOS	F63.9

Adjustment Disorders (Chapter 24)

309.xx	Adjustment Disorder	F43.xx
0	With Depressed Mood	.20
.24	With Anxiety	.28
.28	With Mixed Anxiety and Depressed Mood	.22
.3	With Disturbance of Conduct	.24
.4	With Mixed Disturbance of Emotions and Conduct	.25
.9	Unspecified	.9

Personality Disorders (Chapter 25)

301.0	Paranoid Personality Disorder	F60.0
301.20	Schizoid Personality Disorder	F60.1
301.22	Schizotypal Personality Disorder	F21
301.7	Antisocial Personality Disorder	F60.2
301.83	Borderline Personality Disorder	F60.31
301.50	Histrionic Personality Disorder	F60.4
301.81	Narcissistic Personality Disorder	F60.8
301.82	Avoidant Personality Disorder	F60.6
301.6	Dependent Personality Disorder	F60.7
301.4	Obsessive-Compulsive Personality Disorder	F60.5
301.9	Personality Disorder NOS	F60.9

Other Conditions That May Be a Focus of Clinical Attention (Chapter 26)

PSYCHOLOGICAL FACTORS AFFECTING MEDICAL CONDITION

316	. . . [Specified Psychological Factor] Affecting . . . [Indicate the General Medical Condition]	F54

MEDICATION-INDUCED MOVEMENT DISORDERS

332.1	Neuroleptic-Induced Parkinsonism	G21.0
333.92	Neuroleptic Malignant Syndrome	G21.0
333.7	Neuroleptic-Induced Acute Dystonia	G24.0
333.99	Neuroleptic-Induced Acute Akathisia	G21.1
333.82	Neuroleptic-Induced Tardive Dyskinesia	G24.0
333.1	Medication-Induced Postural Tremor	G25.1
333.90	Medication-Induced Movement Disorder NOS	G25.9

OTHER MEDICATION-INDUCED DISORDER

995.2	Adverse Effects of Medication NOS	T88.7

RELATIONAL PROBLEMS

V61.9	Relational Problem Related to a Mental Disorder or General Medical Condition	Z63.7
V61.20	Parent-Child Relational Problem	Z63.8
V61.1	Partner Relational Problem	Z63.0
V61.8	Sibling Relational Problem	F93.3
V62.81	Relational Problem NOS	Z63.9

PROBLEMS RELATED TO ABUSE OR NEGLECT

V61.21	Physical Abuse of Child	T74.1
V61.21	Sexual Abuse of Child	T74.2
V61.21	Neglect of Child	T74.0
V61.1	Physical Abuse of Adult	T74.1
V61.1	Sexual Abuse of Adult	T74.2

ADDITIONAL CONDITIONS THAT MAY BE A FOCUS OF CLINICAL ATTENTION

V15.81	Noncompliance With Treatment	Z91.1
V65.2	Malingering	Z76.5
V71.01	Adult Antisocial Behavior	Z72.8
V71.02	Child or Adolescent Antisocial Behavior	Z72.8
V62.89	Borderline Intellectual Functioning	R41.8
780.9	Age-Related Cognitive Decline	R41.8
V62.82	Bereavement	Z63.4
V62.3	Academic Problem	Z55.8
V62.2	Occupational Problem	Z56.7
313.82	Identity Problem	F93.8
V62.89	Religious or Spiritual Problem	Z71.8
V62.4	Acculturation Problem	Z60.3
V62.89	Phase of Life Problem	Z60.0

Additional Codes (Chapter 27)

300.9	Unspecified Mental Disorder	F99
V71.09	No Diagnosis or Condition on Axis I	Z03.2
799.9	Diagnosis or Condition Deferred on Axis I	R69
V71.09	No Diagnosis on Axis II	Z03.2
799.9	Diagnosis Deferred on Axis II	R46.8

FOREWORD

It gives me great pleasure to write the foreword to the *DSM-IV Training Guide* authored by two outstanding clinicians, educators, and academicians. William Reid is a noted forensic psychiatrist and medical administrator who has authored or edited eleven other books. He has special expertise in the diagnosis and treatment of patients with antisocial personality disorder and antisocial syndromes. Of particular relevance to this outstanding book is Dr. Reid's special interest in the DSM nomenclature system. Two previous books focused on the treatment of the DSM-III and DSM-III-R psychiatric disorders. This is his second book devoted to training clinicians on the proper use of the DSM. His previous publications have been outstanding and have contributed a great deal to the education of mental health professionals. His national prominence in forensic psychiatry and medical education contributes to the clarity and comprehensiveness of the *DSM-IV Training Guide*.

Michael Wise is one of the country's foremost consultation psychiatrists. A graduate of the stellar Massachusetts General Hospital Consultation Psychiatry Fellowship Program, Dr. Wise has written extensively in many publications on the diagnosis and treatment of patients with delirium and dementia. In addition, he was the co-author with Dr. James Rundell of two editions of the highly popular *Concise Guide to Consultation Psychiatry*. Dr. Wise also served as a member of the PSID Work Group of the DSM-IV Task Force and was responsible for the development of the diagnostic criteria for the "Impulse Control Disorders" section of the DSM-IV.

Both Dr. Reid and Dr. Wise were co-authors of the highly successful *DSM-III-R Training Guide*. This current text, *DSM-IV Training Guide*, is an equally outstanding volume.

The authors divide their book into two sections. The first section, appropriately titled "The Basics," provides a concise yet comprehensive summary of how clinicians should use the DSM-IV. The authors begin with a brief history of the DSM process including a discussion of the multiaxial classification system. They then summarize a number of the unique features of the DSM-IV and discuss how clinicians should approach the diagnostic process. With the use of case vignettes, they guide the reader in the clinical use of Axes I through V. They also provide a primer for clinicians on the appropriate use of the diagnostic codes contained within the DSM-IV text.

The second section is devoted to a discussion of all of the disorders contained in the DSM-IV. These chapters provide the essential information necessary for the clinician to properly diagnose a patient. This includes a general discussion of the disorder along with essential additional information that clinicians may require to make the appropriate diagnosis. Each of the chapters includes one or more case vignettes to highlight those particular issues that are contained in the text. As someone who is quite familiar with the DSM-IV (having served on the DSM-IV Task Force), I found the author's chapters on each of the disorders to be particularly well written and concise. In many cases they help clarify some of the subtle nuances contained in the DSM-IV diagnostic system.

The *DSM-IV Training Guide* written by Drs. Reid and Wise should be essential reading for all clinicians, whether in training or in practice, who wish a cogent summary of the proper diagnosis of mental disorders. The authors' discussions help to illuminate a number of issues that may be somewhat confusing for people less familiar with the DSM system. The cross-referencing to ICD-10 codes and their extensive index are especially helpful. In addition, in the front of the manual they provide a complete listing of all of the DSM-IV disorders and their corresponding ICD-10 codes.

The *DSM-IV Training Guide* is an important text for all mental health professionals' libraries. The added clarity that this book provides to clinicians in properly diagnosing patients is invaluable. This is an outstanding contribution to the field and should help all of us to appropriately diagnose and treat patients suffering from mental disorders.

Robert E. Hales, M.D.
Member, DSM-IV Task Force
American Psychiatric Association
Chairman, Department of Psychiatry
California Pacific Medical Center
Clinical Professor of Psychiatry
University of California, San Francisco

PREFACE

This book is written for the clinician (or student clinician) who needs to understand the complex biopsychosocial concepts of psychiatric diagnosis. Psychiatrists and psychotherapists, as well as medical students, psychiatric residents, and practicing physicians, need a concise, accurate guide to the latest standard of diagnostic nomenclature; this is what we have tried to produce. The *DSM-IV Training Guide* also serves as a valuable resource for counseling students, practicum trainees, psychology interns, and nonmedical psychotherapists.

This book can also be used with *The Complete DSM-IV Training Program*, consisting of a two volume set of videotaped vignettes and either instructional slides or overhead transparencies. The circled numbers you will see in the outside margins refer to those slides or transparencies. For ordering information, see the last page of this volume.

Decades ago, psychiatrists and psychologists often made diagnoses by clinical "feel" or "intuition." A patient "looked" depressed, or one had a "gut feeling" that he or she had a personality disorder. The art of diagnosis is still with us, but research has assumed a more important role in formulating diagnostic criteria. In psychiatry, the "science" of diagnosis is still young. For example, DSM-IV rarely lists physiologic or laboratory criteria, and our understanding of etiologic factors is not yet sufficient to employ them in most DSM-IV diagnoses. Nevertheless, the American Psychiatric Association's Diagnostic and Statistical Manuals have evolved toward reliability of catagorization and nomenclature, thus adding to the validity of studies that move us in the direction of greater understanding of patients and psychopathology. *Accurate diagnosis is the key to effective treatment.*

In our present world of diagnosis-related reimbursement, utilization review, and managed care, a word about diagnostic honesty is in order. Clinicians are often under great pressure to find clinical reasons to treat or not to treat. One may believe that making a particular diagnosis will affect the patient's access to treatment, the treatment itself, reimbursement for that treatment, and eligibility for benefits or entitlements. We strongly encourage the reader to strive for precision and thoroughness of assessment, and to be certain that the factors that influence diagnosis are wholly *clinical*, not economic or organizational ones.

The importance of accuracy, reliability, and completeness of diagnosis goes beyond the individual patient to other mental health and health care arenas. As the reader develops skills with DSM-IV, we encourage him or her to consider the far-reaching implications of patient assessment and diagnosis. The health care administrator needs diagnostic information to make decisions concerning

xxviii • DSM-IV TRAINING GUIDE

staffing and resource allocation. The health care payer, trying to allocate scarce premium or tax dollars, needs it for decisions about individual reimbursement, as well as for broad planning and policy development. Legislators and government managers must have aggregate diagnostic statistics to develop and implement public mental health policy.

Finally, careful reading of this book, and DSM-IV itself, should convince readers that these criteria and the accompanying text do not constitute what some clinicians and laypersons have mistakenly called a "cookbook" approach to diagnosis. DSM-IV contains clear *caveats* about improper uses of the criteria and multiaxial system, the training and experience necessary to use them in clinical settings, and environments in which their use is potentially inappropriate. We hope and believe that this *Training Guide* and its accompanying *Training Program* underscores the correct use of DSM-IV and that it will help the reader-clinician in the assessment and treatment of patients.

William H. Reid, M.D., M.P.H.
Michael G. Wise, M.D., F.A.C.P.

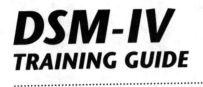

DSM-IV
TRAINING GUIDE

SECTION I
THE BASICS

CHAPTER 1

HISTORY AND EVOLUTION OF *DSM-IV*

Practitioners' desire to classify signs and symptoms of emotional distress into discrete disorders dates back thousands of years. The need to classify mental disorders, which is fundamental to their study, has led to the creation, revision, and demise of numerous classification systems. Fortunately, the mental health professional needs to be familiar with only two current classification systems to properly categorize patients with mental disorders or conditions. The first, published by the American Psychiatric Association (APA), is the *Diagnostic and Statistical Manual of Mental Disorders* (DSM). The latest manual in this series is DSM-IV, published in 1994. The second system is the *International Classification of Diseases* (ICD), which is published by the World Health Organization. The ICD is a worldwide statistical disease classification system for all medical conditions, including mental disorders.

HISTORY

An official U.S. classification for mental disorders was attempted only recently. The 1840 census classified all mental illness in a single category, "Idiocy." This early attempt was expanded in the 1880 census, in which seven mental disorder categories were listed: mania, melancholia, monomania, paresis, dementia, dyssomnia, and epilepsy (APA, DSM-IV, 1994). By the late 1920s, almost every medical teaching center used a different classification system for mental disorders. The result was a diverse nomenclature that often led to meaningless communications and arguments between professionals.

The 1933 Standard Classified Nomenclature of Disease (SCND), which addressed severe neurological and psychiatric disorders, attempted to bring order to the terminology. This nomenclature functioned reasonably well until a crisis in psychiatric terminology was sparked by symptoms seen in World War II veterans. Only 10% of the total cases seen by military psychiatrists could be classified using the SCND (APA, DSM, 1952). In addition, during the postwar period, three separate U.S. nomenclatures existed (the SCND, and those of the

Note: The circled numbers appearing in the margins of this text refer to the overhead transparencies or the instructional slides that are part of the *DMV-IV Training Program.* For more information, contact Brunner/Mazel Publishers, 19 Union Square West, New York, NY 10003. (212) 924-3344 or toll free 1-800-825-3089.

Armed Forces and the Veterans Administration system). None of these nomenclatures was consistent with the ICD.

....
DSM-I

As a result of the aforementioned confusion over terminology, the APA's
Committee on Nomenclature and Statistics proposed a revised classification system. After much deliberation, the first *Diagnostic and Statistical Manual of Mental
Disorders* (DSM) was published in 1952. The manual was later called DSM-I
when it became apparent that revisions were needed. DSM-I was reprinted 20
times, was distributed widely, and did much to stabilize mental health
nomenclature.

....
DSM-II

DSM-II was the result of an international collaborative effort that also
culminated in the mental disorders section in the eighth revision of the *International Classification of Diseases* (ICD-8). Both DSM-II and ICD-8 went into
effect in 1968.

....
DSM-III

Work on DSM-III began in 1974, in anticipation of ICD-9's 1979
scheduled publication date. Unfortunately, the mental disorders section proposed for ICD-9 was not sufficiently detailed for research and clinical work, so
the APA Task Force on Nomenclature and Statistics developed a new classification system. The development process was complicated and included 14 advisory committees, consultants from allied fields, liaison committees with professional organizations, conferences, and field trials. The field trials included
tests of diagnostic reliability, the results of which were published in Appendix F. DSM-III was a dramatic departure from previous DSMs. Innovations
included

> Definition of the term *mental disorder*
> Presentation of diagnostic criteria for each disorder
> Diagnosis according to a multiaxial evaluation system
> Redefinition of major disorders
> Addition of new diagnostic categories
> Hierarchical organization of diagnostic categories
> Systematic description of each disorder
> Decision trees for differential diagnosis
> Glossary of technical terms
> Annotated comparative listing of DSM-II and DSM-III
> Discussion of ICD-9 and ICD-9-CM

Publication of reliability data from field trials
Indices of diagnostic terms and symptoms

DSM-III-R

DSM-III-R's development and stated goals were similar to those of DSM-III. Twenty-six advisory committees were formed, each with membership based on expertise in a particular area. In addition, the experience gained in using the DSM-III diagnostic criteria, particularly in well-conducted research studies, played a significant role in proposed modifications. Two draft proposals of DSM-III-R were made available for critical review, and field trials were conducted. New appendices were added to DSM-III-R; they included proposed diagnostic categories needing further study (e.g., late luteal phase dysphoric disorder, sadistic personality disorder, and self-defeating personality disorder), an alphabetic listing of DSM-III-R diagnoses and codes, a numerical listing of DSM-III-R diagnoses and codes, and an index of selected symptoms.

DSM-IV

In 1988, only one year after DSM-III-R's publication, the APA formed a Task Force to revise DSM-III-R. The Task Force's purpose was to keep DSM diagnostic codes and terminology compatible with ICD-10, scheduled for publication in 1993 (actually published in 1992).

The 27-member Task Force on DSM-IV organized 13 work groups. Each work group, in collaboration with many expert advisers, was then responsible for developing certain sections of DSM-IV. In addition to conducting extensive literature reviews, these work groups reanalyzed existing data and performed numerous field trials to answer important issues regarding diagnoses and diagnostic criteria. (Note: The five-volume *DSM-IV Sourcebook* [APA, 1994 and in press] contains consolidated literature reviews, reports on data reanalyses and field trials, as well as rationale for Work Group decisions.)

This *DSM-IV Training Guide* will discuss specific changes to DSM-III-R that are found in the new edition. The major changes in DSM-IV include

❑ Axis IV is now used to list psychosocial and environmental problems that influence diagnosis, treatment, and prognosis (DSM-III-R Severity of Psychosocial Stressors Scales were eliminated).

❑ Specific Learning Disorders, Motor Skills Disorders, Communications Disorders, and Pervasive Developmental Disorders are listed on Axis I.

❑ Types of information presented for each disorder have changed. Additions include subtypes and/or specifiers, recording procedures, associated laboratory findings, associated physical examination findings, specific cultural features, and course.

❑ The term *organic* was eliminated.

❑ DSM-III-R's Organic Mental Syndromes and Disorders were separated into three sections: (1) "Delirium, Dementia, and Amnestic and Other Cognitive Disorders," (2) "Mental Disorders Due to a General Medical Condition," and (3) "Substance-Related Disorders."

❑ In addition, certain Substance-Induced Disorders were relocated in sections with similar phenomenology (e.g., Substance-Induced Anxiety Disorders is located in the "Anxiety Disorders" section).

❑ Thirteen disorders with diagnostic criteria were added; 56 new Substance-Related Disorders are listed.

❑ Eight disorders were eliminated.

❑ Appendix B, "Criteria Sets and Axes Provided for Further Study," was expanded from 3 to 26.

❑ Appendix G is new; it lists ICD-9-CM codes of selected medical diagnoses and medications.

❑ Appendix I was added: "Outline for Cultural Formulation and Glossary of Culture-Bound Syndromes."

❑ The Symptom Index was eliminated.

INTERNATIONAL CLASSIFICATION OF DISEASES (ICD)

The First Revision Conference of the International List of Causes of Death was held in Paris in 1900. Since the first ICD, which was used strictly for the coding of causes of death, revisions have been made about every 10 years. The ICD did not provide a separate section for mental disorders until the fifth revision (1938); later revisions expanded the classification system to include causes for morbidity. The 1978 revision, ICD-9, was modified for use in the United States for collection of morbidity data, collecting research data, indexing medical records, reviewing cases, and for administrative purposes. This modification, called ICD-9-CM (Clinical Modification), was published in 1979 by the U.S. Department of Health and Human Services. The latest ICD revision, ICD-10, was published in 1992; its official use in the United States is not expected for several years.

Because of close collaboration, DSM-IV codes and terms are fully compatible with ICD-9-CM; ICD-10 codes, which are quite different from current diagnostic codes, are listed in DSM-IV's Appendix 4. In addition, two appendices in DSM-IV are available to aid the clinician in using the ICD: Appendix G, "ICD-9-CM Codes for Selected General Medical Conditions and Medication-Induced Disorders," and Appendix H, "DSM-IV Classification With ICD-10 Codes."

REFERENCES

American Psychiatric Association. (1952). *Diagnostic and Statistical Manual of Mental Disorders* (1st ed.). Washington, D.C.

American Psychiatric Association. (1968). *Diagnostic and Statistical Manual of Mental Disorders* (2nd ed.). Washington, D.C.

American Psychiatric Association. (1980). *Diagnostic and Statistical Manual of Mental Disorders* (3rd ed.). Washington, D.C.

American Psychiatric Association. (1987). *Diagnostic and Statistical Manual of Mental Disorders* (3rd ed., rev.). Washington, D.C.: American Psychiatric Press, Inc.

American Psychiatric Association. (1994). *Diagnostic and Statistical Manual of Mental Disorders* (4th ed.). Washington, D.C.: American Psychiatric Press, Inc.

American Psychiatric Association. (1994). *DSM-IV Sourcebook.* Washington, D.C.: American Psychiatric Press, Inc.

U.S. Department of Health and Human Services. (1979). *The International Classification of Diseases, 9th Revision.* Washington, D.C.

World Health Organization. (1992). *Manual of the International Classification of Diseases and Related Health Problems, Tenth Revision.* Geneva, Switzerland.

CHAPTER 2

MULTIAXIAL CLASSIFICATION

The multiaxial diagnostic system began in 1980 with DSM-III and, with minor modifications, continues as an integral part of DSM-IV. The use of the five axes ensures that information needed for treatment planning, prediction of outcome, and research is recorded. Table 2.1 presents an overview of the multiaxial system.

AXES I AND II

Axis I and Axis II are used to describe the patient's current condition. Axis I lists all clinical syndromes present, except for Personality Disorders or Mental Retardation, which are listed on Axis II. Axis II can also be used to record personality traits or repetitive defense mechanisms that impair the patient's ability to cope. When necessary, multiple diagnoses are made on Axis I; and when necessary, diagnoses on both axes are made.

When more than one disorder is present on Axis I, list first the one which is the reason for the visit. When the Axis II diagnosis is the primary diagnosis or the reason for the visit, note "(Principal Diagnosis)" or "(Reason for Visit)" after the Axis II diagnosis.

If there is *no* diagnosis on either Axis I or II, use DSM-IV code V71.09 (No Diagnosis); if *insufficient information* is available to make the diagnosis on Axis I or II, use DSM-IV code 799.9 (Diagnosis Deferred).

AXIS III

The clinician lists all general medical conditions on this axis. ICD-9-CM codes for selected medical conditions and Medical Disorders are listed in Appendix G. When the general medical condition is the direct cause of a mental disorder, an appropriate diagnosis is made on Axis I. For example, if a patient's hyperthyroidism caused hypomania or mania, a diagnosis of Mood Disorder Due to Hyperthyroidism, With Manic Features is made on Axis I. Other nota-

TABLE 2.1 MULTIAXIAL SYSTEM

Axis I	Clinical Disorders; Other Conditions That May Be a Focus of Clinical Attention
Axis II	Personality Disorders; Mental Retardation
Axis III	General Medical Conditions
Axis IV	Psychosocial and Environmental Problems
Axis V	Global Assessment of Functioning (GAF)

tions, such as "frontal release reflexes present" or "abnormal EEG," are appropriate also. The clinician can also list "None" when appropriate.

AXIS IV

Psychosocial and environmental problems that currently influence the diagnosis, treatment, or prognosis of Axis I or II disorders are listed on Axis IV. These include, for example, problems within the patient's support system (e.g., physical abuse) or employment situation (e.g., unemployment or retirement). Categories to consider are listed on pages 29 and 30 of DSM-IV. A sample report form can be found on page 33 of DSM-IV.

AXIS V

The clinician estimates the patient's level of functioning at the time of evaluation or at any other specified time (e.g., highest level in past year) on Axis V. The Global Assessment of Functioning (GAF) Scale for this purpose is on page 32 of DSM-IV. The assigned codes are self-explanatory; the clinician considers only the psychological, social, and occupational functioning of the patient and not physical or environmental limitations. Appendix B contains several additional scales that might prove useful, including the Defensive Functioning Scale (DSM-IV, pp. 751–757), Global Assessment of Relational Functioning (GARF) Scale (DSM-IV, pp. 758–759) and Social and Occupational Functioning Assessment Scale (SOFAS) (DSM-IV, pp. 760–761).

DIFFERENCES BETWEEN DSM-III-R AND DSM-IV MULTIAXIAL CLASSIFICATION

❑ Specific Learning Disorders, Motor Skills Disorders, Communication Disorders, and Pervasive Developmental Disorders are now listed on Axis I. Only Personality Disorders and Mental Retardation remain on Axis II.

❑ DSM-III-R Severity of Psychosocial Stressor Scale was eliminated. On Axis IV, the clinician simply lists psychosocial and environmental problems.

❑ The Global Assessment of Functioning (GAF) Scale (DSM-IV, p. 32) used for Axis V was modified. The GAF Scale, which in DSM-III-R went from 90 to 1, now goes from 100 to 0.

❑ Several potentially useful scales were added to Appendix B (see specific references in this chapter).

CHAPTER 3
....

SUMMARY OF *DSM-IV* FEATURES

DSM-IV provides a great deal of information to help the clinician understand this diagnostic system. Some highlights are summarized below.

The introduction briefly discusses the history and development of the *Diagnostic and Statistical Manual*, from DSM-I to DSM-IV. DSM-IV defines *mental disorder* as

> a clinically significant behavioral or psychological syndrome or pattern that occurs in an individual and that is associated with present distress (e.g., a painful symptom) or disability (i.e., impairment in one or more important areas of functioning) or with a significantly increased risk of suffering death, pain, disability, or an important loss of freedom. (p. xxi)   (12)

The syndrome or pattern "must not be merely an expectable and culturally sanctioned response to a particular event," nor solely deviant behavior or a conflict with society, unless the latter are symptoms of mental disorder. Persons   (13) with a diagnosis need not be similar in other ways and, in fact, may be dissimilar in ways that might affect treatment.

The introduction discusses other basic features of DSM-IV and mentions several topics that are expanded upon in this book, such as treatment planning, use by nonclinicians, use in nonclinical settings, and use in different cultures. DSM-IV's "Cautionary Statement" on potential for improper use (p. xxvii) is important reading.

Three early sections of DSM-IV are particularly useful. The first section, "Use of the Manual," discusses guidelines for coding, terminology, the organizational plan used for DSM-IV, and an explanation of discussions in the text (see Table 3.1).

The second section, "DSM-IV Classification," is a nonannotated outline of the Axis I and II categories and codes, organized into 16 diagnostic classes and a miscellaneous category called "Other Conditions That May Be a Focus of Clinical Attention."

The third section, "Multiaxial Assessment," discusses the "multiaxial" system. This system provides the clinician with an excellent method for organizing and communicating clinically important information. This section also contains the Global Assessment of Functioning (GAF) Scale and examples of how to record diagnoses.

TABLE 3.1 CATEGORIES OF DISCUSSION IN DSM-III-R AND DSM-IV

DSM-III-R	DSM-IV
Essential features	Diagnostic features
	Subtypes and/or specifiers*
	Recording procedures*
Associated features	Associated features and disorders
Predisposing factors	❑ Associated descriptive features and mental disorders
Impairment	
Predisposing factors	
Complications	❑ Associated laboratory findings*
	❑ Associated physical examination findings and general medical conditions*
Sex ratio	Specific cultural,* age, and gender features
Age at onset	
Prevalence	Prevalence
Course	Course
Familial pattern	Familial pattern
Differential diagnosis	Differential diagnosis

*New catagories

Specific disorders, including diagnostic criteria, are outlined on the next 650 pages of DSM-IV. The categories of discussion on each disorder are listed in Table 3.1, showing the comparison to DSM-III-R's approach.

DSM-IV also contains 10 appendices and an index. Appendix A contains six decision trees, designed to help the clinician eliminate superfluous disorders and narrow the diagnostic focus (although a clinician should not feel pressed to arrive at only one diagnosis, or even one per axis). The *Training Guide* avoids the rote decision tree approach in favor of encouraging clinicians to be more comprehensive in their consideration of history, signs, and symptoms.

Appendix B describes proposed new diagnoses and axes that are not included in the official nomenclature.

Appendix C is a short glossary of technical terms used commonly in DSM-IV. It does not contain many terms used in clinical practice, and its definitions may conflict in part with definitions found elsewhere. There is some overlap with the more comprehensive glossary found at the end of this *Training Guide*.

Appendix D is an annotated comparison of DSM-III-R and DSM-IV.

Appendix E is an alphabetical listing of DSM-IV diagnoses along with diagnostic codes.

Appendix F is a numerical listing of DSM-IV codes along with the diagnoses.

Appendix G contains selected ICD-9-CM codes for general medical conditions and Medication-Induced Disorders. The codes are listed on Axis III.

Appendix H essentially repeats DSM-IV's classification; this time with ICD-10 codes listed for each disorder. As previously mentioned, ICD-10 codes will become official in the United States within several years. This *Training Guide* provides ICD codes with each diagnosis.

Appendix I is new in DSM-IV. The first part discusses a system approach to the assessment of ethnic and cultural factors in individual cases. The second part provides a brief glossary of culture-bound syndromes.

Appendix J lists contributors to DSM-IV by field or area of contribution.

Finally, DSM-IV has an index that lists diagnoses (and some other diagnostic terms) alphabetically with number references; page numbers for diagnostic criteria are listed in parentheses.

CHAPTER 4

THE DIAGNOSTIC PROCESS

Unsophisticated readers of DSM-IV commonly think it is a "cookbook" of psychiatric diagnosis. While its format encourages this misconception and some pseudoclinical computerized diagnosis programs use it to promote sales, DSM-IV is not intended for such use (see "Cautionary Statement," p. xxvii, DSM-IV). Similarly, DSM-IV is sometimes called a phenomenological manual; however, careful reading of the diagnostic criteria and accompanying text encourages a comprehensive clinical approach to evaluation and diagnosis.

Anyone using DSM-IV for clinical, statistical, research, legal, or reimbursement purposes should first be fully trained in the clinical fields relevant to each of the five axes. This implies a biopsychosocial foundation for assessing the medical, emotional, and social characteristics of the patient; interviewing skills; and expertise at obtaining and interpreting information about the patient from other sources (e.g., family interviews, medical records, physical examination, specialty consultation, psychological testing, laboratory procedures). It further suggests, with no prejudice intended, that individuals with incomplete biopsychosocial background or training may be inherently limited in their use of this diagnostic system.

Valid and effective use of DSM-IV almost always requires a clinical setting. Although used in other settings—the social sciences, various reimbursement procedures, legal environments, and so on—DSM-IV's main purpose is to enhance agreement among clinicians and research investigators. A clinician may properly use DSM-IV terminology to help interpret findings to, for example, an insurance company or a court; however, he or she must guard against inappropriate translation of medically relevant information to these and other settings, whose needs, rules, and vocabularies are often quite different from those of psychiatry.

ADDITIONAL KEY DIAGNOSTIC ISSUES

The DSM-IV's text draws attention to several other important concepts which should be discussed before proceeding.

1. *Coexistence of more than one disorder in the same patient.* Although the principle of parsimony—trying to fit all the patient's symptoms and signs into one disorder—is a good clinical rule, the complexities of patients' physical, emo-

tional, and interpersonal lives often lead to more than one diagnosis. DSM-IV decision trees and similarly designed computer programs should not cause one to forego multiple diagnoses.

2. Lack of discrete division between disorders (or between a mental disorder and "normalcy"). The current state of diagnostic art, and the nature of patients themselves, precludes clear-cut borders between closely related syndromes and disorders, and sometimes between normalcy and psychopathology.

3. "Hierarchical" precedence of some diagnoses over others, including pre-empting of some diagnoses when due to general medical disorders or are substance-induced. Hierarchies, as described in DSM-IV, increase clinical accuracy by

- Raising doubt about a second diagnosis when the patient's symptoms are likely caused by the first (e.g., depression in a schizophrenic patient often remits as the thought disorder is adequately treated);

- Encouraging the clinician or treatment team to attend to the most important disorder(s) before devoting time and resources to other problems (e.g., dealing with depression in a patient who is alcohol dependent by achieving abstinence before using antidepressants); and

- Helping guide the clinician through the hierarchy. These are referred to as "forced hierarchies." For example, the diagnostic criteria will state, "Criteria are not met for . . . ," "does not occur exclusively during the course of . . ." or "not better accounted for by. . . ."

4. Limitations in transcultural application of DSM-IV disorders and techniques. Many persons live in, or come from, cultures different from that of the evaluating clinician or those on which most of the DSM-IV criteria are based. A clinician involved in transcultural assessments should understand both normal and psychopathological aspects of individuals in the "foreign" group and be sensitive to the possibility of misunderstanding, even when he or she has considerable clinical experience. This caveat applies even to traditionally distressing symptoms (e.g., certain hallucinations experienced during bereavement in some Native American cultures).

DSM-IV has two features intended to help clinicians better understand cultural and ethnic issues. The text of some disorders discusses "Specific Culture, Age and Gender Features," and Appendix I outlines a method for cultural formulation and presents a brief glossary of culture-bound syndromes.

CHAPTER 5

AXES I AND II

The basic task of the clinician is to describe and record the patient's current mental condition using diagnostic Axes I and II of DSM-IV. In some cases, the patient does not have a mental disorder, or a mental disorder is not the reason for evaluation or treatment. In patients without a mental disorder, special codes or V codes are recorded (see Table 5.1). V codes are located in the section of DSM-IV titled "Other Conditions That May Be a Focus of Clinical Attention."

MULTIPLE DIAGNOSES

Multiple diagnoses are made on Axis I and II whenever necessary and when not specifically preempted by DSM-IV criteria. Axis I is where the clinician lists mental disorders, as well as other conditions that are the focus of clinical attention (e.g., Bereavement or Neuroleptic Malignant Syndrome). Personality Disorders and Mental Retardation are listed on Axis II.

The clinician can also record personality traits or maladaptive defense mechanisms on Axis II. Personality traits and maladaptive defenses are not coded, but are useful in treatment planning and may aid other mental health workers during future contact with the patient.

The "principal diagnosis" or "reason for visit" is presumed to be the first diagnosis on Axis I unless otherwise specified. The clinician can also use other terminology and codes listed in Table 5.1.

DIAGNOSTIC HIERARCHIES

Several general rules limit the use of some DSM-IV diagnoses:

☐ When symptoms are best explained by a Mental Disorder Due to a General Medical Condition or a Substance-Induced Disorder, diagnosis of other mental disorders that could produce similar symptoms is precluded. For example, if a patient with no previous history of depression becomes depressed secondary to hypothyroidism, the correct diagnosis is Mood Disorder Due to Hypothyroidism. Even if the patient meets the other diagnostic criteria for major depression, for example, that diagnosis would not be made.

16

TABLE 5.1

Code	Terminology Used on Axis	Amount of Information Available
799.9	Diagnosis Deferred (Axis I or II)	Insufficient information is available.
*	Axis I or II diagnosis followed by "(provisional)"	Information strongly suggests a diagnosis, but some doubt exists.
300.9	Unspecified Mental Disorder (nonpsychotic)	Enough information is available to rule out a psychotic mental disorder.
298.9	Psychotic Disorder Not Otherwise Specified (NOS)	A psychotic disorder is present, but further specification is not possible.
*	(Class of Disorder) Not Otherwise Specified (NOS)	Enough information is present to indicate a class of disorder (e.g., an anxiety disorder). Either information is insufficient or the disorder does not meet more specific diagnostic criteria.
*	V codes	Specifies the focus of attention of treatment. There may be insufficient information present to specify a disorder.
V71.09	No diagnosis (Axis I or II)	Sufficient information is available to state that no mental disorder exists.

* A specific code for a disorder is entered here.

❑ When a patient has a "major" mental disorder, such as Schizophrenia, associated symptoms (e.g., dysphoria, anxiety, hypochondriacal concerns) are often present. These symptoms are not considered separate disorders (e.g., Dysthymia, Anxiety Disorder, Hypochondriasis). 21

❑ When a patient receives more than one diagnosis, the condition that is chiefly responsible for clinical attention or treatment is labeled the *principal diagnosis* (inpatient) or *reason for visit* (outpatient). The principal diagnosis can be either an Axis I or Axis II disorder. 22

❑ When multiple diagnoses are made on either Axis I or II, disorders are listed from those requiring most clinical attention to those requiring least clinical attention. 23

DIAGNOSTIC CERTAINTY

A clinician's certainty about a diagnosis is directly proportional to the amount of information available. Unfortunately, information is sometimes lacking, particularly early in the evaluative process. DSM-IV allows flexibility in such cases. The clinician has several options, which are contained in Table 5.1.

....

CASE VIGNETTES: AXES I AND II

Case vignettes for diagnosis and coding practice are found at the end of each chapter in this book. Read the vignette, consider the diagnostic and coding possibilities, then check your results against the discussion. Do not be overly concerned if your specific diagnosis is incorrect, as you may not have reviewed the disorders discussed later in the book. The important thing is to consider findings tentative and be aware of the DSM-IV Axis on which it should be coded.

Case Vignette 1

A.L., a 20-year-old man, presents to the emergency room of a local hospital accompanied by his family. He is combative, smells of alcohol, and is obviously quite intoxicated. Three weeks ago he was arrested for driving while intoxicated (DWI). A.L.'s wife reports that he has been drinking increasing amounts of alcohol since marital problems developed 2 months ago. For 3 days he has been tearful and reported to another family member that he "felt hopeless about the marriage." His appetite, concentration, interest and energy levels, and sleep pattern are relatively normal. He denies suicidal ideation. Past history is significant for poor academic performance during high school (i.e., he was enrolled in special-education classes). There is no previous history of alcohol or drug abuse. A.L.'s parents state that no learning disabilities were ever identified, but "his I.Q. is very low."

DIAGNOSIS AND DISCUSSION

A number of clinical problems are present or *potentially* present:

Axis I—303.00 Alcohol Intoxication (ICD-10 code F10.00); 305.00 Alcohol Abuse (ICD-10 code F10.1); V61.1 Partner Relational Problem (ICD-10 code Z63.0) (principal diagnosis); and/or perhaps 309.0 Adjustment Disorder With Depressed Mood (ICD-10 code F43.20)
Axis II—V62.89 Borderline Intellectual Functioning (provisional) (ICD-10 code R41.8) or 317.00 Mild Mental Retardation (provisional) (ICD-10 code F70.9)

A.L. presented to the emergency room in an intoxicated state. He had consumed excessive amounts of alcohol for longer than 2 months, and received a DWI. He meets the diagnostic criteria for Substance Abuse (DSM-IV, pp. 182–183), in this case, Alcohol Abuse. Partner Relational Problem is listed as the "principal diagnosis" because it seems to have led to both the Alcohol Abuse and the Adjustment Disorder. The use of a principal diagnosis also helps identify a major focus for treatment. On Axis II, Mental Retardation is *possibly* present. However, complete information is not available, so "(provisional)" is added to Borderline

Intellectual Functioning to indicate that doubt exists. An alternative diagnosis is Mild Mental Retardation. Further clinical information, specifically I.Q. testing, is needed prior to reaching a final Axis II diagnosis.

Case Vignette 2

C.T. is a 30-year-old male with a history of multiple prior psychiatric hospitalizations. His family brings him in for evaluation. According to the family, he is not sleeping at night and is very suspicious. C.T. reports auditory hallucinations, voices that constantly warn him about the "intentions of people." During the interview C.T. stares intently at you, occasionally becomes angry at your questions, and appears suspicious. His affect varies from appropriate to angry, and his mood is euthymic. He denies depressive symptoms. His associations are not loose; however, he is preoccupied with the idea that the Mafia is going to kill him. At times during the interview he appears quite anxious.

Past history is significant for numerous similar episodes beginning when the patient was 18. C.T. has been psychiatrically hospitalized many times and frequently stops medications following discharge. Between psychotic episodes, he lives with his parents. The family states that he is always suspicious but not this disturbed. He stays by himself and has no motivation to work or do basic household tasks. He has never had a Major Depressive or Manic Episode, and there is no history of substance abuse or medical illness. According to the family, during C.T.'s childhood he was a quiet "loner" who never had any friends. He never dated. The family expresses surprise about C.T.'s angry outbursts in later life because "he never showed any emotions as a child."

DIAGNOSIS AND DISCUSSION

Axis I—295.30 Schizophrenia, Paranoid Type, Episodic With Interepisode Residual Symptoms, With Prominent Negative Symptoms (ICD-10 code F20.02)
Axis II—301.20 Schizoid Personality Disorder (Premorbid) (ICD-10 code F60.1)

This patient presents a classic history. The course of the disorder is long-standing, and the patient is experiencing an acute exacerbation. After the patient has had symptoms for more than 1 year, the longitudinal course of Schizophrenia is specified according to diagnostic criteria found in DSM-IV (pp. 285–286), in this case, Episodic With Interepisode Residual Symptoms, With Prominent Negative Symptoms.

Although the patient is anxious, separate Axis I diagnoses such as Anxiety Disorder are not made because symptoms commonly associated with a major psychiatric disorder are not listed as separate disorders. Premorbid personality characteristics are listed on Axis II. Simply write "(premorbid)" following the Personality Disorder diagnosis if the criteria were met prior to the onset of Schizophrenia.

CHAPTER 6

AXIS III

Axis III is where the clinician lists all the patient's medical disorders or conditions. ICD-9-CM (chap. 1) contains an exhaustive list of medical conditions, along with appropriate classification codes. Appendix G in DSM-IV also contains codes for certain general medical conditions and Medication-Induced Disorders. Axis III ensures that medical or physical conditions that can directly or indirectly influence management and treatment are not forgotten.

At times, the Axis III disorder causes an Axis I or II abnormality. For example, if a patient with Alcohol Dependence develops signs and symptoms of a Delirium (acute confusional state), it is likely that the patient's Delirium is caused by the alcohol (e.g., Alcohol Withdrawal or Wernicke's encephalopathy). Sometimes the Axis III condition does not directly cause the psychiatric disorder, but knowledge of the medical problem is essential for proper management of the case (e.g., a pregnant woman who is severely depressed, suicidal, and is also an insulin-dependent diabetic). Failure to properly manage the medical condition during treatment of the mental disorder could have disastrous consequences. The clinician can also list other observations on Axis III, such as "frontal release signs present" or "abnormal EEG." If no significant medical or physical disorders are present, state "None" or "None Known" on Axis III.

ICD-9-CM also lists E codes for accidental injuries, poisonings, and suicide attempts; some of these codes are listed in DSM-IV's Appendix G.

The combination of Axes I, II, and III presents an overview of the patient's mental and physical condition. For example:

Axis I	295.30	Schizophrenia, Paranoid Type
	305.00	Alcohol Abuse
Axis II	301.20	Schizoid Personality Disorder (premorbid)
Axis III	571.2	Cirrhosis, alcoholic

In this example, we know the patient is a chronic paranoid schizophrenic, with a significant problem with alcohol. The patient has liver cirrhosis, in all likelihood caused by the alcohol. The ICD-9-CM diagnostic code 571.2 ("cirrhosis, alcoholic") was found in DSM-IV's Appendix G. This patient had a schizoid personality prior to developing Schizophrenia, thus "(premorbid)" is noted.

CHAPTER 7

AXIS IV

The clinician lists on Axis IV the psychosocial and environmental stressors encountered by the patient during the 12 months prior to evaluation. The
clinician can note stressors that occur prior to the previous year if they significantly contribute to the mental disorder.

List all relevant psychosocial and environmental problems on Axis IV.
Occasionally, this is the primary reason for clinical attention. In such cases, use
the appropriate diagnosis and code from the category "Other Conditions That
May Be a Focus of Clinical Attention" (DSM-IV, pp. 675–686). For example,
if a 19-year-old college student presents for evaluation because of failing grades,
and no mental disorder was found to account for this problem, "V62.3 Academic
Problem" may be entered on Axis I.

Stressors that may be considered include, but are not limited to, problems or difficulties in the individual's primary support group; social environment;
educational situation; occupational, housing, economic, or financial situation;
access to health care services; interaction with the legal system and/or crime-
related situation; or other psychosocial and environmental factors.

CASE VIGNETTES: AXIS IV

Case Vignette 1

B.G. is a 39-year-old, never-married man who works as an accountant in a retail
business. He has a long history of poor self-esteem and his mood is usually mildly
dysphoric. His coworkers describe him as a dependable, quiet man. For the past
9 months the business has slowly declined and bankruptcy is a remote possibility.
Since the downturn in business, B.G.'s mood is more dysphoric and he blames
himself for the financial condition of the company. He presents for evaluation
after his boss insists that he seek assistance.

List the patient's known stressors.

DIAGNOSIS AND DISCUSSION
Axis IV—Possibility of job loss

The only environmental stressor evident from this history is a change in B.G.'s work situation. It is likely that B.G.'s individual vulnerability (his poor self-esteem) magnifies the impact of this stressor so that his response is greater than that expected of the "average" individual.

Case Vignette 2

E.W. is a 14-year-old girl who is the only child currently living with her parents. She is a good student and is known as an outgoing child. Five months ago her maternal grandfather, who had been living with the family for 10 years, died. E.W.'s mother has had difficulty with the loss of her father and is quite depressed, but she will not seek professional assistance.

Three months ago, E.W.'s school performance began to decline and she began coming home early from school because of stomach pain. E.W., the identified patient, presents for evaluation.

List the patient's known psychosocial and environmental problems. (If necessary, refer to p. 34 of DSM-IV).

DIAGNOSIS AND DISCUSSION
Axis IV—Death of maternal grandfather, mother's bereavement/depression, academic problems

E.W. has two stresses that are crucial in her declining academic performance and abdominal pain. These are the death of her grandfather, who lived with her, and her mother's depression. Although E.W. is the identified patient, evaluation and treatment of her mother may be a major focus of treatment.

CHAPTER 8

AXIS V

The clinician rates the individual's overall or global level of functioning on Axis V of DSM-IV. The specific scale used is the Global Assessment of Functioning (GAF) Scale (DSM-IV, p. 32). The GAF Scale is a composite index that considers psychological, social, and occupational functioning. The clinician is warned "Do not include impairment in functioning due to physical (or environmental) limitations." GAF Scale ratings are continuous and range from 0 (inadequate information) to 1 (persistent severe difficulties) to 100 (superior functioning).

In most instances, the clinician rates the patient's current level of functioning. The period used for rating is recorded in parentheses behind the GAF score, for example, GAF = 41 (current). The current GAF establishes a baseline so that results of therapeutic interventions can be measured.

Additional GAF ratings, for example, the highest level of functioning during the year prior to evaluation, can be made on Axis V. The previous example would be listed on Axis V as GAF = 85 (highest level in past year). The highest GAF during the past year may have prognostic significance because the person may return to at least that level of functioning after treatment.

RATING THE LEVEL OF ADAPTIVE FUNCTION

Rating the patient's level of functioning according to the GAF Scale is relatively easy if adequate information is available. Simply locate a description that accurately portrays the individual by referring to page 32 of DSM-IV. Each description has an associated range of numbers or codes (e.g., the person with serious impairment is rated from 41 to 50). The clinician selects a number in that range which best represents the patient's level of functioning. For example, a 29-year-old male presents for evaluation in a catatonic state. He is mute and will not follow any commands. According to the GAF Scale, a person who has gross impairment in communication falls into a rating range between 11 and 20. The clinician would rate the patient's current level of functioning within the appropriate range. An individual who is unable to maintain minimal personal hygiene is rated between 1 and 10. (See Table 8.1 for an abbreviated GAF Scale.)

23

TABLE 8.1 ABBREVIATED GLOBAL ASSESSMENT OF FUNCTIONING (GAF) SCALE

Rating	Range of Level of Functioning in Social, Occupational, or School Situations
91–100	Superior functioning, no symptoms
81–90	Absent or minimal symptoms, only everyday problems and concerns
71–80	Only slight impairment, symptoms are transient
61–70	Mild symptoms but generally functioning well
51–60	Moderate symptoms (e.g., occasional panic attacks)
41–50	Serious symptoms (e.g., thoughts of suicide, unable to keep job)
31–40	Some impairment in reality testing or communications, or major impairment in several areas, such as work or school, family relations, judgment, thinking, or mood
21–30	Behavior is considerably influenced by delusions and hallucinations, or serious impairment in communications or judgment, or inability to function in almost all areas
11–20	Some danger of harming self or others, or occasionally fails to maintain minimal personal hygiene, or gross impairment in communication
1–10	Persistent danger of harming self or others, or persistent inability to maintain minimal personal hygiene, or serious suicidal act with clear expectation of death
0	Inadequate information

DIFFERENCES BETWEEN DSM-III-R AND DSM-IV AXIS V

The GAF Scale in DSM-III-R went from 90 to 1; whereas in DSM-IV the GAF Scale goes from 100 to 0. DSM-IV added a 91–100 range to the scale, defined as "superior functioning" and "no symptoms," and a 0, defined as inadequate information available. Otherwise, the rating scale and associated descriptors did not change.

DSM-III-R stated that the clinician should rate two time periods, current and the highest level of functioning "for at least a few months during the past year." DSM-IV suggests only rating the current level of functioning, with the option to use the GAF Scale for other periods of time (e.g., at discharge from the hospital).

In Appendix B, DSM-IV lists several additional rating scales for further study: the Defensive Functioning Scale (pp. 751–754); the Global Assessment of Relational Functioning (GARF) (pp. 758–759); and the Social and Occupational Functioning scale (SOFAS) (pp. 760–761).

Case Vignettes: Axis V

Case Vignette 1

M.J. is a 39-year-old, married, female clerical worker with three children. Her problems began about 6 months ago, after her husband had an affair with a neighborhood woman. Since that time, M.J. has experienced increasing paranoid ideation and during the past 2 months, her job performance has deteriorated. She recently started withdrawing from friends but continues her role as a mother without obvious difficulty. She is not suicidal. Prior to her husband's affair she reportedly had "lifelong" mild anxiety, long-standing insomnia, and a good work record. She is brought for evaluation by her husband because of worsening problems.

Diagnosis and Discussion
Axis V—GAF = 32
    GAF = 70 (Highest level past year)

M.J. has significant impairment in many areas. Her paranoid ideation impairs her psychologically, she is isolating herself from friends (social dysfunction), and her job performance is declining (occupational difficulty). According to the GAF Scale, her adaptive function is in the range of 31–40. If on examination she is quite paranoid and she is about to lose her job, one might rate her current level of function on Axis V as 31 or 32. Her level of functioning during the past 12 months was clearly higher than her current level, probably at least in the 61–70 range. If her anxiety level before the current episode was very mild, or intermittent, and she had only minimal insomnia, a rating of 70 on Axis V is appropriate.

Case Vignette 2

A.K. is a 10-year-old boy who is brought by his mother for evaluation. According to the mother, A.K. was an excellent student (mostly A's with a few B's) until about 2 months ago, when his parents separated. Since the father's departure, the boy has complained of stomach pains associated with going to school. According to A.K.'s teacher, A.K.'s conduct in school has changed from "excellent" to "needs improvement." During the past 2 months the father visited the boy once and telephoned him two times. The mother describes the previous relationship between the father and son as "very close." The mother reports that prior to the father's departure, A.K. occasionally fell behind in his schoolwork but responded quickly to encouragement. The mother believes that the earlier lapses in schoolwork occurred during times of increased marital discord.

Diagnosis and Discussion
Axis V—GAF = 54 (Current)
    GAF = 80 (Two months ago)

A.K.'s history indicates that his level of functioning 2 months ago was relatively good. He had symptoms prior to his father's departure, but the symptoms were transient and understandable given the marital discord. Therefore, 2 months ago his GAF Scale rating would be in the 71–80 range. Whether the evaluator places an individual at the top or the bottom of a particular range depends on the specifics of the case. With A.K.'s history, a rating of 80 seems appropriate. His current level of functioning is obviously lower, although his symptoms are moderate and understandable given the close relationship he had previously with his father. The appropriate GAF Scale range is 51–60. The specific code given by this examiner was 54.

CHAPTER 9

DIAGNOSTIC CODES

DSM-IV diagnostic codes provide a method for recording diagnoses for administrative, reimbursement, and statistical purposes. Each diagnosis has a code number. DSM-IV lists these code numbers in several locations: DSM-IV Classification (pp. 13–24), Appendix E (alphabetic listing, pp. 793–802), Appendix F (numeric listing, pp. 803–812), and Appendix H (with ICD-10 codes) (pp. 829–841).

Besides the diagnostic codes, other codes (including V codes) are available for particular clinical situations. Fourth- and fifth-digit codes are used in several diagnostic categories to achieve further specification. For example, the diagnostic code for Dementia of the Alzheimer's Type, With Early Onset is 290.xx. The .xx is replaced by .10 in uncomplicated cases, .11 if delirium is prominent, .12 if delusions are prominent, and .13 if depressed mood is prominent.

DSM-IV's Axes III and V are also coded. Axis III, which lists physical conditions or other pertinent medical information, is coded according to ICD-9-CM. DSM-IV's Appendix G (pp. 813–828) contains a selected number of commonly used ICD-9-CM codes. The mental health clinician usually writes medical diagnoses or information on Axis III, and medical-records personnel code that information. Axis V lists the individual's level of functioning in accordance with the Global Assessment Functioning (GAF) Scale (DSM-IV, p. 32). Chapters 5 through 8 in this book discuss DSM-IV's five axes.

Additional codes (DSM-IV, p. 687) are used when insufficient diagnostic information is available. For example, code 799.9 on Axis I and/or Axis II signifies that the diagnosis is deferred.

V CODES*

V codes (DSM-IV, pp. 680-686) specify conditions that are not mental disorders but are a focus of attention or treatment. For example, a male adolescent is brought by his parents for evaluation after several heated arguments over his choice of friends. The clinician evaluates the adolescent and finds no mental disorder. The issue, and the focus for treatment, may be a Parent-Child Relational Problem (V61.20).

*Do not confuse V ("vee") codes with Axis V ("five").

27

The V codes in DSM-IV are taken from a large list found in ICD-9-CM. With the exception of V71.09 (No Diagnosis), which can be used on either Axis I or II, V codes are listed on Axis I when the problem is the focus of clinical attention, or may be listed on Axis IV when it is not.

....

FOURTH- AND FIFTH-DIGIT CODES

An *x* in the fourth and/or fifth digit(s) of a diagnostic code indicates that additional information is required. The following is a list of diagnoses requiring a fourth- or fifth-digit designation, as well as the meaning of the appended code.

Attention-Deficit and Disruptive Behavior Disorders

314.xx Attention Deficit/Hyperactivity Disorder
    .01   Combined Type
    .00   Predominantly Inattentive Type
    .01   Predominantly Hyperactive-Impulsive Type

Dementias

290.xx Dementia of the Alzheimer's Type, With Early Onset
    .10   Uncomplicated
    .11   With Delirium
    .12   With Delusions
    .13   With Depressed Mood

290.xx Dementia of the Alzheimer's Type, With Late Onset
    .0   Uncomplicated
    .3   With Delirium
    .20   With Delusions
    .21   With Depressed Mood

290.xx Vascular Dementia
    .40   Uncomplicated
    .41   With Delirium
    .42   With Delusions
    .43   With Depressed Mood

Substance-Related Disorders

292.xx Amphetamine-Induced Psychotic Disorder
    .11   With Delusions
    .12   With Hallucinations

Schizophrenia and Other Psychotic Disorders

295.xx Schizophrenia
    .10   Disorganized Type

.20	Catatonic Type
.30	Paranoid Type
.60	Residual Type
.90	Undifferentiated Type

293.xx Psychotic Disorder Due to . . . [Indicate the General Medical Condition]

.81	With Delusions
.82	With Hallucinations

Mood Disorders

Code "x" in fifth digit: 1 = Mild; 2 = Moderate; 3 = Severe, Without Psychotic Features; 4 = With Psychotic Features (specify whether Mood-Congruent or Mood-Incongruent); 5 = In Partial Remission; 6 = In Full Remission; 0 = Unspecified.

296.0x	Single Manic Episode
296.2x	Major Depression, Single Episode
296.3x	Major Depression, Recurrent
296.4x	Most Recent Episode Manic
296.5x	Most Recent Episode Depressed
296.6x	Bipolar Disorder, Mixed

Somatoform Disorders

307.xx Pain Disorder

.80	Associated With Psychological Factors
.89	Associated With Both Psychological Factors and a General Medical Condition

Factitious Disorders

300.xx Factitious Disorder

.16	With Predominantly Psychological Signs and Symptoms
.19	With Predominantly Physical Signs and Symptoms
.19	With Combined Psychological and Physical Signs and Symptoms

Sexual and Gender Identity Disorders

302.xx Gender Identity Disorder

.6	In Children
.85	In Adolescents or Adults

Sleep Disorders

780.xx Sleep Disorder Due to . . . [Indicate the General Medical Condition]

.52	Insomnia Type

.54	Hypersomnia Type
.59	Parasomnia Type
.59	Mixed Type

Adjustment Disorders

309.xx Adjustment Disorder

.0	With Depressed Mood
.24	With Anxiety
.28	With Mixed Anxiety and Depressed Mood
.3	With Disturbance of Conduct
.4	With Mixed Disturbance of Emotions and Conduct
.9	Unspecified

....

DIFFERENCES BETWEEN DSM-IV AND DSM-III-R FOURTH- AND FIFTH-DIGIT CODES

❑ New fifth-digit specifiers were created for Attention-Deficit/Hyperactivity Disorder, Substance-Induced Psychotic Disorders, Pain Disorder, Factitious Disorder, Gender Identity Disorder, and Sleep Disorders Due to General Medical Condition.

❑ Axis IV is no longer coded; psychosocial and environmental stressors are simply listed.

❑ Axis III codes for specific general medical conditions and Medication-Induced Disorders are listed in Appendix G (DSM-IV, pp. 813–828).

SECTION II

THE DISORDERS

CHAPTER 10

DISORDERS USUALLY FIRST DIAGNOSED IN INFANCY, CHILDHOOD, OR ADOLESCENCE

This large classification describes disorders that usually begin or become evident in infancy, childhood, or adolescence. Any clinician using this category in children or adolescents should have a basic knowledge of child development in order to be able to distinguish true clinical syndromes from normal variations for age or developmental stage.

Most DSM-IV disorders may be diagnosed in adults, adolescents, or children. Although this section should be consulted when evaluating children or adolescents, disorders described elsewhere in DSM-IV should also be considered, provided there is no proscription against their use before adulthood.

Note the "usually" in the section title. Several of the diagnoses may be applied to adult symptoms (e.g., stuttering). In addition, adults with histories of childhood symptoms (e.g., Attention-Deficit/Hyperactivity Disorder) may be diagnosed as having disorders listed in this section, sometimes In Partial Remission.

MENTAL RETARDATION
(Code on Axis II)

> **Mild Mental Retardation**
> **Moderate**
> **Severe**
> **Profound**
> **Severity Unspecified**

NOTE: The reader may wish to consult the classification system of the American Association on Mental Retardation (AAMR) where level, functioning, and needed supports are addressed more completely. Also, the term *developmental disability*, while often implying Mental Retardation, is not limited to it.

ESSENTIAL FEATURES. Essential features are significantly subaverage general intellectual functioning and significant deficits or impairments in adaptive functioning, both of which present before the age of 18. Although a valid and reliable intelligence quotient (IQ) measurement is a major indicator of retardation, the IQ should be treated with some flexibility in order to allow for additional deficits or acknowledge unusually good adaptation. When a known biological factor is present, it should be coded on Axis III.

For persons under the age of 18 who become functionally retarded after a period of normal intelligence, both Dementia and Mental Retardation are diagnosed if both criteria are met.

COMPLICATIONS. Mental retardation is accompanied by mental illness at a rate several times that of the general population. Although often difficult to diagnose in persons with Mental Retardation, one may discover Mood Disorders, Attention-Deficit/Hyperactivity Disorder (AD/HD), some Developmental Disorders, Stereotypic Movement Disorder, Impulse Control Disorders, and—less commonly—Psychotic Disorders. Symptoms related to the Mental Retardation should be separated from other disorders. Behaviors thought to be symptoms may actually be due to frustration or attempts to communicate.

When social or legal competency is an issue, one should note that persons with Mild Mental Retardation may be more competent than assumed. Well-meaning efforts to limit competency can create unnecessary limitations on activities or individual rights.

ASSOCIATED PHYSICAL, LABORATORY, AND GENERAL MEDICAL FINDINGS. Most borderline or Mild Mental Retardation is associated more with social and environmental deprivation than with physical findings. More significant deficits are associated with a wide variety of genetic, intrauterine, perinatal, and childhood problems and insults. Physical stigmata, including congenital deformity and/or serious, progressive medical illness, often accompany Moderate, Severe, and Profound Mental Retardation. Down's syndrome is associated with increased incidence, and early presentation, of Dementia of the Alzheimer's Type.

DIFFERENTIAL DIAGNOSIS. Mental Retardation should be diagnosed when the criteria are met, regardless of other diagnoses. Learning Disorders reflect a delay or failure of development in a specific area, in contrast to Mental Retardation's general developmental delays. Pervasive Developmental Disorders reflect *abnormal* development, as contrasted with Mental Retardation's *delay* in development. A V-code finding of Borderline Intellectual Functioning does not imply Mental Retardation.

DIAGNOSTIC CRITERIA FOR MENTAL RETARDATION (317–319)

(ICD-10 codes F70.9–F79.9)

A. Significantly subaverage intellectual functioning: an IQ of approximately 70 or below on an individually administered IQ test (for infants, a clinical judgment of significantly subaverage intellectual functioning).

B. Concurrent deficits or impairments in present adaptive functioning (i.e., the person's effectiveness in meeting the standards expected for his or her age by his or her cultural group) in at least two of the following skill areas: communication, self-care, home living, social/interpersonal skills, use of community resources, self-direction, functional academic skills, work, leisure, health and safety.

C. The onset is before age 18 years.

Code based on degree of severity reflecting level of intellectual impairment:

317	**Mild Mental Retardation:** IQ 50–55 to approximately 70	*(ICD-10 code F70.9)*
318.0	**Moderate:** IQ 35–40 to 50–55	*(ICD-10 code F71.9)*
318.1	**Severe:** IQ 20–25 to 35–40	*(ICD-10 code F72.9)*
318.2	**Profound:** IQ below 20 or 25	*(ICD-10 code F73.9)* ⑶⑺
319	**Severity Unspecified:** When there is strong presumption of Mental Retardation but the person's intelligence is not testable by standard instruments	*(ICD-10 code F79.9)*

❏ ❏ ❏ ❏

LEARNING DISORDERS
(Specific Developmental Disorders in DSM-III-R)

Reading Disorder
Mathematics Disorder
Disorder of Written Expression
Learning Disorder Not Otherwise Specified (NOS)

NOTE: Speech, language and motor skills disorders coded as Specific Developmental Disorders in DSM-III-R are generally found in Communication Disorders and Motor Skills Disorders in DSM-IV. They are now coded on Axis I.

ESSENTIAL FEATURES. These disorders are characterized by inadequate development of specific academic, language, speech, and/or motor skills not due to demonstrable physical or neurological disorders, Pervasive Developmental Disorder, Mental Retardation, or lack of educational opportunity. Diagnosis ordinarily depends on standardized, individually administered tests which show achievement *substantially (usually two standard deviations) below* that of peers of similar age, education, and intelligence. Significant discrepancy between IQ and abilities suggests Learning Disorder. The evaluation should correct for known culture bias.

COMPLICATIONS. Complications can include other developmental deficits, such as Communication Disorders or Disruptive Behavior Disorders. Depression and other Axis I disorders may be seen. Lowered self-esteem and problems in social functioning are common.

PREDISPOSING FACTORS. Predisposing factors are similar to those for Pervasive Developmental Disorders.

DIFFERENTIAL DIAGNOSIS. Inadequate testing, lack of educational opportunity, and cultural factors can mimic a Learning Disorder. Learning deficits caused solely by vision or hearing problems should not be considered Learning Disorders. Learning Disorders should not be diagnosed in the presence of Mental Retardation or Pervasive Developmental Disorder unless a specific deficiency (e.g., reading, mathematics) is below the norm for persons of similar IQ, education, or development. A separate diagnosis should be made for each Learning Disorder for which diagnostic criteria are met.

315.00 Reading Disorder (ICD-10 code F81.0)
(Developmental Reading Disorder
in DSM-III-R, Dyslexia)

ESSENTIAL FEATURES. Reading Disorder is a Learning Disorder (see features above) with markedly decreased reading accuracy and/or comprehension, as measured by standardized, individual testing, sufficient to impair academic progress or daily activities.

COMPLICATIONS, ASSOCIATED FEATURES, DIFFERENTIAL DIAGNOSIS. See above. Other Learning Disorders are often present as well. Incidence in first-degree relatives is statistically higher than in the general population.

DIAGNOSTIC CRITERIA FOR (ICD-10 code F81.0)
READING DISORDER (315.00)

A. Reading achievement, as measured by individually administered standardized tests of reading accuracy or comprehension, is substantially below that expected given the person's chronological age, measured intelligence, and age-appropriate education.

B. The disturbance in Criterion A significantly interferes with academic achievement or activities of daily living that require reading skills.

C. If a sensory deficit (e.g., vision or hearing problem) is present, the reading difficulties are in excess of those usually associated with it.

CODING NOTE: If a general medical condition or sensory deficit is present, it should be coded on Axis III.

❑ ❑ ❑ ❑

315.1 Mathematics Disorder (ICD-10 code F81.2)
(Developmental Arithmetic Disorder in DSM-III-R)

ESSENTIAL FEATURES. This is a Learning Disorder (see features above) with markedly decreased arithmetic skills, as measured by standardized, individual testing, sufficient to impair academic progress or daily activities.

COMPLICATIONS, ASSOCIATED FEATURES, DIFFERENTIAL DIAGNOSIS. Similar to Reading Disorder, above. Reading Disorder or Disorder of Written Expression commonly accompanies Mathematics Disorder.

DIAGNOSTIC CRITERIA FOR (ICD-10 code F81.2)
MATHEMATICS DISORDER (315.1)

A. Mathematical ability, as measured by individually administered standardized tests, is substantially below that expected given the person's chronological age, measured intelligence, and age-appropriate education.

B. The disturbance in Criterion A significantly interferes with academic achievement or activities of daily living that require mathematical ability.

C. If a sensory deficit (e.g., vision or hearing problems) is present, the difficulties with mathematical ability are in excess of those usually associated with it.

CODING NOTE: If a general medical (e.g., neurological) condition or sensory deficit is present, code the condition on Axis III.

❑ ❑ ❑ ❑

315.2 Disorder of Written Expression (ICD-10 code F81.8)
(Developmental Expressive Writing Disorder
in DSM-III-R)

ESSENTIAL FEATURES. This is a Learning Disorder (see features above) with markedly decreased writing skills, as measured by standardized, individual testing, sufficient to impair academic progress or daily activities.

COMPLICATIONS, ASSOCIATED FEATURES, DIFFERENTIAL DIAGNOSIS. Similar to Reading Disorder, above. It may be accompanied by language and perceptual-motor deficits.

DIAGNOSTIC CRITERIA FOR   (ICD-10 code F81.8)
DISORDER OF WRITTEN EXPRESSION (315.2)

A. Writing skills, as measured by individually administered standardized tests (or functional assessment of writing skills), are substantially below those expected given the person's chronological age, measured intelligence, and age-appropriate education.

B. The disturbance in Criterion A significantly interferes with academic achievement or activities of daily living that require the composition of written text (e.g., writing grammatically correct sentences and organized paragraphs).

C. If a sensory deficit (e.g., vision or hearing problem) is present, the difficulties with writing skills are in excess of those usually associated it.

> **CODING NOTE: If a general medical (e.g., neurological) condition or sensory deficit is present, code the condition on Axis III.**

▢ ▢ ▢ ▢

315.9 Learning Disorder Not Otherwise   (ICD-10 code F81.9)
Specified (NOS)

This category is for syndromes that do not meet criteria for any specific Learning Disorder (e.g., spelling skills substantially below those expected for chronological age, measured intelligence, and age-appropriate education).

▢ ▢ ▢ ▢

MOTOR SKILLS DISORDER

315.4 Developmental Coordination Disorder   (ICD-10 code F82)

ESSENTIAL FEATURES. There is marked impairment in the development of motor coordination without Pervasive Developmental Disorder, not completely explainable by Mental Retardation or known physical disorder.

ASSOCIATED FEATURES. Communication Disorders (see following) and delays in nonmotor developmental milestones are common.

DIFFERENTIAL DIAGNOSIS. Symptoms caused by general medical conditions are considered. The carelessness or recklessness of AD/HD may cloud diagnosis; if criteria for both are present, both may be diagnosed. The disorder may be diagnosed in persons with Mental Retardation if coordination deficits exceed those expected or associated with Mental Retardation. The diagnosis is preempted by Pervasive Developmental Disorder.

DIAGNOSTIC CRITERIA FOR DEVELOPMENTAL COORDINATION DISORDER (315.4)

(ICD-10 code F82)

A. Performance in daily activities that require motor coordination is substantially below that expected given the person's chronological age and measured intelligence. This may be manifested by marked delays in achieving motor milestones (e.g., walking, crawling, sitting), dropping things, "clumsiness," poor performance in sports, or poor handwriting.

B. The disturbance in Criterion A significantly interferes with academic achievement or activities of daily living.

C. The disturbance is not due to a general medical condition (e.g., cerebral palsy, hemiplegia, or muscular dystrophy) and does not meet criteria for a Pervasive Developmental Disorder.

D. If Mental Retardation is present, the motor difficulties are in excess of those usually associated with it.

> **CODING NOTE: If a general medical (e.g., neurological) condition or sensory deficit is present, code the condition on Axis III.**

▢ ▢ ▢ ▢

COMMUNICATION DISORDERS

(Generally Language and Speech Disorders, under Specific Developmental Disorders, in DSM-III-R)

Expressive Language Disorder
Mixed Receptive-Expressive Language Disorder
Phonological Disorder
Stuttering
Communication Disorder Not Otherwise Specified (NOS)

▢ ▢ ▢ ▢

315.31 Expressive Language Disorder

(ICD-10 code F80.1)

(Developmental Expressive Language Disorder in DSM-III-R)

ESSENTIAL FEATURES. There is marked impairment in expressive language development, substantially below nonverbal intelligence and receptive language development for age and education.

ASSOCIATED FEATURES AND COMPLICATIONS. These include stuttering and cluttering (especially in younger children), Learning Disorders, other developmental delays, other Axis I disorders, neurological signs and symptoms. The disorder may be developmental or acquired; however, children whose impairment can be explained solely by living in a bilingual home should not receive this diagnosis.

DIFFERENTIAL DIAGNOSIS. If receptive language skills are significantly impaired, one should diagnose Mixed Receptive-Expressive Language Disorder. Autistic Disorder should be differentiated by its representative impairments (see following). Several other developmental, trauma-related, general medical, emotional, and environmental (e.g., deprivation) conditions may impair expressive and/or receptive language development; a concurrent diagnosis of Language Disorder should be made only if the language symptoms/signs exceed those expected by the primary condition or persist after recovery. Disorder of Written Expression does not include oral (or signing) deficits. Selective Mutism can be differentiated by the presence of normal language in some settings.

DIAGNOSTIC CRITERIA FOR (ICD-10 code F80.1)
EXPRESSIVE LANGUAGE DISORDER (315.31)

A. The scores obtained from standardized, individually administered measures of expressive language development are substantially below those obtained from standardized measures of both nonverbal intellectual capacity and receptive language development. The disturbance may be manifested clinically by symptoms that include having a markedly limited vocabulary, making errors in tense, or having difficulty recalling words or producing sentences with developmentally appropriate length or complexity.

B. The difficulties with expressive language interfere with academic or occupational achievement, or with social communication.

C. Criteria are not met for Mixed Receptive-Expressive Language Disorder or a Pervasive Developmental Disorder.

D. If Mental Retardation, a speech-related motor or sensory deficit, or environmental deprivation is present, the language difficulties are in excess of those usually associated with these problems.

> CODING NOTE: If a speech-related motor or sensory deficit or a neurological condition is present, code it on Axis III.

❏ ❏ ❏ ❏

315.31 Mixed Receptive-Expressive (ICD-10 code F80.2)
Language Disorder
(Generally subsumes DSM-III-R Developmental Receptive Language Disorder)

ESSENTIAL FEATURES. There is marked impairment in *both* receptive and expressive language development, substantially below nonverbal intelligence and receptive language development for age, education, and intelligence.

ASSOCIATED FEATURES AND COMPLICATIONS. See Expressive Language Disorder (above) for general linguistic features and complications. The receptive aspects of this disorder vary with age, and can be mistaken for deafness, attention problems, or simple confusion. Social communication is generally poor, often appearing odd and inappropriate.

DIFFERENTIAL DIAGNOSIS. Similar to Expressive Language Disorder (preceding).

DIAGNOSTIC CRITERIA FOR   (ICD-10 code F80.2)
MIXED RECEPTIVE-EXPRESSIVE LANGUAGE DISORDER (315.31)

A. Scores obtained from a battery of standardized, individually administered measures of both receptive and expressive language development are substantially below those obtained from standardized measures of nonverbal intellectual capacity. Symptoms include those for Expressive Language Disorder as well as difficulty understanding words, sentences, or specific types of words, such as spatial terms.

B. The difficulties with receptive and expressive language significantly interfere with academic or occupational achievement, or with social communication.

C. Criteria are not met for a Pervasive Developmental Disorder.

D. If Mental Retardation, a speech-related motor or sensory deficit, or environmental deprivation is present, the language difficulties are in excess of those usually associated with these problems.

> **CODING NOTE: If a speech-related motor or sensory deficit or a neurological condition is present, code it on Axis III.**

❏ ❏ ❏ ❏

315.39 Phonological Disorder   (ICD-10 code F80.0)
(Developmental Articulation Disorder in DSM-III-R)

ESSENTIAL FEATURES. There is consistent failure to make correct articulations of speech sounds, given age and dialect. Symptoms may include articulation or cognition/categorization deficits involving phonation, sound production, omission, ordering, and/or substitution.

ASSOCIATED FEATURES. There may be delayed onset of speech development, and causative or concomitant neurological or anatomical deficit.

DIFFERENTIAL DIAGNOSIS. Physical abnormalities causing misarticulation, hearing impairment, dysarthria, or apraxia are considered in the differential diagnosis. Phonological Disorder may be cited in addition to sensory deficit, Mental Retardation, Pervasive Developmental Disorders, or severe environmental deprivation only if phonological symptoms exceed those expected for the other syndrome. Rhythm and voice disorders are not diagnosed here.

DIAGNOSTIC CRITERIA FOR PHONOLOGICAL DISORDER (315.39)

(ICD-10 code F80.0)

A. Failure to use developmentally expected speech sounds that are appropriate for age and dialect (e.g., errors in sound production, use, representation, or organization such as, but not limited to, substitutions of one sound for another [use of /t/ for target /k/ sound] or omissions of sounds such as final consonants).

B. The difficulties in speech sound production interfere with academic or occupational achievement, or with social communication.

C. If Mental Retardation, a speech-related motor or sensory deficit, or environmental deprivation is present, the speech difficulties are in excess of those usually associated with these problems.

> CODING NOTE: If a speech-related motor or sensory deficit or a neurological condition is present, code it on Axis III.

❑ ❑ ❑ ❑

307.0 Stuttering
(significantly modified from DSM-III-R)

(ICD-10 code F98.5)

> NOTE: DSM-III-R's Cluttering was deleted.

ESSENTIAL FEATURES. There is marked impairment in speech fluency characterized by frequent repetitions or prolongations of sounds or syllables. Other speech dysfluencies may be involved, and the disturbance is more severe when there is special pressure to communicate. Stuttering may be absent during oral reading, singing, or talking to non-human objects. Stammering is not distinguished from Stuttering in the United States.

ASSOCIATED FEATURES. The speaker may initially be unaware of the problem but later anticipate it fearfully. Anxiety, frustration, and low self-esteem may limit adult social and occupational choice. Other Communication Disorders, AD/HD, and Anxiety Disorders are commonly associated in childhood. Motor tics or other movements, unusual breathing, or clenching of fists may accompany stuttering.

PREDISPOSING FACTORS. Predisposing factors include other Communication Disorders or a family history of them. Stress and anxiety often exacerbate Stuttering but are not thought to cause it.

DIFFERENTIAL DIAGNOSIS. Normal childhood dysfluency (usually intermittent) and spastic dysphonia (distinguished by abnormal breathing pattern) are considered. If a speech-related motor or sensory deficit is present, Stuttering should be diagnosed only if the symptom exceeds those usually associated with these problems.

DIAGNOSTIC CRITERIA FOR
STUTTERING (307.0)

(ICD-10 code F98.5)

A. Disturbance in the normal fluency and time patterning of speech (inappropriate for the individual's age), characterized by frequent occurrences of one or more of the following:
   (1) sound and syllable repetitions
   (2) sound prolongations
   (3) interjections
   (4) broken words (e.g., pauses within a word)
   (5) audible or silent blocking (filled or unfilled pauses in speech)
   (6) circumlocutions (word substitutions to avoid problematic words)
   (7) words produced with an excess of physical tension
   (8) monosyllabic whole word repetitions (e.g., "I-I-I-I see him.")

B. The disturbance in fluency interferes with academic or occupational achievement, or with social communication.

C. If a speech-related motor or sensory deficit is present, the speech difficulties are in excess of those usually associated with these problems.

> **CODING NOTE: If a speech-related motor or sensory deficit or a neurological condition is present, code it on Axis III.**

❑ ❑ ❑ ❑

307.9 Communication Disorder Not Otherwise Specified (NOS)

(ICD-10 code F80.9)

This category is for disorders in communication that do not meet criteria for any specific Communication Disorder—for example, a voice disorder (abnormality of vocal pitch, loudness, quality, tone, or resonance).

❑ ❑ ❑ ❑

PERVASIVE DEVELOPMENTAL DISORDERS

Autistic Disorder
Rett's Disorder
Childhood Disintegrative Disorder
Asperger's Disorder
Pervasive Developmental Disorder Not Otherwise Specified (NOS)

> NOTE: Pervasive Developmental Disorders are now coded on Axis I.

ESSENTIAL FEATURES. These disorders are characterized by severe, qualitative impairment in the development of reciprocal social interaction, verbal and nonverbal communication skills, and/or a severely restricted repertoire of activities and interests, which may be stereotyped and repetitive. The impairments are clearly out of consonance with developmental level or mental age. These disorders are ordinarily apparent by early childhood.

ASSOCIATED FEATURES AND COMPLICATIONS. When Mental Retardation is associated with these disorders, it is coded on Axis II. Severity of Pervasive Developmental Disorders often increases with severity of handicap and younger age of the child. Complications may include uneven abnormalities in development of cognitive skills, stereotypies and other abnormalities of posture and motor behavior, odd or absent responses to sensory input, abnormalities in preferred diet or sleep pattern, anxiety, abnormalities of mood, and self-injurious behavior. Other mental disorders frequently occur but are often difficult to diagnose because of communication deficits. Schizophrenia is considered separately from Pervasive Developmental Disorders, although some patients develop Schizophrenia or schizophreniform psychosis later in life.

PREDISPOSING FACTORS. A great many pre-, peri-, and postnatal organic conditions appear to predispose infants to development of Pervasive Developmental Disorders. Mental Retardation may appear to be predisposing, but this relationship is not clear.

DIFFERENTIAL DIAGNOSIS. Mental Retardation (which may coexist with it), Schizophrenia (rare in childhood), hearing or visual impairment, and Communication Disorders are considered in the differential diagnosis. Tic Disorders and Stereotypic Movement Disorder are characterized by stereotyped body movements, without qualitative impairments in reciprocal social interaction.

▫ ▫ ▫ ▫

299.00 Autistic Disorder
(Early Infantile Autism, Childhood Autism, Kanner's Autism)
(significantly modified from DSM-III-R)

(ICD-10 code F84.0)

ESSENTIAL FEATURES. Beginning before age 3, there is markedly impaired development of social interaction and communication, with a greatly restricted repertoire of activities and interests. Social interaction is profoundly and lastingly affected. Even simple awareness of others may be absent. Repetitive and stereotyped behaviors are the rule, and preoccupation with particular patterns, rituals, objects, or object parts is common. In those patients who have some normal developmental periods, they do not extend beyond 3 years of age.

ASSOCIATED FEATURES AND DISORDERS. Mental Retardation is usual but not universal, and should be diagnosed and coded on Axis II. Cognitive skills and communication development are uneven and/or impaired. Behavioral symptoms are common and may include decreased attention span, poor impulse control, hyperactivity, abnormal aggression, or self-injury. Response to sensory stimuli may be unusual or bizarre (e.g., apathy during pain or great fearfulness in seemingly benign situations). Mood Disorders may develop, perhaps in response to the patient's awareness of his or her impairment.

ASSOCIATED PHYSICAL, LABORATORY, AND GENERAL MEDICAL FINDINGS. Nonspecific neurological signs are not uncommon. Genetic, prenatal, or perinatal concomitants may be found, but none is considered specifically causative or pathognomonic. Seizures are common, usually developing after childhood, as are EEG abnormalities (with or without seizures). About 80% of patients are male.

DIFFERENTIAL DIAGNOSIS. Rett's Disorder is present only in females and has a distinctive pattern of deficits (see below). Childhood Disintegrative Disorder has a long period of normal development followed by regression. Autistic Disorder preempts Asperger's Disorder, which spares language development. Schizophrenia is routinely preceded by a period of normal development but may be separately diagnosed. Selective Mutism lacks the completeness of deficit and developmental abnormality, as do Communication Disorders. Autistic Disorder should not be diagnosed in addition to Mental Retardation unless the specific social and communicative deficits and characteristic behaviors are present. Autistic Disorder preempts Stereotypic Movement Disorder unless the autism does not better account for the stereotypy. Deafness should be ruled out.

DIAGNOSTIC CRITERIA FOR AUTISTIC DISORDER (299.00)

(ICD-10 code F84.0)

A. A total of six (or more) items from sections (1), (2), and (3), with at least two from (1), and one each from (2) and (3):
   (1) qualitative impairment in social interaction, as manifested by at least two of the following:
      (a) marked impairment in the use of multiple nonverbal behaviors such as eye-to-eye gaze, facial expression, body postures, and gestures to regulate social interaction
      (b) failure to develop peer relationships appropriate to developmental level
      (c) lack of spontaneous seeking to share enjoyment, interests, or achievements with other people (e.g., by a lack of showing, bringing, or pointing out objects of interest)
      (d) lack of social or emotional reciprocity
   (2) qualitative impairments in communication as manifested by at least one of the following:
      (a) delay in, or total lack of, the development of spoken language (not

accompanied by an attempt to compensate through alternative modes of communication such as gesture or mime)

    (b) in individuals with adequate speech, marked impairment in the ability to initiate or sustain a conversation with others

    (c) stereotyped and repetitive use of language or idiosyncratic language

    (d) lack of varied, spontaneous make-believe play or social imitative play appropriate to developmental level

(3) restricted repetitive and stereotyped patterns of behavior, interests, and activities, as manifested by at least one of the following:

    (a) encompassing preoccupation with one or more stereotyped and restricted patterns of interest that is abnormal either in intensity or focus

    (b) apparently inflexible adherence to specific, nonfunctional routines or rituals

    (c) stereotyped and repetitive motor mannerisms (e.g., hand or finger flapping or twisting, or complex whole-body movements)

    (d) persistent preoccupation with parts of objects

B. Delays or abnormal functioning in at least one of the following areas, with onset prior to age 3 years: (1) social interaction, (2) language as used in social communication, or (3) symbolic or imaginative play.

C. The disturbance is not better accounted for by Rett's Disorder or Childhood Disintegrative Disorder.

❑ ❑ ❑ ❑

299.80 Rett's Disorder
(new in DSM-IV)
    (ICD-10 code F84.2)

ESSENTIAL FEATURES. There is appearance in a female of multiple developmental deficits after a period of normal development and functioning. Psychomotor development is normal for at least 5 months after birth. Maturation slows and some skills deteriorate during the first 30–48 months of life. Decreased rate of head growth and loss of hand skills are characteristic. Communication is severely affected. Coordination is impaired and social deficits are generally severe.

ASSOCIATED FEATURES. Severe or Profound Mental Retardation is typical. Seizure disorder and/or abnormal EEG may be seen.

DIFFERENTIAL DIAGNOSIS. Other Pervasive Developmental Disorders, such as Autistic Disorder, may appear similar. Children with Childhood Disintegrative Disorder appear normal for at least 2 years after birth. Asperger's Disorder lacks severe cognitive and communication deficits.

DIAGNOSTIC CRITERIA FOR
RETT'S DISORDER (299.80)

(ICD-10 code F84.2)

A. All of the following:
   (1) apparently normal prenatal and perinatal development
   (2) apparently normal psychomotor development through the first 5 months after birth
   (3) normal head circumference at birth

B. Onset of all of the following after the period of normal development:
   (1) deceleration of head growth between ages 5 and 48 months
   (2) loss of previously acquired purposeful hand skills between ages 5 and 30 months with the subsequent development of stereotyped hand movements (e.g., hand-wringing or hand washing)
   (3) loss of social engagement early in the course (although often social interaction develops later)
   (4) appearance of poorly coordinated gait or trunk movements
   (5) severely impaired expressive and receptive language development with severe psychomotor retardation

NOTE: Rett's Disorder afflicts females only.

CODING NOTE: Code Mental Retardation, typically present, on Axis II.

□ □ □ □

299.10 Childhood Disintegrative Disorder
(Disintegrative Psychosis, Heller's Syndrome, Dementia Infantalis) (new in DSM-IV)

(ICD-10 code F84.3)

ESSENTIAL FEATURES. There is conspicuous deterioration in multiple areas of development and functioning following at least 2 years of seemingly normal development.

ASSOCIATED FEATURES. Severe Mental Retardation is usual. Nonspecific neurological findings and EEG changes may be present, as may seizures. Other serious medical conditions may be present but are not typical, and causative links are not established.

DIFFERENTIAL DIAGNOSIS. Other Pervasive Developmental Disorders, such as Autistic Disorder (see detailed discussion above), may be considered. The relatively late onset and loss of previously acquired development differentiates this disorder from most. Asperger's Disorder lacks delay in language development. Dementias caused by infection, trauma, or other general medical conditions preempt the diagnosis.

DIAGNOSTIC CRITERIA FOR CHILDHOOD DISINTEGRATIVE DISORDER (299.10)

(ICD-10 code F84.3)

A. Apparently normal development for at least the first 2 years after birth as manifested by the presence of age-appropriate verbal and nonverbal communication, social relationships, play, and adaptive behavior.

B. Clinically significant loss of previously acquired skills (before age 10 years) in at least two of the following areas:
  (1) expressive or receptive language
  (2) social skills or adaptive behavior
  (3) bowel or bladder control
  (4) play
  (5) motor skills

C. Abnormalities of functioning in at least two of the following areas:
  (1) qualitative impairment in social interaction (e.g., impairment in nonverbal behaviors, failure to develop peer relationships, lack of social or emotional reciprocity)
  (2) qualitative impairments in communication (e.g., delay or lack of spoken language, inability to initiate or sustain a conversation, stereotyped and repetitive use of language, lack of varied make-believe play)
  (3) restricted, repetitive, and stereotyped patterns of behavior, interests, and activities, including motor stereotypies and mannerisms

D. The disturbance is not better accounted for by another specific Pervasive Developmental Disorder or by Schizophrenia.

> **NOTE: Code associated Mental Retardation on Axis II, and accompanying general medical conditions on Axis III.**

□ □ □ □

299.80 Asperger's Disorder
(new in DSM-IV)

(ICD-10 code F84.5)

ESSENTIAL FEATURES. There is marked and sustained impairment in the development of social interaction and development of restricted, repetitive behaviors, interests and activities, similar to symptoms of Autistic Disorder but in the absence of serious delays in communication or cognitive devlelopment.

ASSOCIATED FEATURES. Nonspecific neurological findings and/or general medical conditions may be present.

DIFFERENTIAL DIAGNOSIS. Other specific Pervasive Developmental Disorders, such as Autistic Disorder (see discussions above), preempt this diagnosis, as does Schizophrenia. Obsessive-Compulsive Disorder is not as restricting, nor does it qualitatively impair social interaction as does Asperger's Disorder. Primitive Personality Disorders (e.g., schizoid) involve less severe social impairments and lack marked stereotypy.

Diagnostic Criteria for Asperger's Disorder (299.80)

(ICD-10 code F84.5)

A. Qualitative impairment in social interaction, as manifested by at least two of the following:
   (1) marked impairment in the use of multiple nonverbal behaviors such as eye-to-eye gaze, facial expression, body postures, and gestures to regulate social interaction
   (2) failure to develop peer relationships appropriate to developmental level
   (3) Lack of spontaneous seeking to share enjoyment, interests, or achievements with other people (e.g., by a lack of showing, bringing, or pointing out objects of interest to other people)
   (4) Lack of social or emotional reciprocity

B. Restricted repetitive and stereotyped patterns of behavior, interests, and activities, as manifested by at least one of the following:
   (1) encompassing preoccupation with one or more stereotyped and restricted patterns of interest that is abnormal in either intensity or focus
   (2) apparently inflexible adherence to specific, nonfunctional routines or rituals
   (3) stereotyped and repetitive motor mannerisms (e.g., hand or finger flapping or twisting, or complex whole-body movements)
   (4) persistent preoccupation with parts of objects

C. The disturbance causes clinically significant impairment in social, occupational, or other important areas of functioning.

D. There is no clinically significant general delay in language (e.g., single words used by age 2 years, communicative phrases used by age 3 years).

E. There is no clinically significant delay in cognitive development or in the development of age-appropriate self-help skills, adaptive behavior (other than in social interaction), and curiosity about the environment in childhood.

F. Criteria are not met for another specific Pervasive Developmental Disorder or Schizophrenia.

□ □ □ □

299.80 Pervasive Developmental Disorder Not Otherwise Specified (NOS)

(ICD-10 code F84.9)

This is a residual category for patients with severe and pervasive impairment in development of reciprocal social interaction or verbal and nonverbal communication skills, or presentations of marked stereotyping of behavior or interests, but for whom criteria are not met for Autistic Disorder, Schizophrenia, or Avoidant, Schizoid, or Schizotypal Personality Disorder. Atypical autism, in which the patient does not meet all criteria for Autistic Disorder (e.g., because of late onset or atypical symptomatology) should be coded here.

□ □ □ □

··

ATTENTION-DEFICIT AND DISRUPTIVE BEHAVIOR DISORDERS

Attention-Deficit/Hyperactivity Disorder (AD/HD)
Conduct Disorder
Oppositional Defiant Disorder
Disruptive Behavior Disorder Not Otherwise Specified (NOS)

These disorders are characterized by socially disruptive behavior, which may be more distressing to others than to the patient.

314.xx Attention-Deficit/Hyperactivity Disorder (AD/HD)
(significantly modified from DSM-III-R)

314.01 Combined Type	*(ICD-10 code F90.0)*
314.00 Predominantly Inattentive Type	*(ICD-10 code F98.8)*
314.01 Predominantly Hyperactive-Impulsive Type	*(ICD-10 code F90.0)*
314.9 AD/HD NOS	*(ICD-10 code F90.9)*

ESSENTIAL FEATURES. There is developmentally inappropriate inattention, impulsiveness, and hyperactivity beginning before age 7 years, appearing at various levels in more than one setting (e.g., home, school, work), and significantly interfering with social, academic, or occupational functioning. In some patients either inattention or hyperactivity-impulsivity predominates, temporarily or indefinitely.

Symptoms usually become more subtle with age. In early childhood, hyperactivity, inattention, and impulsivity are obvious (although they may be difficult to distinguish from normal behavior before age 4 or 5). By adolescence, hyperactivity is the exception; behavior problems or poor school performance may be the primary presenting symptoms. In adults, job failure, impulsive behavior, or antisocial activity may predominate.

ASSOCIATED FEATURES. Associated features vary with age, and may include poor self-esteem, lability of mood, poor frustration tolerance, and temper outbursts. Academic underachievement and conflict with authority are characteristic. Symptoms of Oppositional Defiant Disorder, Conduct Disorder, and specific developmental disorders are often seen and should be separately diagnosed. "Functional" Encopresis or Enuresis is occasionally seen. In clinical samples, Tourette's Disorder is often accompanied by AD/HD.

Predisposing Factors. The history often suggests physical abuse, neglect, multiple foster placements, toxic exposure (e.g., environmental or in utero), perinatal complications, severe infection, or Mental Retardation. Seventy-five to 90% of patients are male.

Differential Diagnosis. Age-appropriate overactivity (generally better organized and less random than that seen in AD/HD) is considered. If the symptoms can be accounted for by Mental Retardation, AD/HD should not be diagnosed. Social reaction or Adjustment Disorders related to inadequate, disorganized, or chaotic environments may cause similar behavior. Pervasive Developmental Disorders and Psychotic Disorders preempt AD/HD, as do other mental disorders, if they better explain the symptoms.

DIAGNOSTIC CRITERIA FOR ATTENTION-DEFICIT/HYPERACTIVITY DISORDER

A. Either (1) or (2):

(1) *Inattention:* Six (or more) of the following symptoms of *inattention* have persisted for at least 6 months to a degree that is maladaptive and inconsistent with developmental level:

   (a) often fails to give close attention to details or makes careless mistakes in schoolwork, work, or other activities

   (b) often has difficulty sustaining attention in tasks or play activities

   (c) often does not seem to listen when spoken to directly

   (d) often does not follow through on instructions and fails to finish schoolwork, chores, or duties in the workplace (not due to oppositional behavior or failure to understand instructions)

   (e) often has difficulties organizing tasks and activities

   (f) often avoids, dislikes, or is reluctant to engage in tasks that require sustained mental effort (such as schoolwork or homework)

   (g) often loses things necessary for tasks or activities (e.g., toys, school assignments, pencils, books, or tools)

   (h) is often easily distracted by extraneous stimuli

   (i) is often forgetful in daily activities

(2) *Hyperactivity-impulsivity:* Six (or more) of the following symptoms of *hyperactivity–impulsivity* have persisted for at least 6 months to a degree that is maladaptive and inconsistent with developmental level:
Hyperactivity

   (a) often fidgets with hands or feet or squirms in seat

   (b) often leaves seat in classroom or in other situations in which remaining seated is expected

(c) often runs about or climbs excessively in situations in which it is in-appropriate (in adolescents or adults, may be limited to subjective feelings of restlessness)

(d) often has difficulty playing or engaging in leisure activities quietly

(e) is often "on the go" or acts as if "driven by a motor"

(f) often talks excessively

Impulsivity

(g) often blurts out answers before questions have been completed

(h) often has difficulty awaiting turn

(i) often interrupts or intrudes on others (e.g., butts into conversations or games)

B. Some hyperactive-impulsive or inattention symptoms that caused impairment were present before age 7 years.

C. Some impairment from the symptoms is present in two or more settings (e.g., at school [or work] and at home).

D. There must be clear evidence of clinically significant impairment in social, aca-demic, or occupational functioning.

E. The symptoms do not occur exclusively during the course of a Pervasive De-velopmental Disorder, Schizophrenia, or other Psychotic Disorder and are not better accounted for by another mental disorder (e.g., Mood Disorder, Anxi-ety Disorder, Dissociative Disorder, or a Personality Disorder).

Code based on type:
314.01 Combined Type: if both Criteria A1 and A2 are met for the past 6 months (ICD-10 F90.0)

314.00 Predominantly Inattentive Type: if Criterion A1 is met but Criterion A2 is not met for the past 6 months (ICD-10 F98.8)

314.01 Predominantly Hyperactive-Impulsive Type: if Criterion A2 is met but Criterion A1 is not met for the past 6 months (ICD-10 F90.0)

314.9 AD/HD NOS: symptoms are prominent but do not quite meet above criteria (ICD-10 F90.9)

CODING NOTE: For individuals (especially adolescents and adults) who currently have symptoms that no longer meet full criteria, "In Partial Remission" should be specified.

❏ ❏ ❏ ❏

312.8 Conduct Disorder   (ICD-10 code F91.8)
(significantly modified from DSM-III-R)

ESSENTIAL FEATURES. There is a persistent pattern of conduct in which the basic rights of others and/or major age-appropriate societal norms or rules are violated. The criteria provide for four kinds of antisocial behavior. The diagnosis may be made in adults but is preempted by Antisocial Personality Disorder (APD, 301.7) if APD criteria are met. Information from the patient should not be regarded as reliable; outside informants should be sought. As in AD/HD, symptoms are generally seen in more than one setting. The disorder is likely to persist into adulthood, and is considered a predisposing factor for APD.

In the Childhood-Onset Type, at least one symptom or criterion is present before age 10 years, and the full syndrome usually develops before puberty. Males predominate and aggression is the norm.

The Adolescent-Onset Type has no known symptoms prior to age 10 and is less likely to be associated with severe aggression. Females with Conduct · Disorder are much more likely to present with this type.

ASSOCIATED FEATURES. In the Childhood-Onset Type, previous Oppositional Defiant Disorder is common. Substance use/abuse or sexual behavior may begin unusually early for the child's peer group. Lack of concern for the feelings and well-being of others, lack of guilt or remorse, low self-esteem (although the patient may appear "tough"), poor frustration tolerance, temper outbursts, provocative recklessness, anxiety, depression, and/or low academic achievement (which may justify additional diagnoses) are common.

PREDISPOSING FACTORS. Attention-Deficit/Hyperactivity Disorder (AD/HD) and Oppositional Defiant Disorder have been implicated as possible precursors of Conduct Disorder, as have parental rejection, inconsistent parenting, early institutional placement, paternal absence or social deviance, large family size, and association with delinquent subgroups.

DIFFERENTIAL DIAGNOSIS. The differential diagnosis includes Child or Adolescent Antisocial Behavior (V71.02) and Oppositional Defiant Disorder (following). AD/HD per se does not imply Conduct Disorder; if criteria for AD/HD are met, both may be diagnosed. Behavior solely associated with a particular setting or stressor should be coded as an Adjustment Disorder. Antisocial Personality Disorder cannot be diagnosed before age 18; it preempts Conduct Disorder. Conduct symptoms associated with Mood Disorders should not be confused with Conduct Disorder. If criteria for both are present, both should be diagnosed.

DIAGNOSTIC CRITERIA FOR   (ICD-10 code F91.8)
CONDUCT DISORDER (312.8)

A. A repetitive and persistent pattern of behavior in which the basic rights of others or major age-appropriate societal norms or rules are violated, as manifested by the presence of three (or more) of the following criteria in the past 12 months, with at least one criterion present in the past 6 months:

Aggression toward people and animals
 (1) often bullies, threatens, or intimidates others
 (2) often initiates physical fights
 (3) has used a weapon that can cause serious physical harm to others (e.g., a bat, brick, broken bottle, knife, gun)
 (4) has been physically cruel to people
 (5) has been physically cruel to animals
 (6) has stolen while confronting a victim (e.g., mugging, purse snatching, extortion, armed robbery)
 (7) has forced someone into sexual activity

Destruction of property
 (8) has deliberately engaged in fire setting with the intention of causing serious damage
 (9) has deliberately destroyed others' property (other than by fire setting)

Deceitfulness or theft
 (10) has broken into someone else's house, building, or car
 (11) often lies to obtain goods or favors or to avoid obligations (i.e., "cons" others)
 (12) has stolen items of nontrivial value without confronting a victim (e.g., shoplifting, but without breaking and entering; forgery)

Serious violations of rules
 (13) often stays out at night despite parental prohibitions, beginning before age 13 years
 (14) has run away from home overnight at least twice while living in parental or parental surrogate home (or once without returning for a lengthy period)
 (15) is often truant from school, beginning before age 13 years

B. The disturbance in behavior causes clinically significant impairment in social, academic, or occupational functioning.

C. If the individual is age 18 years or older, criteria are not met for Antisocial Personality Disorder.

Specify type based on age of onset:
Childhood-Onset Type: onset of at least one criterion characteristic of Conduct Disorder prior to age 10 years

Adolescent-Onset Type: absence of any criteria characteristic of Conduct Disorder prior to age 10 years

Specify severity:
Mild: few if any conduct problems in excess of those required to make the diagnosis and conduct problems cause only minor harm to others

Moderate: number of conduct problems and effect on others intermediate between mild and severe

Severe: many conduct problems in excess of those required to make the diagnosis *or* conduct problems cause considerable harm to others

❑ ❑ ❑ ❑

313.81 Oppositional Defiant Disorder   *(ICD-10 code F91.3)*
(significantly modified from DSM-III-R)

ESSENTIAL FEATURES. There is a pattern of negativistic, hostile, and defiant behavior toward authority figures but without the serious aggression or violations of others' rights seen in Conduct Disorder. The disorder may not be manifest in school or outside the family but is almost always seen at home. Rationalization of the unacceptable behavior is usual.

ASSOCIATED FEATURES. Associated features include low self-esteem, mood lability, low frustration tolerance, temper outbursts, and substance abuse, varying with age. Attention-Deficit/Hyperactivity Disorder (AD/HD) is often present. A history of interrupted or inconsistent parenting is common, and it is tempting to infer a causal link with repeated changes of the primary caregiver. Learning and Communication Disorders are commonly seen.

DIFFERENTIAL DIAGNOSIS. Conduct Disorder and adults with Antisocial Personality Disorder have more severe antisocial and aggressive symptoms; they preempt the diagnosis. Oppositional Defiant Disorder should not be diagnosed separately when the symptoms are observed with a Psychotic or Mood Disorder. Oppositional behavior can be part of a normal developmental stage or Mental Retardation, or arise from frustration associated with sensory or language impairment.

DIAGNOSTIC CRITERIA FOR   (ICD-10 code F91.3)
OPPOSITIONAL DEFIANT DISORDER (313.81)

A. A pattern of negativistic, hostile, and defiant behavior lasting at least 6 months, during which four (or more) of the following are present:
    (1) often loses temper
    (2) often argues with adults
    (3) often actively defies or refuses to comply with adults' requests or rules
    (4) often deliberately annoys people
    (5) often blames others for his or her mistakes or misbehavior
    (6) is often touchy or easily annoyed by others
    (7) is often angry and resentful
    (8) is often spiteful or vindictive

NOTE: Consider a criterion met only if the behavior occurs more frequently than is typically observed in individuals of comparable age and developmental level.

B. The disturbance in behavior causes clinically significant impairment in social, academic, or occupational functioning.

C. The behaviors do not occur exclusively during the course of a Psychotic or Mood Disorder.

D. Criteria are not met for Conduct Disorder, and, if the individual is age 18 years or older, criteria are not met for Antisocial Personality Disorder.

❑ ❑ ❑ ❑

312.9 Disruptive Behavior Disorder Not Otherwise Specified (NOS) *(ICD-10 code F91.9)*

This category is for clinically significant conditions that are similar to, but below threshold criteria for, Oppositional Defiant Disorder and Conduct Disorder.

❑ ❑ ❑ ❑

....

FEEDING AND EATING DISORDERS OF INFANCY OR EARLY CHILDHOOD
(Eating Disorders in DSM-III-R)

Pica
Rumination Disorder
Feeding Disorder of Infancy or Early Childhood

NOTE: Anorexia Nervosa, Bulimia Nervosa, and Eating Disorder Not Otherwise Specified (NOS) are no longer described among Disorders First Diagnosed in Infancy, Childhood, or Adolescence. See Eating Disorders, pp 539–550.

These are gross disturbances in feeding or eating behavior typically (but not always) beginning in infancy. Simple obesity is coded as a physical disorder and is not included in this section unless emotional symptoms merit inclusion under Psychological Factor Affecting Physical Condition (316).

307.52 Pica *(ICD-10 code F98.3)*
(significantly modified from DSM-III-R)

ESSENTIAL FEATURES. There is persistent eating of one or more nonnutritive, sometimes bizarre substances, separate from any culturally accepted ritual or context. In older children and adults, it is often hidden from observers and may not be diagnosed until medical complications appear.

ASSOCIATED FEATURES AND DISORDERS. Pica is not uncommon in persons with Moderate or Severe Mental Retardation (and should be separately diagnosed). It is sometimes seen in pregnant women. Pica is not associated with aversion to food, nor generally with any dietary deficiency or attempt to replace, for example, minerals absent from the diet.

COMPLICATIONS. Poisoning, infection, gastrointestinal obstruction, and perforation are the most common complications. The condition is occasionally life threatening, particularly among mentally retarded persons.

PREDISPOSING FACTORS. In addition to the conditions mentioned above, parental neglect appears to predispose children to Pica. Pica is rare in otherwise normal adults.

DIFFERENTIAL DIAGNOSIS. Occasional normal mouthing or sometimes swallowing nonfood items in infancy or early childhood, Pervasive Developmental Disorders, delusional ritual or belief, and certain physical disorders (e.g., Kleine-Levin syndrome) are considered in the differential diagnosis. Pica should not be additionally coded in these disorders unless it merits special clinical attention.

DIAGNOSTIC CRITERIA FOR (ICD-10 code F98.3)
PICA (307.52)

A. Persistent eating of nonnutritive substances for a period of at least 1 month.

B. The eating of nonnutritive substances is inappropriate to the developmental level.

C. The eating behavior is not part of a culturally sanctioned practice.

D. If the eating behavior occurs exclusively during the course of another mental disorder (e.g., Mental Retardation, Pervasive Developmental Disorder, Schizophrenia), it is sufficiently severe to warrant independent clinical attention.

❑ ❑ ❑ ❑

307.53 Rumination Disorder (ICD-10 code F98.2)
(Rumination Disorder of Infancy in DSM-III-R)
(significantly modified from DSM-III-R)

ESSENTIAL FEATURES. There is repeated regurgitation and rechewing of food without associated general medical (e.g., gastrointestinal) disorder. The symptom develops after a period of normal function and lasts at least a month. Nausea, retching, disgust, or associated gastrointestinal disorders are not present. The food may be ejected or chewed and reswallowed. There is a characteristic straining and arching position, with the head held back. The infant appears to experience satisfaction from this activity. Onset is in infancy, except in some cases of mentally retarded persons.

ASSOCIATED FEATURES. Associated features include weight loss or failure to gain. The disorder usually appears between 3 and 12 months of age, occasionally later in mentally retarded children. Caretakers are often frustrated, sometimes to the point of alienation from the child. On the other hand, inadequate caretaking or neglect may contribute to the development of the disorder.

ASSOCIATED PHYSICAL, LABORATORY, AND GENERAL MEDICAL FINDINGS. Findings consistent with malnutrition may be seen.

COMPLICATIONS. Complications include slowed growth, failure to gain, and death from malnutrition.

DIFFERENTIAL DIAGNOSIS. Normal regurgitation found in early infancy and congenital abnormalities, including pyloric stenosis, esophageal reflux, and gastrointestinal infections, are considered. If the activity occurs exclusively during bouts of Anorexia Nervosa or Bulimia Nervosa, it should not be diagnosed. If part of a Pervasive Developmental Disorder or Mental Retardation, it should not be diagnosed unless special clinical attention is merited.

DIAGNOSTIC CRITERIA FOR RUMINATION DISORDER (307.53) (ICD-10 code F98.2)

A. Repeated regurgitation and rechewing of food for a period of at least 1 month following a period of normal functioning.

B. The behavior is not due to an associated gastrointestinal or other general medical condition (e.g., esophageal reflux).

C. The behavior does not occur exclusively during the course of Anorexia Nervosa or Bulimia Nervosa. If the symptoms occur exclusively during the course of Mental Retardation or a Pervasive Developmental Disorder, they are sufficiently severe to warrant independent clinical attention.

□ □ □ □

307.59 Feeding Disorder of Infancy or Early Childhood (ICD-10 code F98.2)
(new in DSM-IV)

ESSENTIAL FEATURES. There is persistent failure to eat adequately, with significant weight loss or failure to gain, beginning before age 6 years. The syndrome is not explained by a general medical condition, nor better explained by another mental disorder.

ASSOCIATED FEATURES. Irritability, apathy, and/or developmental delays are sometimes seen. Inadequate parenting, such as not presenting food appropriately, is common, as are problems with parent-child interaction (often exacerbated by the infant's rejection of food). Parental psychopathology, abuse, or neglect should be considered. Improved feeding or weight gain after changing the care-giver should suggest this feeding disorder.

ASSOCIATED PHYSICAL, LABORATORY, AND GENERAL MEDICAL FINDINGS. Findings consistent with malnutrition may be seen, including laboratory abnormalities and growth delays.

DIFFERENTIAL DIAGNOSIS. Ordinary infant feeding problems (that do not lead to weight loss or failure to gain) are considered. General medical conditions that either cause feeding disturbances or make it harder for the infant to feed preempt this diagnosis, unless the signs and symptoms are greater than expected for the accompanying condition.

DIAGNOSTIC CRITERIA FOR FEEDING DISORDER OF INFANCY OR EARLY CHILDHOOD (307.59)

(ICD-10 code F98.2)

A. Feeding disturbance as manifested by persistent failure to eat adequately with significant failure to gain weight or significant loss of weight over at least 1 month.

B. The disturbance is not due to an associated gastrointestinal or other general medical condition (e.g., esophageal reflux).

C. The disturbance is not better accounted for by another mental disorder (e.g., Rumination Disorder) or by lack of available food.

D. The onset is onset before age 6 years.

❑ ❑ ❑ ❑

....

TIC DISORDERS

Tourette's Disorder
Chronic Motor or Vocal Tic Disorder
Transient Tic Disorder
Tic Disorder Not Otherwise Specified (NOS)

Tics are involuntary, sudden, rapid, recurrent, nonrhythmic, stereotyped motor movements or vocalizations. They are experienced as irresistible but usually can be temporarily suppressed. They are frequently exacerbated by stress and usually markedly diminished during sleep (and sometimes during absorbing activities such as reading).

Simple tics are primitive and uncomplicated (e.g., grunts, jerks, blinking). *Complex tics* involve more complicated, often pseudopurposeful movements (e.g., gestures, grooming, smelling things) or vocalizations (e.g., complete words or phrases). *Vocal tics* may manifest as echolalia (immediately repeating

44

others' words), palilalia (repeating one's own words), or coprolalia (using unacceptable or obscene language), although not all such expressions are the result of tics.

Tic Disorders must be differentiated from other sources of abnormal movements, such as primary neurological disorders, sequelae of head trauma, and medication effects or toxicities (including those from neuroleptic drugs). Tics are not rhythmic, do not have the stereotypic appearance of Pervasive Developmental Disorders or Stereotypic Movement Disorder, and do not have the complexity or driven quality of compulsions. Their involuntary nature is usually obvious and aids in diagnosis.

□ □ □ □

307.23 Tourette's Disorder (ICD-10 code F95.2)
(significantly modified from DSM-III-R)

ESSENTIAL FEATURES. Essential features include multiple motor and one or more vocal tics, which may appear simultaneously or at different periods during the illness. They occur frequently, often many times a day, over at least a year. The tics typically involve the head. The vocal tics are generally guttural and primitive, and may uncommonly include coprolalia. The first symptoms to appear are often single tics, perhaps eye blinking or tongue protrusion.

ASSOCIATED FEATURES. Associated features can include occasional intrusive, socially unacceptable, or obscene thoughts or behaviors, which may reach the level of obsessions or compulsions. Social difficulties, either because of embarrassment or misunderstanding by others, are common. Other disorders, such as Attention-Deficit/Hyperactivity Disorder or Obsessive-Compulsive Disorder, may be seen. Genetic transmission occurs via autosomal dominance with high penetrance, although the presentation varies from generation to generation; some patients have no family history of the disorder.

DIFFERENTIAL DIAGNOSIS. The differential diagnosis of tics in general includes other movement disturbances (e.g., choreiform, dystonic, athetoid, myoclonic, hemiballismic), muscle spasms, synkinesias, dyskinesias, stereotyped movements and compulsions (see introduction above). Other items in the differential diagnosis include amphetamine intoxication (which can exacerbate symptoms of Tourette's Disorder when present), several neurological disorders, general medical conditions, Schizophrenia, and Tardive Dyskinesia. Chronic Motor or Vocal Tic Disorder exhibits motor or vocal tics but not both, and is generally milder. Transient Tic Disorder is usually milder and is differentiated by its shorter duration (less than 12 consecutive months). Tourette's Disorder preempts both.

DIAGNOSTIC CRITERIA FOR (ICD-10 code F95.2)
TOURETTE'S DISORDER (307.23)

A. Both multiple motor and one or more vocal tics have been present at some time during the illness, although not necessarily concurrently. (A *tic* is a sudden, rapid, recurrent, nonrhythmic, stereotyped motor movement or vocalization.)

B. The tics occur many times a day (usually in bouts) nearly every day or intermittently throughout a period of more than 1 year, and during this period there was never a tic-free period of more than 3 consecutive months.

C. The disturbance causes marked distress or significant impairment in social, occupational, or other important areas of functioning.

D. The onset is before age 18 years.

E. The disturbance is not due to the direct physiological effects of a substance (e.g., stimulants) or a general medical condition (e.g., Huntington's disease or postviral encephalitis).

□ □ □ □

307.22 Chronic Motor or Vocal Tic Disorder (ICD-10 code F95.1)
(significantly modified from DSM-III-R)

ESSENTIAL FEATURES. Either motor or vocal tics are present, but not both. Otherwise similar to Tourette's Disorder, except that the severity and functional impairment are usually much less.

DIFFERENTIAL DIAGNOSIS. (See differential diagnosis of tics under Tourette's Disorder, above.) Transient Tic Disorder (see following) and Tourette's Disorder are considered. Tourette's Disorder preempts the diagnosis.

DIAGNOSTIC CRITERIA FOR (ICD-10 code F95.1)
CHRONIC MOTOR OR VOCAL TIC
DISORDER (307.22)

A. Single or multiple motor or vocal tics (i.e., sudden, rapid, recurrent, nonrhythmic, stereotyped motor movements or vocalizations), but not both, have been present at some time during the illness.

B. The tics occur many times a day nearly every day or intermittently throughout a period of more than 1 year, and during this period there was never a tic-free period of more than 3 consecutive months.

C. The disturbance causes marked distress or significant impairment in social, occupational, or other important areas of functioning.

D. The onset is before age 18 years.

E. The disturbance is not due to the direct physiological effects of a substance (e.g., stimulants) or a general medical condition (e.g., Huntington's disease or postviral encephalitis).

F. Criteria have never been met for Tourette's Disorder.

❑ ❑ ❑ ❑

307.21 Transient Tic Disorder   *(ICD-10 code F95.0)*
(significantly modified from DSM-III-R)

ESSENTIAL FEATURES. There are motor and/or vocal tics that occur many times a day, nearly every day, for at least 4 weeks, but not longer than 1 year. Eye blinking or other facial tics are most common, but other parts of the body may be involved. Otherwise similar to Tourette's Disorder.

DIFFERENTIAL DIAGNOSIS. (See differential diagnosis of tics under Tourette's Disorder, preceding.) Tourette's Disorder and Chronic Motor or Vocal Tic Disorder (either of which preempts the diagnosis) are considered.

DIAGNOSTIC CRITERIA FOR   *(ICD-10 code F95.0)*
TRANSIENT TIC DISORDER (307.21)

A. Single or multiple motor and/or vocal tics (i.e., sudden, rapid, recurrent, non-rhythmic, stereotyped motor movements or vocalizations).

B. The tics occur many times a day, nearly every day for at least 4 weeks, but for no longer than 12 consecutive months.

C. The disturbance causes marked distress or significant impairment in social, occupational, or other important areas of functioning.

D. The onset is before age 18 years.

E. The disturbance is not due to the direct physiological effects of a substance (e.g., stimulants) or a general medical condition (e.g., Huntington's disease or postviral encephalitis).

F. Criteria have never been met for Tourette's Disorder or Chronic Motor or Vocal Tic Disorder.

Specify if:
Single Episode or **Recurrent**

❑ ❑ ❑ ❑

307.20 Tic Disorder Not Otherwise Specified (NOS) (ICD-10 code F95.9)

This is a residual category for tic disorders that do not meet the above criteria for a specific Tic Disorder (e.g., duration, age of onset). It should not be used for tics that are the result of neurological injury, illness, or other medical conditions.

❏ ❏ ❏ ❏

ELIMINATION DISORDERS

Encopresis With Constipation and Overflow Incontinence
Encopresis Without Constipation and Overflow Incontinence
Enuresis (not due to a general medical condition)

787.6, 307.7 Encopresis (ICD-10 codes R15, F98.1)
(includes "Functional Encopresis" in DSM-III-R)
(significantly modified from DSM-III-R)

ESSENTIAL FEATURES. There is repeated defecating in inappropriate places (e.g., into clothing or onto floor). It may be involuntary (most common) or voluntary. Age and duration criteria must be met, and there is no causative substance (e.g., laxative) or general medical condition other than one associated with constipation. Informal labeling as "primary" (no previous period of fecal continence) or "secondary" (symptoms arising after a period of continence) may be useful. The course may be intermittent, but the disorder rarely persists for many years.

ASSOCIATED FEATURES. Shame, embarrassment, and avoidance of potentially embarrassing situations such as school or camp are common. Adverse effects on the child's self-esteem, social ostracism, and adverse reactions by caretakers may be seen. Many children also have Enuresis. Smearing of feces should be differentiated from attempts to clean or hide feces accidentally passed. Intentional Encopresis is often associated with Conduct Disorders and other psychopathology, which should be separately diagnosed.

PREDISPOSING FACTORS. Inadequate, inconsistent toilet training and severe psychosocial stress (but sometimes as little as starting school or acquiring a sibling) are considered predisposing factors.

DIFFERENTIAL DIAGNOSIS. Encopresis may be diagnosed in the presence of a general medical condition that involves constipation (e.g., aganglionic megacolon), but should not be diagnosed when due to other medical disorders (e.g., diarrhea).

DIAGNOSTIC CRITERIA FOR
ENCOPRESIS (787.6, 307.7)

(ICD-10 codes
R15, F98.1)

A. Repeated passage of feces into inappropriate places (e.g., clothing or floor) whether involuntary or intentional.

B. At least one such event a month for at least 3 months.

C. Chronological age at least 4 years (or equivalent developmental level).

D. The behavior is not due exclusively to the direct physiological effects of a substance (e.g., laxatives) or a general medical condition except through a mechanism involving constipation.

> **Code as follows:**
> **787.6 With Constipation and Overflow Incontinence**
> (ICD-10 R15)
>
> **307.7 Without Constipation and Overflow Incontinence**
> (ICD-10 F98.1)

□ □ □ □

307.6 Enuresis (not due to a general medical condition)

(ICD-10 code F98.0)

(Functional Enuresis in DSM-III-R)
(significantly modified from DSM-III-R)

ESSENTIAL FEATURES. There is repeated involuntary or intentional urination, during day or night, into bed or clothes, after a mental age at which continence is expected. Frequency and duration criteria may be waived if clinically significant distress or impairment is present. There is no causative substance (e.g., a diuretic) or general medical condition.

The *nocturnal* subtype, most common, typically involves the first third of the night's sleep. Urination usually takes place during deep, non-REM sleep but may be associated with dreaming. The *diurnal* (daytime) subtype is sometimes related to preoccupation with other activities or anxiety about public toilets, and is more common in females than males. It rarely persists beyond age 8 or 9. The DSM-III-R concepts of "primary" (the person has never had a full year of urinary continence) and "secondary" (symptoms arising after at least 1 year of continence) may be clinically useful.

ASSOCIATED FEATURES. Shame, embarrassment, and avoidance of potentially embarassing situations such as school or camp are common. Most children do not have a coexisting mental disorder, although Encopresis, Sleepwalking, and Sleep Terrors may be seen (and should be separately diagnosed). The incidence of other mental disorders is higher in people with a history of Enuresis. Social or mental impairment is often related to effects on self-esteem, social ostracism, and adverse reactions by caretakers.

PREDISPOSING FACTORS. Predisposing factors include delay in development of bladder musculature and causes of lowered bladder volume, delayed or lax toilet training, and psychological stress such as hospitalization, entering school, or birth of a sibling. Although the condition may be diagnosed in association with urinary tract infections (either existing before infection or persisting after appropriate treatment), potential neurological, anatomic, and infectious etiologies should be sought before making this "functional" diagnosis.

DIFFERENTIAL DIAGNOSIS. General medical conditions that predispose one to polyuria, urgency, or inability to control the urinary sphincter (e.g., neurogenic bladder, diabetes, seizure disorder, urinary tract infection), and intentional urination which is part of Oppositional Defiant Disorder or a similar condition are considered in the differential diagnosis.

DIAGNOSTIC CRITERIA FOR ENURESIS (307.6)   (ICD-10 code F98.0)

A. Repeated voiding of urine into bed or clothes (whether involuntary or intentional).

B. The behavior is clinically significant as manifested by either a frequency of twice a week for at least 3 consecutive months or the presence of clinically significant distress or impairment in social, academic (occupational), or other important areas of functioning.

C. Chronological age is at least 5 years (or equivalent developmental level).

D. The behavior is not due exclusively to the direct physiological effect of a substance (e.g., a diuretic) or a general medical condition (e.g., diabetes, spina bifida, a seizure disorder).

> **Specify type:**
> Nocturnal Only
> Diurnal Only
> Nocturnal and Diurnal

❑ ❑ ❑ ❑

OTHER DISORDERS OF INFANCY, CHILDHOOD, OR ADOLESCENCE

Separation Anxiety Disorder
Selective Mutism
Reactive Attachment Disorder of Infancy or Early Childhood
Stereotypic Movement Disorder
Disorder of Infancy, Childhood, or Adolescence Not Otherwise Specified (NOS)

309.21 Separation Anxiety Disorder   (ICD-10 code F93.0)
(significantly modified from DSM-III-R)

ESSENTIAL FEATURES. Excessive anxiety concerning separation from home or from those to whom the child is attached, beyond that expected for the person's developmental level. Symptoms begin before age 18 years, are present for at least 4 weeks, and cause clinically significant distress or impairment. Children often show fears of real or imaginary objects, or exhibit extreme homesickness. Older children and adolescents, especially boys, may deny their overconcern, yet exhibit anxiety. Although similar to a phobia, it is not included among the phobic disorders. When no demands for separation are made, symptoms are typically absent. Onset before age 6 may be specified as Early Onset; this is associated with the development of Panic Disorder in adulthood.

ASSOCIATED FEATURES. Fears (e.g., of the dark, accidents, danger to family or home), depressed mood or Mood Disorder, need for constant attention, or aggressive behavior when removed from home or family is seen. Specific manifestations vary with age and culture.

PREDISPOSING FACTORS. The disorder frequently is associated with a life stress, typically a loss (e.g., a death, divorce, family move, or other environmental change). Children from close-knit families are overrepresented, while neglected children are underrepresented.

DIFFERENTIAL DIAGNOSIS. Normal separation anxiety of early childhood and overanxious disorder (in which the anxiety is not focused on separation) are considered. Pervasive Developmental Disorders, Schizophrenia and other Psychotic Disorders, Panic Disorder With Agoraphobia, and Agoraphobia Without History of Panic Disorder preempt this diagnosis. Other Anxiety Disorders and Mood Disorders should be differentiated, but are diagnosed concomitantly if both criteria are met. In Conduct Disorder, the child may stay away from home as well as school but usually does not show signs of anxiety about separation.

DIAGNOSTIC CRITERIA FOR   (ICD-10 code F93.0)
SEPARATION ANXIETY DISORDER (309.21)

A. Developmentally inappropriate and excessive anxiety concerning separation from home or from those to whom the individual is attached, as evidenced by three (or more) of the following:
   (1) recurrent excessive distress when separation from home or major attachment figures occurs or is anticipated
   (2) persistent and excessive worry about losing, or about possible harm befalling, major attachment figures
   (3) persistent and excessive worry that an untoward event will lead to separation from a major attachment figure (e.g., getting lost or being kidnapped)
   (4) persistent reluctance or refusal to go to school or elsewhere because of fear of separation

    (5) persistent and excessive fear or reluctance to be alone or without major attachment figures at home or without significant adults in other settings

    (6) persistent reluctance or refusal to go to sleep without being near a major attachment figure or to sleep away from home

    (7) repeated nightmares involving the theme of separation

    (8) repeated complaints of physical symptoms (such as headaches, stomachaches, nausea, or vomiting) when separation from major attachment figures occurs or is anticipated

B. Duration of the disturbance is at least 4 weeks.

C. The onset is before age 18 years.

D. The disturbance causes clinically significant distress or impairment in social, academic (occupational), or other important areas of functioning.

E. The disturbance does not occur exclusively during the course of a Pervasive Developmental Disorder, Schizophrenia, or other Psychotic Disorder and, in adolescents and adults, is not better accounted for by Panic Disorder With Agoraphobia.

> **Specify if:**
> **Early Onset:** if onset occurs before age 6 years

❑ ❑ ❑ ❑

313.23 Selective Mutism   (ICD-10 code F94.0)
(Elective Mutism in DSM-III-R)
(significantly modified from DSM-III-R)

ESSENTIAL FEATURES. Persistent refusal to talk in one or more specific social situations in which speaking is expected, such as school, despite speaking in other settings. The mutism is not a symptom of Social Phobia, Mood Disorder, or Psychotic Disorder. Communication may be by gestures or short utterances. The child often will not speak at school, but talks normally at home.

ASSOCIATED FEATURES. Sometimes a result of teasing or scapegoating from peers, symptoms can include excessive shyness, social isolation or withdrawal, clinging, school refusal, compulsiveness, or controlling or oppositional behavior (including tantrums). Although most children with Selective Mutism have normal language development, occasional Communication Disorders or abnormalities of articulation may be present. School and social functioning may be severely impaired.

PREDISPOSING FACTORS. Predisposing factors include maternal overprotection, Communication Disorders, and marked social or environmental change (e.g., immigration, early childhood hospitalization or trauma). Some Anxiety Disorders, such as Social Phobia, or Mental Retardation may be either associated or predisposing.

DIFFERENTIAL DIAGNOSIS. Mental Retardation, Pervasive Developmental Disorders, and Communication Disorders, which produce an *inability* to speak rather than *refusal* to do so, are considered. Selective Mutism should not be diagnosed in persons who have immigrated to a country with a different language, unless one is sure they speak the new language fluently. Schizophrenia and other Psychotic Disorders preempt the diagnosis. When Selective Mutism is part of Social Phobia, both diagnoses may be made.

DIAGNOSTIC CRITERIA FOR (ICD-10 code F94.0)
SELECTIVE MUTISM (313.23)

A. Consistent failure to speak in specific social situations in which there is an expectation for speaking (e.g., at school), despite speaking in other situations.

B. The disturbance interferes with educational or occupational achievement or with social communication.

C. The duration is at least 1 month (not limited to the first month of school).

D. The failure to speak is not due to a lack of knowledge of, or comfort with, the spoken language required in the social situation.

E. The disturbance is not better accounted for by a Communication Disorder (e.g., Stuttering), and does not occur exclusively during the course of a Pervasive Developmental Disorder, Schizophrenia, or other Psychotic Disorder.

❑ ❑ ❑ ❑

313.89 Reactive Attachment Disorder of (ICD-10 code
Infancy or Early Childhood F94.1, F94.2)

ESSENTIAL FEATURES. There is marked disturbance of social relatedness in most or all social and interpersonal contexts, related to grossly inadequate or pathogenic care by the primary caregivers. The disturbance may be manifested either by persistent failure to initiate or respond to social interactions in an age-appropriate manner, such as with severe inhibition, hypervigilance, or extreme ambivalence (Inhibited Type), or by indiscriminate, nonselective familiarity with or attachment to others (Disinhibited Type). Similar syndromes have been called "failure to thrive" or "hospitalism."

Infants with this disorder present with poor social responsiveness. They may exhibit little (or late-to-develop) visual tracking of others' eyes and faces, or little response to the voice of the parent or caregiver (both of which should be developed by 2 months of age). In order to confirm or rule out the diagnosis, the examiner may observe the caregiver and child together extensively, perhaps in their home environment. Adequate infant or child care, in or out of the hospital, causes substantial improvement, unless physical complications (e.g., starvation, dehydration) are severe.

ASSOCIATED FEATURES. Associated features include developmental delays and feeding disturbances (e.g., Pica, Rumination, regurgitation, vomiting). The child may be apathetic, with a weak cry and ineffectual motor responses, excessive sleep, and disinterest in the environment. Physical and laboratory signs of abuse, malnutrition, or dehydration may be present.

PREDISPOSING FACTORS. Parental psychopathology or substance abuse, family poverty, prolonged hospitalization, and parental inexperience are among the predisposing factors.

DIFFERENTIAL DIAGNOSIS. Reactive Attachment Disorder should not be diagnosed in the presence of significant Mental Retardation unless the retardation does not account for the attachment symptoms. Pervasive Developmental Disorders preempt the diagnosis. The Disinhibited Type may be confused with Attention Deficit/Hyperactivity Disorder. Some severe neurological deficits or chronic physical illnesses may partially mimic this disorder; however, the marked disturbance in social relatedness found in Reactive Attachment Disorder is generally absent. Grossly pathogenic caretaking which does not result in all criteria being met should be cited as a V code with focus on the victim (e.g., Child Neglect or Abuse [V61.21/995.5] or Parent-Child Relational Problem [V61.20]).

DIAGNOSTIC CRITERIA FOR REACTIVE ATTACHMENT DISORDER OF INFANCY OR EARLY CHILDHOOD (313.89)

(ICD-10 code F94.1, F94.2)

A. Markedly disturbed and developmentally inappropriate social relatedness in most contexts, beginning before age 5 years, as evidenced by either (1) or (2):
   (1) persistent failure to initiate or respond in a developmentally appropriate fashion to most social interactions, as manifest by excessively inhibited, hypervigilant, or highly ambivalent and contradictory responses (e.g., the child may respond to caregivers with a mixture of approach, avoidance, and resistance to comforting, or may exhibit frozen watchfulness)
   (2) diffuse attachments as manifest by indiscriminate sociability with marked inability to exhibit appropriate selective attachments (e.g., excessive familiarity with relative strangers or lack of selectivity in choice of attachment figures)

B. The disturbance in Criterion A is not accounted for solely by developmental delay (as in Mental Retardation) and does not meet criteria for a Pervasive Developmental Disorder.

C. Pathogenic care as evidenced by at least one of the following:

(1) persistent disregard for the child's basic emotional needs for comfort, stimulation, and affection

(2) persistent disregard for the child's basic physical needs

(3) repeated changes of primary caregiver that prevent formation of stable attachments (e.g., frequent changes in foster care)

D. There is a presumption that the care in Criterion C is responsible for the disturbed behavior in Criterion A (e.g., the disturbances in Criterion A began following the pathogenic care in Criterion C).

Specify type:
Inhibited: if Criterion A1 predominates in the clinical presentation (ICD-10 code F94.1)

Disinhibited: if Criterion A2 predominates in the clinical presentation (ICD-10 code F94.2)

❑ ❑ ❑ ❑

307.3 Stereotypic Movement Disorder (ICD-10 code F98.4)
(Stereotypy/Habit Disorder in DSM-III-R)
(significantly modified from DSM-III-R)

ESSENTIAL FEATURES. The patient exhibits voluntary and repetitive behaviors, often appearing driven, that serve no constructive or social purpose except self-stimulation (e.g., rocking, other rhythmic behaviors, head banging, picking at oneself, vocalizations). The disorder interferes considerably with normal activities and/or leads to significant physicial injury.

ASSOCIATED FEATURES. Associated features frequently include Mental Retardation, sensory deprivation (e.g., as once found in some institutions for persons with Mental Retardation), self-restraining behaviors (e.g., keeping one's hands inside his shirt), or complications of self-injury. Injury is sometimes severe, especially when associated with Moderate or Severe Mental Retardation and neuropsychiatric disorder such as Lesch-Nyhan syndrome.

PREDISPOSING FACTORS. Mental Retardation, multiple handicaps, sensory deficit or deprivation, and certain neurological disorders (e.g., Lesch-Nyhan syndrome, fragile-X syndrome) are among the predisposing factors. The behavior may begin as a means of communicating, or dealing with, physical pain or illness (e.g., ear infection leading to head banging in a mentally retarded person who cannot otherwise describe or cope with his or her discomfort). The disorder may be separately diagnosed if it coexists with severe psychiatric disorders or Substance-Induced Disorders (other than a Pervasive Developmental Disorder or Tic Disorder).

DIFFERENTIAL DIAGNOSIS. Normal self-stimulation in young children or that related to simple sensory deprivation (neither of which usually results in injury), and Tic Disorders (in which the behavior appears less driven and is not intentional) must be differentiated. Stereotypic Movement Disorder should not be diagnosed if the symptoms are better accounted for by a Pervasive Developmental Disorder, nor should it be diagnosed in addition to Mental Retardation unless the stereotypic behavior or self-injury is significant enough to become a focus of treatment. Obsessive-Compulsive Disorder is generally more complex and ritualistic. Trichotillomania is limited to pulling one's hair. Factitious Disorder has a conscious motivation. Self-mutilation associated with primitive Personality Disorders and Psychotic Disorders is sometimes difficult to differentiate from this diagnosis, but the premeditation, complexity, or delusional context of the former is generally inconsistent with Stereotypic Movement Disorder. Involuntary movements associated with some general medical conditions (e.g., Huntington's disease, Tardive Dyskinesia) usually follow typical patterns and lack the intentionality of this disorder.

DIAGNOSTIC CRITERIA FOR (ICD-10 code F98.4)
STEREOTYPIC MOVEMENT DISORDER (307.3)

A. Repetitive, seemingly driven, nonfunctional motor behavior (e.g., hand shaking or waving, body rocking, head banging, mouthing of objects, self-biting, picking at skin or bodily orifices, hitting own body).

B. The behavior markedly interferes with normal activities or results in self-inflicted bodily injury that requires medical treatment (or would result in an injury if preventive measures were not used).

C. If Mental Retardation is present, the stereotypic or self-injurious behavior is of sufficient severity to become a focus of treatment.

D. The behavior is not better accounted for by a compulsion (as in Obsessive-Compulsive Disorder), a tic (as in Tic Disorder), a stereotypy that is part of a Pervasive Developmental Disorder, or hair pulling (as in Trichotillomania).

E. The behavior is not due to the direct physiological effects of a substance or a general medical condition.

F. The behavior persists for 4 weeks or longer.

> **Specify if:**
> **With Self-Injurious Behavior:** if the behavior results in bodily damage that requires medical treatment (or that would result in bodily damage if protective measures were not used)

□ □ □ □

313.9 Disorder of Infancy, Childhood, (ICD-10 code F98.9)
or Adolescence Not Otherwise Specified (NOS)

This is a residual category for disorders with onset in infancy, childhood, or adolescence that do not meet criteria for any specific disorder in the classification.

□ □ □ □

....

Differences Between DSM-III-R and DSM-IV
Disorders Usually First Diagnosed in Infancy, Childhood, or Adolescence

49

❑ Four new disorders are introduced in this section of DSM-IV: **Rett's Disorder, Childhood Disintegrative Disorder, Asperger's Disorder** (all Pervasive Developmental Disorders), and **Feeding Disorder of Infancy or Early Childhood.** All are coded on Axis I.

❑ Several DSM-III-R childhood disorders were shifted to other sections in DSM-IV (e.g., **Anorexia** and **Bulimia** are now in a separate category called Eating Disorders; **Anxiety Disorders** diagnosed in childhood are now found in the Anxiety Disorders section).

❑ The disorders in this section have a new criterion, seen throughout DSM-IV, which limits diagnosis to those conditions which cause clinically significant distress or impairment in social, academic, occupational, or other areas of functioning.

❑ DSM-III-R Overanxious Disorder of Childhood and Avoidant Disorder of Childhood were moved from this section and included under Anxiety Disorders. Their symptoms are now coded as **Generalized Anxiety Disorder** (300.02) and **Social Phobia** (300.23) respectively.

❑ **Developmental Reading Disorder, Mathematics Disorder,** and **Disorder of Written Expression** are now coded on Axis I. Known general medical etiology does not preempt these diagnoses.

❑ **Expressive Language Disorder, Mixed Receptive/Expressive Language Disorder,** and **Phonological Disorder** are not specifically developmental; they may be acquired. Receptive Language Disorder is no longer diagnosed without an expressive component. **Phonological Disorder** (Developmental Articulation Disorder in DSM-III-R) is not limited to articulation problems. Vowel sounds may be affected.

❑ **Stuttering** now has diagnostic criteria.

❑ Cluttering was eliminated. DSM-IV implies (but does not specifically state) that cluttering may be considered under **Stuttering.**

❑ **Pervasive Developmental Disorders** are now coded on Axis I.

❑ **Autistic Disorder** now specifies age criteria, eliminating the childhood onset subtype; requires fewer specific criteria (A1, A2, A3); and introduces Rett's and Childhood Disintegrative Disorders as preempting Autistic Disorder. DSM-IV asks for at least 6 symptoms from 3 groups; DSM-III-R required 8 of 16 specified symptoms.

❑ **Attention-Deficit/Hyperactivity Disorder (AD/HD)** criteria are more complex and differentiated by type. Symptoms must be present in two or more settings. Severity specifiers were omitted. Undifferentiated AD/HD was deleted.

❑ **Conduct Disorder** has slightly broader behavioral criteria and the type structure is different: Group, Solitary Aggressive, and Undifferentiated are deleted; **Childhood Onset** and **Adolescent Onset** were added. Time criteria are different (now 12 months). "Clinically significant impairment" is required.

❑ **Oppositional Defiant Disorder** now requires only four A criteria. Swearing and obscene language are no longer separate items among the A criteria. Clinical significance is stressed. Antisocial Personality Disorder is preempting after age 18. A severity rating is no longer specified.

❑ **Pica** now specifically exempts cultural ritual and limits diagnosis in the presence of other mental illness. The eating behavior must be inappropriate for the person's developmental level.

❑ In **Rumination Disorder,** weight loss or failure to gain is no longer a specific criterion. Exemptions for general medical disorders, Pervasive Developmental Disorder, Mental Retardation, Anorexia and Bulimia are now more specific.

❑ In **Tourette's Disorder, Chronic Motor or Vocal Tic Disorder,** and **Transient Tic Disorder,** onset must be before age 18 rather than 21.

❑ In **Tourette's Disorder** and **Chronic Motor or Vocal Tic Disorder,** there now must be no tic-free period greater than 3 months. Transient Tic Disorder requires a duration of at least 4 weeks. **Tourette's Disorder** no longer requires a change in location of tics. A diagnosis of **Tourette's Disorder** in the patient's history preempts **Motor or Vocal Tic Disorder.**

❑ **Encopresis** is no longer limited to functional encopresis. Medical conditions causing constipation do not preempt the diagnosis. The duration criterion is shorter (3 months). It is no longer necessary to specify "primary" or "secondary." The two subtypes—**With** and **Without Constipation and Overflow Incontinence**—are new. DSM-IV now clarifies that the symptoms must not be due to the direct physiological effects of a substance.

❑ In **Enuresis,** the presence of significant distress or impairment can override frequency and duration criteria. Frequency criteria are different and are now the same for older and younger children. Mental age is raised to 5 years. It is no longer necessary to specify "primary" or "secondary." DSM-IV now clarifies that the symptoms must not be due to the direct physiological effects of a substance.

❑ In **Separation Anxiety Disorder,** there is less emphasis on early childhood in the general criteria, but a new **Early Onset** specifier has been added. Anticipation of separation and its actual occurrence are now combined into one criterion. A clinical significance criterion was added. The duration criterion was increased from 2 to 4 weeks. Panic Disorder With Agoraphobia is now preempting.

❑ In **Selective Mutism,** clinical significance, duration criteria (1 month), and more specific separation from other disorders was added.

❑ **Reactive Attachment Disorder of Infancy or Early Childhood** now specifies two types (**Inhibited** and **Disinhibited**).

❑ **Stereotypic Movement Disorder** has considerably expanded differential diagnosis and preemptive diagnoses, and a new duration requirement (4 weeks).

❑ ❑ ❑ ❑

CASE VIGNETTES
(Disorders Usually First Diagnosed in Infancy, Childhood, or Adolescence)

Case Vignette 1

G.R., a 13-year-old boy, often refuses to talk to his mother, a single parent, for days at a time. He talks to his teachers and siblings. There is no diagnosable Communication Disorder, and G.R. is obviously capable of speaking when he wants to do so. His grades have declined significantly during the past 2 years. During the past year he has often started fights with peers, stolen from his mother's purse several times, and often lied to cover his indiscretions or get things he wants. The behavior started around age 8 or 9, and has escalated to the point at which he has been arrested several times (usually for curfew violations) since age 12. G.R. was referred to the mental health clinic by a juvenile court judge after recently vandalizing several cars and threatening the drivers with a knife.

DIAGNOSIS AND DISCUSSION
Axis I—312.8 Conduct Disorder, Childhood Onset, Moderate (ICD-10 F91.8)

G.R. does not meet criteria for Selective Mutism; the occasional refusal to talk seems related to the Conduct Disorder. He does not meet criteria for Antisocial Personality Disorder. The behavior problem exceeds the level of V-code Child or Adolescent Antisocial Behavior. Consideration of Oppositional Defiant Disorder is preempted by the Conduct Disorder diagnosis.

Case Vignette 2

T.P., a fourth grader from a middle-class family, has had difficulty with arithmetic since kindergarten. Now that he is taking science classes, the deficit affects more than his math grade, which is always failing or near-failing. His performance in other subjects, such as writing and reading, is satisfactory. T.P. scored in the lowest 3 or 4% on standardized, individual math tests but is in the normal range on verbal measures. He complains that his math grades are low because he can't see the blackboard well, although he sits in the first row and wears glasses to correct his considerable nearsightedness. T.P.'s mother reports that he avoids math homework and becomes irritable when forced to do it. He recently had an episode of bedwetting while spending the night with a friend.

DIAGNOSIS AND DISCUSSION
Axis I—315.1 Mathematics Disorder (ICD-10 F81.2)

The symptoms are too narrowly focused for other developmental disorders. There is little indication that nearsightedness causes the problem. T.P. does not meet the criteria for Enuresis.

Case Vignette 3

S.J. is 26-year-old mentally retarded woman with social functioning consistent with her measured IQ of about 50. She has a long history of swallowing small objects. S.J. knows that she has been told not to do this, but she will grab crayons and plastic utensils when she believes others are not watching and either quickly swallow or hide them, somewhat unsophisticatedly, for later ingestion. On one occasion, she complained of abdominal pain and was found to have the remnants of a leather belt in her stomach. Surgery was required, and the belt was removed without permanent sequelae. S.J. once accused another resident of her group home of stealing from her. The food in the home is not very palatable, and the operator has been suspected of not providing adequate food and other services.

DIAGNOSIS AND DISCUSSION
Axis I—307.52 Pica (ICD-10 F98.3)
Axis II—318.0 Mental Retardation, probably Moderate (ICD-10 F71.9)

S.J.'s eating behavior is sufficiently significant to merit a diagnosis of Pica in addition to the Mental Retardation (which is separately coded). There is no reason to believe that the eating behavior is related to dietary deficiency, which may or may not be present, or a Psychotic Disorder.

Case Vignette 4

N.R. is a 5-month-old infant, an only child. He was brought to the pediatrics clinic by his mother, who was concerned about frequent vomiting for several weeks. Pediatric examination revealed nothing of physical importance, and further testing ruled out pyloric stenosis and other gastrointestinal abnormality. The mother had not noticed anything more than occasional spitting up during the first 3 months of life, but stated that the child had recently vomited small amounts after feeding, especially since she had increased the volume of N.R.'s feedings. There was no characteristic posturing. The mother was uncertain about whether or not N.R. rechewed the regurgitated food, and was unable to determine whether or not the episodes were pleasurable for the infant. The vomiting continued two to three times a week for about 8 weeks, then gradually disappeared. Weight gain was not affected.

DIAGNOSIS AND DISCUSSION
No apparent psychiatric diagnosis. N.R. does not meet criteria for Rumination Disorder. A V code might be considered.

Case Vignette 5

After 2 or 3 months of apparently normal development, J.T.'s parents noticed that she didn't seem to react to their smiles and vocalizations. She did not hold their gaze, and, unlike her siblings, failed to develop facial expressiveness or expected responses to her environment. As the months passed, she seemed to withdraw into her own world. J.T. had not learned to speak by age 3, although she later would often repeat nonsense syllables in constant patterns. At age 8, she now engages in almost no social interaction, focusing instead on certain toys and other objects in an obsessive, sometimes ritualistic way. Her EEG is abnormal but nonspecific; no seizures have been observed. Weight gain, growth and physical measurements, including head size, have always been normal for her chronological age. Because of her marked social detachment, intelligence is difficult to test. Other functioning is generally consistent with tests that estimate her IQ at about 45, although she sometimes appears brighter.

DIAGNOSIS AND DISCUSSION
Axis I—299.00 Autistic Disorder (ICD-10 F84.0)
Axis II—318.0 Moderate Mental Retardation (provisional) (ICD-10 F71.9)

Rett's Disorder is associated with a few more months of normal development and with slowing of head growth. Childhood Disintegrative Disorder is associated with at least 2 years of normal development. Asperger's Disorder spares language development.

Case Vignette 6

P.B. is a young man of 25 who had difficulty completing high school and has drifted from job to job for years. He seems to have every intention of keeping jobs and succeeding socially, but his impulsivity and propensity for minor antisocial behavior (such as swearing at his boss, stealing tools from a job site, skipping work and taking a company pickup to the beach) undermine his progress. P.B. is genuinely puzzled by his repeated failures. He has had several scrapes with the law, but no serious criminal activity. He has not married but once lived with a woman for about 2 months. He sometimes calls on his parents for financial support. There is no indication of intellectual deficit, psychosis, or Mood Disorder.

P.B.'s parents describe no significant developmental delays. They recall that even before the first grade he had trouble focusing his attention on tasks or activities, including pleasurable ones. In school, he was repeatedly cited for not sitting still, leaving his seat and walking about the classroom without permission, forgetting simple assignments, and the like. His mother remembers telling some of P.B.'s many therapists that he was "like a whirlwind" from the time he learned to walk. He would talk incessantly, routinely intrude on others' conversations, and monopolize discussions or activities to the extent that others avoided him at school and in other settings. His early schoolwork suffered considerably until he was provided with small classes and tutoring. He became less active in adolescence, but school continued to be a problem and he developed more antisocial behavior.

DIAGNOSIS AND DISCUSSION
Axis I—314.01 Attention-Deficit/Hyperactivity Disorder, Predominantly Hyperactive-Impulsive Type (ICD-10 F90.0)

A diagnosis of mixed type may be appropriate. In Partial Remission is an acceptable qualifier as well. There is insufficient information to diagnose Conduct Disorder or a Personality Disorder.

CHAPTER 11

DELIRIUM, DEMENTIA, AND AMNESTIC AND OTHER COGNITIVE DISORDERS

This chapter contains many of the disorders that were called Organic Mental Syndromes and Disorders in DSM-III-R. The term *organic* is not used in DSM-IV because it implies that other mental disorders do not have a biologic basis (i.e., are not organic).

The shared clinical feature of these disorders is brain dysfunction. This dysfunction manifests itself through cognitive deficits. The clinical presentation is multifaceted, as seen in Delirium or Dementia, or the clinical abnormalities are limited to certain areas of cognitive function, such as the memory impairment seen in Amnestic Disorders.

DELIRIUM
(significantly modified from DSM-III-R)

ESSENTIAL FEATURES. A key feature in Delirium is a disturbance in consciousness that is accompanied by widespread brain dysfunction. The cognitive impairments cannot be better explained by Dementia. Delirious patients have difficulty maintaining attention; the individual is usually easily distracted. The onset of symptoms is usually rapid (i.e., hours to days), and the severity of dysfunction may fluctuate widely over the course of a day. The patient who is delirious has cognitive changes, such as memory (e.g., disorientation) or language dysfunction, and perceptual disturbances, such as hallucinations or illusions. There is evidence that the Delirium resulted from a general medical condition, is substance related (e.g., related to intoxication or withdrawal), or is caused by a combination of these factors.

ASSOCIATED FEATURES. Concomitant emotional disturbances, such as fear, anxiety, depression, anger, and apathy, are common. Neurological signs, such as dysgraphia (difficulty writing), constructional apraxia (difficulty drawing), and

78

dysnomia (difficulty naming objects), are often present. Tremor, symmetrical increase or decrease in reflexes, and signs of autonomic hyperactivity (sweating, flushed face, increased heart rate and blood pressure, and dilated pupils) may also be seen. The EEG is typically abnormal and typically shows slowing or, more rarely, fast activity. The sleep-wake cycle is often disturbed and may even be reversed (i.e., daytime sleepiness and nighttime restlessness). Psychomotor behavior is often disturbed with agitation, retardation, or shifts from one to the other. Advanced age (>60 years), young age (children), Substance Withdrawal, cardiotomy, and preexisting brain injury (e.g., Dementia or stroke) increase the risk for developing Delirium.

COURSE. Delirium can begin abruptly (e.g., with head trauma) or, more typically, evolves over hours to days. The resolution of the Delirium depends on rapid identification and correction of underlying etiological factors. Delirium usually resolves within days, although it can persist for weeks to months (e.g., after anoxic insults). Complete recovery is common, although residual deficits do occur. Approximately 10 to 15% of individuals over the age of 65 who are hospitalized for a medical condition have Delirium at the time of admission, and another 10 to 15% develop Delirium during hospitalization.

DIFFERENTIAL DIAGNOSIS. There are a number of psychotic disorders that must be ruled out prior to a diagnosis of Delirium. These include Brief Psychotic Disorder and a Mood Disorder With Psychotic Features. Schizophrenia, which requires a duration of at least 6 months, and Schizophreniform Disorder, which requires a duration of from 1 to 6 months, typically occur in young individuals; Delirium is quite uncommon in young people except as a symptom of severe drug withdrawal. Demented patients are at high risk for developing a delirium and can do so as a result of physiologic or severe environmental stress. Malingering and Factitious Disorder also are considered in the differential diagnosis. When more than one etiology for the Delirium exists, which is often the case, the correct diagnosis is Delirium Due to Multiple Etiologies. Patients with some symptoms of Delirium but not meeting all DSM-IV criteria (so-called "subsyndromal presentation") are diagnosed as Cognitive Disorder Not Otherwise Specified.

DIAGNOSTIC CRITERIA FOR DELIRIUM DUE TO . . . [INDICATE GENERAL MEDICAL CONDITION] (293.0)   (ICD-10 code F05.0)

A. Disturbance of consciousness (i.e., reduced clarity of awareness of the environment) with reduced ability to focus, sustain, or shift attention.

B. A change in cognition (such as memory deficit, disorientation, language disturbance) or the development of a perceptual disturbance that is not better accounted for by a preexisting, established, or evolving Dementia.

C. The disturbance develops over a short period of time (usually hours to days) and tends to fluctuate during the course of the day.

D. There is evidence from the history, physical examination, or laboratory findings that the disturbance is caused by the direct physiological consequences of a general medical condition.

CODING NOTE: If delirium is superimposed on a preexisting Dementia of the Alzheimer's Type or Vascular Dementia, indicate by coding the appropriate subtype of the dementia, e.g., 290.3 Dementia of the Alzheimer's Type, With Late Onset, With Delirium.

CODING NOTE: Include the name of the general medical condition on Axis I, e.g., 293.0 Delirium Due to Hepatic Encephalopathy; also code the general medical condition on Axis III (see DSM-IV Appendix G for selected ICD-9-CM codes).

▢ ▢ ▢ ▢

DIAGNOSTIC CRITERIA FOR   (see specific
SUBSTANCE INTOXICATION DELIRIUM   codes below)

A, B, & C. Criteria same as Delirium Due to a General Medical Condition (preceding).

D. There is evidence from the history, physical examination, or laboratory findings of either (1) or (2):
(1) The symptoms in Criteria A and B developed during Substance Intoxication.
(2) Medication use is etiologically related to the disturbance.

NOTE: This diagnosis is made instead of a diagnosis of Substance Intoxication only when the cognitive symptoms are in excess of those usually associated with the intoxication syndrome and when the symptoms are sufficiently severe to warrant independent clinical attention.

NOTE: The diagnosis is recorded as Substance-Induced Delirium if related to medication use. Refer to DSM-IV Appendix G for selected ICD-9-CM E codes indicating specific medications.

Code [Specific Substance] Intoxication Delirium:
291.0 Alcohol (ICD-10 F10.03); 292.81 Amphetamine or Amphetamine-Like Substance (ICD-10 F15.03); 292.81 Cannabis (ICD-10 F12.03); 292.81 Cocaine (ICD-10 14.03); 292.81 Hallucinogen (ICD-10 F16.03); 292.81 Inhalant (ICD-10 F18.03); 292.81 Opioid (ICD-10 F11.03); 292.81 Phencyclidine [or Phencyclidine-Like Substance] (ICD-10 F19.03); 292.81 Sedative, Hypnotic, or Anxiolytic (ICD-10 F13.03); 292.81 Other [or Unknown] Substance [e.g., cimetidine, digitalis, benztropine] (ICD-10 F19.03)

▢ ▢ ▢ ▢

DIAGNOSTIC CRITERIA FOR SUBSTANCE WITHDRAWAL DELIRIUM

(see specific codes below)

A, B, C. Criteria same as Delirium Due to a General Medical Condition (preceding).

D. There is evidence from the history, physical examination, or laboratory findings that the symptoms in Criteria A and B developed during, or shortly after, a withdrawal syndrome.

> NOTE: This diagnosis is made instead of a diagnosis of Substance Withdrawal only when the cognitive symptoms are in excess of those usually associated with the withdrawal syndrome and when the symptoms are sufficiently severe to warrant independent clinical attention.

> **Code [Specific Substance] Withdrawal Delirium:**
> **291.0** Alcohol (ICD-10 F10.4); **292.81** Sedative, Hypnotic, or Anxiolytic (ICD-10 F13.4); **292.81** Other [or Unknown] Substance (ICD-10 F19.4)

◻ ◻ ◻ ◻

DIAGNOSTIC CRITERIA FOR DELIRIUM DUE TO MULTIPLE ETIOLOGIES

(see specific codes below)

A, B, C. Criteria same as Delirium Due to a General Medical Condition (preceding).

D. There is evidence from the history, physical examination, or laboratory findings that the delirium has more than one etiology (e.g., more than one etiological general medical condition, or a general medical condition plus Substance Intoxication or medication side effect).

> CODING NOTE: Use multiple codes reflecting specific delirium and specific etiologies, e.g., 293.0 Delirium Due to Viral Encephalitis (ICD-10 F05.0); 291.0 Alcohol Withdrawal Delirium (ICD-10 F10.4).

◻ ◻ ◻ ◻

780.09 Delirium Not Otherwise Specified (NOS)

(ICD-10 code F05.9)

This diagnosis is used when Delirium is present but without sufficient clinical evidence to establish a specific etiology *or* when Delirium is believed to be caused by etiologies other than those listed (e.g., sensory deprivation).

◻ ◻ ◻ ◻

DEMENTIA

Dementia of the Alzheimer's Type
Vascular Dementia
Dementia Due to Other General Medical Conditions
Substance-Induced Persisting Dementia
Dementia Due to Multiple Etiologies
Dementia Not Otherwise Specified (NOS)

ESSENTIAL FEATURES. Individuals who have Dementia, like Delirium, exhibit signs and symptoms of global brain dysfunction. There is impairment of both recent and remote memory, and impairment of at least one other brain function (e.g., aphasia, apraxia, agnosia). The cumulative effects of these impairments must interfere with work, social activities, or relationships; and there must be a decline from a higher level of function.

ASSOCIATED FEATURES. Awareness of cognitive deficits varies among individuals. Early in a progressive dementing illness the individual is sometimes aware of deficits; however, that awareness usually fades as the Dementia progresses. Anxiety, depression, or sleep disturbance may accompany Dementia. Increased physiological, psychological, or environmental stress can aggravate deficits. Hallucinations, most commonly visual, can occur. Delirium occurs commonly in patients with Dementia.

Computerized tomography (CT) or magnetic resonance imaging (MRI) may show cerebral atrophy or other reasons for declining cognitive functions, such as hydrocephalus, tumors, subdural hematoma, or stroke. Single photon emission computed tomography (SPECT) or positron-emission tomography (PET) can provide evidence of functional defects. The prevalence of Dementia of the Alzheimer's Type and Vascular Dementia increase with advancing age (i.e., 20% or more of individuals over age 85 years are demented).

COURSE. Dementia can progress, remain stable, or improve.

DIFFERENTIAL DIAGNOSIS. Mental Retardation is not necessarily associated with memory impairment and occurs before the age of 18; dementia is, by definition, associated with memory impairment. Dementia almost always begins late in life. Normal aging often gives rise to "forgetfulness" and a decline in the speed of cognitive function (e.g., decreased speed of performance on timed tasks) best described as Age-Related Cognitive Decline (Code 780.9). Schizophrenia has an early age of onset and is associated with less severe cognitive decline (*dementia praecox*).

In Delirium, the onset of confusion is typically fairly acute and the degree of obtundation varies rapidly over short periods of time. The individual who is demented has reasonably constant, yet significantly decreased, cognitive function. (**Note:** individuals who have a dementia are at increased risk for developing a superimposed delirium.) Major Depressive Disorder, especially in elderly individuals, can be confused with Dementia. Major Depression is sometimes associated with marked cognitive slowing (depressive pseudodementia) that is reversed when the depressive disorder is appropriately treated. Individuals with Malingering and Factitious Disorder present inconsistent clinical signs and symptoms, and often have atypical findings on clinical examination.

Once the clinician has diagnosed Dementia, the question of etiology is important. Considerations include Dementia Due to Multiple Etiologies, Vascular Dementia, Dementia Due to Other General Medical Disorders (e.g., head trauma, Parkinson's disease), Substance-Induced Persisting Dementia (e.g., alcohol, inhalants, lead) and, last (because it is a diagnosis of exclusion) Dementia of the Alzheimer's Type.

▢ ▢ ▢ ▢

290.xx Dementia of the Alzheimer's Type (DAT)
(ICD-10 code F00.xx)
(see specific codes, following)

ESSENTIAL FEATURES. A definite diagnosis of DAT requires either a brain biopsy or postmortem brain analysis. Therefore, DAT is a diagnosis made after other etiologies are ruled out. Among demented patients, DAT is the most common diagnosis and occurs in 2 to 4% of individuals older than age 65. The prevalence of DAT increases with age, with Down's syndrome, and following head trauma. Brain atrophy is usually present on CT or MRI.

The cognitive deficits in DAT develop slowly and the deterioration is progressive. The average life expectancy from onset to death is 8 to 10 years, although the variance is great. Memory and other cognitive deficits (i.e., aphasia, apraxia, agnosia) typically occur early, and motor dysfunction (e.g., gait) occurs late. First-degree relatives of individuals who develop DAT before age 65 (Early Onset) are at increased risk to develop this disorder.

DIAGNOSTIC CRITERIA FOR DEMENTIA OF THE ALZHEIMER'S TYPE
(see specific codes below)

A. The development of multiple cognitive deficits manifested by *both*
    (1) memory impairment (impaired ability to learn new information or to recall previously learned information) *and*
    (2) one (or more) of the following cognitive disturbances:
        (a) aphasia (language disturbance despite intact articulation)

       (b) apraxia (impaired ability to carry out motor activities despite intact motor function)

       (c) agnosia (failure to recognize or identify objects despite intact sensory function)

       (d) disturbance in executive functioning (i.e., planning, organizing, sequencing, abstracting)

B. The cognitive deficits in Criteria Al and A2 each cause significant impairment in social or occupational functioning and represent a significant decline from a previous level of functioning.

C. The course is characterized by gradual onset and continuing cognitive decline.

D. The cognitive deficits in Criteria Al and A2 are not due to any of the following:

    (1) other central nervous system conditions that cause progressive deficits in memory and cognition (e.g., cerebrovascular disease, Parkinson's disease, Huntington's disease, subdural hematoma, normal-pressure hydrocephalus, brain tumor)

    (2) systemic conditions that are known to cause dementia in some patients (e.g., hypothyroidism, vitamin B_{12} or folic acid deficiency, niacin deficiency, hypercalcemia, neurosyphilis, HIV infection)

    (3) substance-induced conditions

E. The deficits do not occur exclusively during the course of a delirium.

F. The disturbance is not better accounted for by another Axis I disorder (e.g., Major Depressive Disorder, Schizophrenia).

> **Code based on type of onset and predominant features:**
> **290.xx With Early Onset:** if onset is at age 65 years or below (ICD-10 F00.xx)
>> **290.11 With Delirium:** if delirium is superimposed on the dementia
>> **290.12 With Delusions:** if delusions are the predominant feature (ICD-10 F00.01)
>> **290.13 With Depressed Mood:** if depressed mood (including presentations that meet full symptom criteria for a Major Depressive Episode) is the predominant feature (ICD-10 F00.03). A separate diagnosis of Mood Disorder Due to a General Medical Condition is not given.
>> **290.10 Uncomplicated:** if none of the above predominates in the current clinical presentation (ICD-10 F00.00)
>
> **290.xx With Late Onset:** if onset is after age 65 years (ICD-10 F00.xx)
>> **290.3 With Delirium:** if delirium is superimposed on the dementia
>> **290.20 With Delusions:** if delusions are the predominant feature (ICD-10 F00.11)

290.21 With Depressed Mood: if depressed mood (including presentations that meet full symptom criteria for a Major Depressive Episode) is the predominant feature (ICD-10 F00.13). A separate diagnosis of Mood Disorder Due to a General Medical Condition is not given.

290.0 Uncomplicated: if none of the above predominates in the current clinical presentation (ICD-10 F00.10)

Specify if:
With Behavioral Disturbance

CODING NOTE: Also code 331.0 Alzheimer's Disease on Axis III. (ICD-10 G30.0 [Early Onset] or G30.1 [Late Onset])

❏ ❏ ❏ ❏

290.xx Vascular Dementia   *(ICD-10 Code F01.xx)*
(Multi-Infarct Dementia in DSM-III-R)
(significantly modified from DSM-III-R)

ESSENTIAL FEATURES. The A and B diagnostic criteria for Vascular Dementia (VD) are the same as those for Dementia of the Alzheimer's Type (DAT). However, patients with VD typically have focal neurological deficits as a result of vascular brain lesions. These lesions are visible on CT or MRI, and the EEG can show focal abnormalities. The history often is positive for past strokes, hypertension, and/or diseases of the heart valves. Although the clinical course occasionally is similar to DAT, a more typical pattern is sudden decline from a vascular lesion (e.g., a stroke) followed by a gradual recovery.

DIAGNOSTIC CRITERIA FOR   (see specific
VASCULAR DEMENTIA   codes below)

A, B. Criteria as in Dementia of the Alzheimer's Type.

C. Focal neurological signs and symptoms (e.g., exaggeration of deep tendon reflexes, extensor plantar response, pseudobulbar palsy, gait abnormalities, weakness of an extremity) or laboratory evidence indicative of cerebrovascular disease (e.g., multiple infarctions involving cortex and underlying white matter) that are judged to be etiologically related to the disturbance.

D. The deficits do not occur exclusively during the course of a delirium.

Code based on predominant features:
290.41 With Delirium: if delirium is superimposed on the dementia

290.42 With Delusions: if delusions are the predominant feature (ICD-10 F01.81)

290.43 With Depressed Mood: if depressed mood (including presentations that meet full symptom criteria for a Major Depressive

Episode) is the predominant feature (ICD-10 F01.83). A separate diagnosis of Mood Disorder Due to a General Medical Condition is not given.

290.40 Uncomplicated: if none of the above predominates in the current clinical presentation (ICD-10 F01.80)

Specify if:
With Behavioral Disturbance

CODING NOTE: Also code cerebrovascular condition on Axis III.

□ □ □ □

290.xx, 294.x Dementia Due to Other General Medical Conditions   *(ICD-10 code F02.x)*
(new in DSM-IV)

Criteria A and B are the same as for other dementias. The main factors in making this diagnosis are the history, physical examination, or laboratory findings, which reveal a medical condition that "is etiologically related to the Dementia." DSM-IV describes briefly the clinical features of several different dementias, for example, Dementia Due to HIV Disease (see DSM-IV, pp. 148–151).

DIAGNOSTIC CRITERIA FOR   (see coding below)
DEMENTIA DUE TO OTHER
GENERAL MEDICAL CONDITIONS

A, B. Criteria same as for Dementia of the Alzheimer's Type.

C. There is evidence from the history, physical examination, or laboratory findings that the disturbance is the direct physiological consequence of one of the general medical conditions listed below.

D. The deficits do not occur exclusively during the course of a delirium.

Code according to etiology:
294.9 Due to HIV Disease (ICD-10 F02.4)

294.1 Due to Head Trauma (ICD-10 F02.8)

294.1 Due to Parkinson's Disease (ICD-10 F02.3)

294.1 Due to Huntington's Disease (ICD-10 F02.2)

290.10 Due to Pick's Disease (ICD-10 F02.0)

290.10 Due to Creutzfeldt-Jakob Disease (ICD-10 F02.1)

294.1 Dementia Due to . . . (indicate the General Medical Condition not listed above) (ICD-10 F02.8) (e.g., normal-pressure hydrocephalus, hypothyroidism, brain tumor, vitamin B$_{12}$ deficiency, intracranial radiation)

CODING NOTE: Also code the general medical condition on Axis III (see DSM-IV Appendix G for selected ICD-9-CM codes).

❑ ❑ ❑ ❑

___.___ Substance-Induced Persisting Dementia (code according to substance)

Criteria A and B are the same as for other dementias; however, the symptoms are caused by the persisting (not intoxicant) effects of a substance (e.g., drug of abuse, medication).

DIAGNOSTIC CRITERIA FOR   (see coding below)
SUBSTANCE-INDUCED PERSISTING DEMENTIA

A, B. Same as Dementia of the Alzheimer's Type.

C. The deficits do not occur exclusively during the course of a delirium and persist beyond the usual duration of Substance Intoxication or Withdrawal.

D. There is evidence from the history, physical examination, or laboratory findings that the deficits are etiologically related to the persisting effects of substance use (e.g., a drug of abuse, a medication).

> **Code according to specific etiological substance:**
> **291.2 Alcohol** (ICD-10 F10.73); **292.82 Inhalant** (ICD-10 F18.73); **292.82 Sedative, Hypnotic, or Anxiolytic** (ICD-10 F13.73); **292.82 Other (or Unknown) Substance** (ICD-10 F19.73)

❑ ❑ ❑ ❑

___.___ Dementia Due to Multiple Etiologies (code each etiology)

Criteria A and B are the same as for other dementias; however, the symptoms appear to be caused by more than one source.

DIAGNOSTIC CRITERIA FOR   (see coding below)
DEMENTIA DUE TO MULTIPLE ETIOLOGIES

A, B. Same as Dementia of the Alzheimer's Type.

C. There is evidence from the history, physical examination, or laboratory findings that the disturbance has more than one etiology (e.g., head trauma plus chronic alcohol use, Dementia of the Alzheimer's Type with the subsequent development of Vascular Dementia).

D. The deficits do not occur exclusively during the course of a delirium.

> CODING NOTE: Use multiple codes based on specific dementias and specific etiologies, e.g., 290.0 Dementia of the Alzheimer's Type, With Late Onset, Uncomplicated (ICD-10 F00.10); 290.40 Vascular Dementia, Uncomplicated (ICD-10 F01.80).

❑ ❑ ❑ ❑

....

AMNESTIC DISORDERS

(53)

ESSENTIAL FEATURES. Impairment is limited to short- and long-term memory. Immediate recall, usually measured by the ability to repeat immediately a series of digits, is unimpaired. The memory deficits are not part of a Delirium or a Dementia.

ASSOCIATED FEATURES. Because an individual with Amnestic Disorder cannot form memory for recent events, disorientation and amnesia are nearly always present. Confabulation (fabrication of events that are not remembered) is common, particularly early in the disorder. Individuals with Amnestic Disorder often are unconcerned about these deficits and may exhibit apathy, lack of initiative, disinterest, and emotional blandness. Chronic alcohol use that results in thiamine deficiency is commonly associated with Amnestic Disorder.

The onset and course of Amnestic Disorders are quite variable. Certain types of injury, such as head trauma or delayed resuscitation following a cardiac arrest, can result in an acute Amnestic Disorder, whereas continued excessive use of a substance such as alcohol can result in an insidious onset.

DIFFERENTIAL DIAGNOSIS. Memory impairment is an important element in a number of mental disorders. In Delirium, the individual has rapidly varying confusion and has problems maintaining attention. In Dementia, there are additional signs of brain dysfunction, such as aphasia, apraxia, agnosia, or poor executive function. Individuals who have certain Dissociative Disorders cannot remember significant events; however, they do not have a physiologic reason for memory difficulties, can learn new information, and have circumscribed memory deficits that are traceable to a traumatic event. Substance Abusers have "blackouts" during intoxication and can experience Substance-Induced Persisting Amnestic Disorder (e.g., Wernicke-Korsakoff Syndrome). Individuals with Age-Related Cognitive Disorder have "forgetfulness," but this does not lead to significant impairment or include loss of identity. Malingering and Factitious Disorder are also considered in the differential diagnosis.

> NOTE: If the Amnestic Disorder is caused by a general medical disorder, including head trauma, the diagnosis is Amnestic Disorder Due to a General Medical Condition. If the disorder is caused by a medication, drug, or toxic substance, the diagnosis is Substance-Induced Persistent Amnestic Disorder. If both play a role in the memory dysfunction, both diagnoses are given. If the clinician is unsure of the reason for the amnesia, a diagnosis of Amnestic Disorder Not Otherwise Specified (Code 294.8) is made.

DIAGNOSTIC CRITERIA FOR AMNESTIC DISORDER DUE TO . . . [INDICATE THE GENERAL MEDICAL CONDITION] (294.0)

(ICD-10 code F04)

A. The development of memory impairment as manifested by impairment in the ability to learn new information or the inability to recall previously learned information.

B. The memory disturbance causes significant impairment in social or occupational functioning and represents a significant decline from a previous level of functioning.

C. The memory disturbance does not occur exclusively during the course of a delirium or a dementia.

D. There is evidence from the history, physical examination, or laboratory findings that the disturbance is the direct physiological consequence of a general medical condition (including physical trauma).

Specify if:
Transient: if memory impairment lasts for 1 month or less

Chronic: if memory impairment lasts for more than 1 month

CODING NOTE: Include the name of the general medical condition on Axis I, e.g., 294.0 Amnestic Disorder Due to Head Trauma. Also code the general medical condition on Axis III (see DSM-IV Appendix G for selected ICD-9-CM general medical codes).

❑ ❑ ❑ ❑

DIAGNOSTIC CRITERIA FOR SUBSTANCE-INDUCED PERSISTING AMNESTIC DISORDER

(see coding following)

A, B. Same as Amnestic Disorder Due to a General Medical Condition (preceding).

C. The memory disturbance does not occur exclusively during the course of a delirium or a dementia and persists beyond the usual duration of Substance Intoxication or Withdrawal.

D. There is evidence from the history, physical examination, or laboratory findings that the memory disturbance is etiologically related to the persisting effects of substance use (e.g., a drug of abuse, a medication).

Code according to specific etiologic substance:
291.1 Alcohol (ICD-10 F10.6); **292.83 Sedative, Hypnotic, or Anxiolytic** (ICD-10 F13.6); **292.83 Other (or Unknown) Substance** (ICD-10 F19.6)

NOTE: If more than one substance is likely to have caused the amnesia, list each separately.

▢ ▢ ▢ ▢

294.8 Amnestic Disorder Not Otherwise Specified (NOS)   *(ICD-10 code R41.3)*

This is a residual category for Amnestic Disorders that appear to be the result of a physiological event but do not meet any of the above diagnostic criteria. Amnesias of unknown etiology should be coded here.

▢ ▢ ▢ ▢

294.9 Cognitive Disorder Not Otherwise Specified (NOS)   *(ICD-10 Code F06.9)*

This diagnosis is used when a cognitive dysfunction is the direct result of a physiological event but the disorder does not meet the diagnostic criteria for other disorders in this section (Dementia, Delirium, Amnesia).

....

DIFFERENCES BETWEEN *DSM-III-R* and *DSM-IV* DELIRIUM, DEMENTIA, AND AMNESTIC DISORDERS

General

- The DSM-III-R section titled "Organic Mental Syndromes and Disorders" was divided into three sections in DSM-IV: **Delirium, Dementia, and Amnestic and Other Cognitive Disorders; Mental Disorders Due to a General Medical Condition;** and **Substance-Related Disorders.** The word "organic" was eliminated from DSM-IV.

- DSM-III-R diagnoses such as Organic Mood Disorder, Organic Hallucinosis, and Organic Delusional Syndrome were moved to other sections in DSM-IV that share their phenomenology. For example, the former Organic Mood Disorder is now called **Mood Disorder Due to a General Medical Condition,** and is located in the Mood Disorders category.

- DSM-III-R made a strong distinction between Organic Mental *Syndromes* (i.e., meets criteria but etiology unknown) and Organic Mental

54

Disorders (i.e., etiology known or presumed). This is not the case in DSM-IV.

Delirium

- Diagnostic criteria for **Delirium** were modified in several ways. DSM-III-R's criterion requiring disorganized thinking was eliminated, as were disturbed sleep cycle and increased or decreased psychomotor activity.

- **Delirium Due to Multiple Etiologies** is new in DSM-IV.

(55)

Dementia

- The diagnostic criteria for **Dementia** were changed in DSM-IV; personality change was eliminated from the criteria. Criteria for severity were also deleted. Multi-Infarct Dementia was renamed **Vascular Dementia.**

- **Substance-Induced Persisting Dementia** and **Dementia Due to Multiple Etiologies** and **Dementias Due to Other General Medical Conditions** (e.g., HIV, head trauma, Parkinson's disease, Huntington's disease, Pick's disease, and Creutzfeldt-Jakob disease) are new in DSM-IV.

Amnestic Disorders

- DSM-IV reorganized the Amnestic Disorders category, made the memory criterion more concise, and lists two new diagnoses: **Amnestic Disorder Due to a General Medical Condition and Substance-Induced Persisting Amnestic Disorders.**

▫ ▫ ▫ ▫

....

CASE VIGNETTES: DELIRIUM, DEMENTIA, AND AMNESTIC DISORDERS

Case Vignette 1

The family of a 70-year-old man, A.R., brings him in for evaluation because he has had increasing difficulty caring for himself. His memory is poor and he has gotten lost several times in his own neighborhood. Police assistance was needed to find him. A.R. believes that his neighbors are stealing things from his house. Further history reveals that A.R.'s memory problems first began about 2 years ago. His memory problems slowly progressed, and he has gotten more irritable and suspicious over the past 6 months. According to his children, "He is like a different person." His four married children have alternated staying with him for the past month, but they are unable to continue this effort. A.R. has been in good physical health, is on no medication, and has no history of mental disorders or inappropriate substance use.

A.R. appears disheveled and is somewhat hostile. He is alert and does not cooperate with the examiner. When asked to perform memory tasks, he says, "I'm not going to answer your dumb questions." He believes his wife, who died 5 years ago, is alive and is being held captive. His handwriting is unreadable and he is unable to copy even simple designs. Physical examination, laboratory results, radiographic findings and MRI are all normal.

DIAGNOSIS AND DISCUSSION

Axis I—290.20 Dementia of the Alzheimer's Type, With Late Onset, With Delusions (ICD-10 code F00.11)
Axis II—V71.09 No diagnosis or 799.9 Diagnosis Deferred (ICD-10 code Z03.2 or R46.8)
Axis III—331.0 Alzheimer's Dementia (ICD-10 code G30.1)

A.R. presents with short- and long-term memory impairment, impaired judgment, dysgraphia, constructional apraxia, delusional thinking, and a personality change. The clinical course is one of slow deterioration and increasing impairment. A thorough medical evaluation failed to reveal a specific cause for his declining cognitive function. There is no history of a Mood Disorder and he does not appear depressed. The most likely diagnosis is Dementia, specifically Dementia of the Alzheimer's Type (DAT). The onset was approximately 2 years ago, when the patient was 68, and the DAT is complicated by delusions.

Case Vignette 2

The police bring B.D. to the emergency department of a local hospital because of belligerent behavior. B.D. is well known to the staff because of prior evaluations caused by chronic heavy use of alcohol. On this particular evening, B.D. was staggering down the street yelling at passersby and threatening them.

B.D. is dirty, unshaven, and difficult to arouse. At times, he attempts to get up from the stretcher and is combative when told to lie down. He does not respond coherently to questions and mumbles his answers. His neurological examination is abnormal for a positive Babinski reflex of the right great toe. His blood alcohol level is zero, and toxic screen for other drugs is negative. His pulse rate, temperature, and blood pressure are all normal. His blood chemistries are all normal, except for a mild elevation in his liver enzymes.

DIAGNOSIS AND DISCUSSION

Axis I—(293.0) Delirium Due to an Acute Subdural Hematoma (provisional) (ICD-10 F05.0) 303.90 Alcohol Dependence (ICD-10 F10.2x)
Axis II— 799.9 Diagnosis Deferred (ICD-10 R46.8)
Axis III—(852.20) Subdural Hematoma (provisional) (ICD-9-CM E825.20)

B.D. has a Delirium. He is confused, combative, and mumbling incoherently. In someone with B.D.'s history, there are a number of possible reasons for his Delirium. These include Alcohol Withdrawal Delirium, although his vital signs would be elevated, and Alcohol Intoxication Delirium. However, his blood alcohol level is zero, and his liver enzymes are only mildly elevated.

The most likely cause of the Delirium in the individual is an acute subdural hematoma. Individuals with Alcohol Dependence and Alcohol Abuse frequently fall and are injured. He has probably fallen, hit his head, and subsequently developed a hematoma. The hematoma causes the abnormal Babinski reflex and the Delirium. The clinician should immediately request a CT or MRI to verify the diagnosis, as well as administer thiamine and folate.

> NOTE: The "(provisional)" is added to indicate a strong suspicion about the diagnosis; it would be removed if a hematoma is seen on further examination (e.g., CT or MRI). This individual may also have an Alcohol-Induced Persisting Dementia or an Alcohol-Induced Persisting Amnestic Disorder. These diagnoses cannot be made during an ongoing Delirium. After the Delirium has completely cleared, clinical reassessment would establish whether additional diagnoses are warranted.

CHAPTER 12

MENTAL DISORDERS DUE TO A GENERAL MEDICAL CONDITION

CODING NOTE: The causative medical disorder is coded on Axis III (see DSM-IV Appendix G).

In DSM-III-R, the section titled "Organic Mental Syndromes and Disorders" included mental disorders caused by general medical conditions and Substance-Induced Disorders. DSM-IV eliminated the word *organic* and distributed the disorders into a number of sections, including "Delirium, Dementia, and Amnestic and Other Cognitive Disorders," "Substance-Related Disorders," and "Mental Disorders Due to a General Medical Condition."

This section contains the diagnostic criteria for three disorders: Catatonic Disorder Due to a General Medical Condition, Personality Change Due to a General Medical Condition, and Mental Disorder Not Otherwise Specified Due to a General Medical Condition. Other Mental Disorders Due to a General Medical Condition are located in sections with similar phenomenology (e.g., Mood Disorder Due to a General Medical Condition is found in the DSM-IV section titled "Mood Disorders").

Several aspects of clinical presentation may raise the suspicion that a general medical condition is playing a causal role in the mental disorder. These are (1) an atypical presentation (e.g., a 40-year-old man who develops rapid cognitive decline); (2) a temporal relationship between the onset of the medical illness and the onset of the mental disorder; and (3) the elimination of "primary" mental disorder and Substance-Induced Disorders in the differential diagnosis.

NOTE: "Primary" mental disorder is differentiated from that which occurs "secondary" to a medical disorder or substance.

293.89 Catatonic Disorder Due to a General Medical Condition (ICD-10 Code F06.1)
(new in DSM-IV)

A wide variety of medical conditions can cause catatonia. An electroencephalogram (EEG) will help distinguish catatonia that is caused by medical illness from that caused by a psychiatric disorder such as Schizophrenia, Catatonic Type, or a Mood Disorder With Catatonic Features. Another diagnosis to consider is a Neuroleptic-Induced Movement Disorder.

DIAGNOSTIC CRITERIA FOR CATATONIC DISORDER DUE TO . . . [INDICATE THE GENERAL MEDICAL CONDITION] (293.89)

(ICD-10 code F06.1)

A. The presence of catatonia as manifested by motoric immobility, excessive motor activity (that is apparently purposeless and not influenced by external stimuli), extreme negativism or mutism, peculiarities of voluntary movement, or echolalia or echopraxia.

B. There is evidence from the history, physical examination, or laboratory findings that the disturbance is the direct physiological consequence of a general medical condition.

C. The disturbance is not better accounted for by another mental disorder (e.g., a Manic Episode).

D. The disturbance does not occur exclusively during the course of a delirium.

> CODING NOTE: Include the name of the general medical condition on Axis I (e.g., 293.89 Catatonic Disorder Due to Hepatic Encephalopathy). Also code the general medical condition on Axis III (see DSM-IV Appendix G for codes).

❑ ❑ ❑ ❑

310.1 Personality Change Due to a General Medical Condition
(significantly modified from DSM-III-R)

(ICD-10 Code F07.0)

When a medical condition, such as head trauma or a stroke, produces a persistent change in an individual's personality, this diagnosis is appropriate. Eight different subtypes are described. Other psychiatric disorders are considered when a personality change occurs, especially Dementia and Delirium. In addition, chronic medical conditions and Substance Dependence, especially when long-standing, can cause personality alteration. Schizophrenia is also associated with a change in personality.

DIAGNOSTIC CRITERIA FOR PERSONALITY CHANGE DUE TO . . . [INDICATE THE GENERAL MEDICAL CONDITION] (310.1)

(ICD-10 Code F07.0)

A. A persistent personality disturbance that represents a change from the individual's previous characteristic personality pattern. (In children, the disturbance involves a marked deviation from normal development or a significant change in the child's usual behavior patterns lasting at least 1 year.)

B. There is evidence from the history, physical examination, or laboratory findings that the disturbance is the direct physiological consequence of a general medical condition.

C. The disturbance is not better accounted for by another mental disorder (including other Mental Disorders Due to a General Medical Condition).

D. The disturbance does not occur exclusively during the course of a delirium and does not meet criteria for a dementia.

E. The disturbance causes clinically significant distress or impairment in social, occupational, or other important areas of functioning.

Specify Type:
Labile Type: if the predominant feature is affective lability

(58)

Disinhibited Type: if the predominant feature is poor impulse control as evidenced by sexual indiscretions, etc.

Aggressive Type: if the predominant feature is aggressive behavior

Apathetic Type: if the predominant feature is marked apathy and indifference

Paranoid Type: if the predominant feature is suspiciousness or paranoid ideation

Other Type: if the predominant feature is not one of the above, e.g., personality change associated with a seizure disorder

Combined Type: if more than one feature predominates in the clinical picture

Unspecified Type

CODING NOTE: Include the name of the general medical condition on Axis I, for example, 310.1 Personality Change Due to Temporal Lobe Epilepsy. Also code the general medical condition on Axis III (see DSM-IV Appendix G for codes).

❑ ❑ ❑ ❑

293.9 Mental Disorder Not Otherwise Specified Due to a General Medical Condition (ICD-10 Code F09)

This is a residual category without specific criteria.

❑ ❑ ❑ ❑

DIFFERENCES BETWEEN DSM-III-R AND DSM-IV MENTAL DISORDERS DUE TO A GENERAL MEDICAL CONDITION

❑ Disorders caused by general medical conditions were located in the Organic Mental Syndromes and Disorders section of DSM-III-R. DSM-IV created a new section.

❑ **Catatonia Due to a General Medical Condition** is new in DSM-IV.

❑ **Personality Change Due to a General Medical Condition** was called Organic Personality Disorder in DSM-III-R. DSM-III-R had one subtype (explosive), whereas DSM-IV has eight.

CASE VIGNETTE: MENTAL DISORDERS DUE TO A GENERAL MEDICAL CONDITION

Case Vignette

W.J. is a 27-year-old man who was discharged 2 months ago from the hospital following a prolonged stay. The hospitalization was the result of a serious automobile accident 5 months ago in which he suffered numerous facial fractures and lacerations.

He was brought for evaluation by his wife of 9 years. She states, "He isn't the same." She describes his behavior since the accident: "He doesn't seem to care about anything anymore." This description stood in stark contrast to his previous behavior: "He was a hard worker," "always busy," "outgoing and friendly." She reports that he eats and sleeps well, and has not been observed crying. Both W.J. and his wife deny any substance use, including prescribed medications. His physicians feel that he has recovered physically.

On examination, W.J. is pleasant, attentive, and very cooperative. He seems bland and makes no spontaneous comments, but does respond appropriately to questions. He denies feeling depressed or anxious: "I'm fine." His mood is euthymic and his affect is appropriate to that mood. Cognitive tests reveal normal memory function and no evidence of apraxia, agnosia, or agraphia. His style throughout examination appears slightly slower than expected, given his wife's description.

DIAGNOSIS AND DISCUSSION

Axis I—310.1 Personality Change Due to Head Trauma, Apathetic Type (ICD-10 code F07.0)

Axis II—V71.09 No Diagnosis (ICD-10 code Z03.2)

Axis III—Suspected Contusion, Cerebral; Multiple Fractures (ICD-9-CM code 851.80)

W.J. was involved in a serious automobile accident and suffered extensive body and head trauma. As a result of the head trauma, his personality has changed; he was transformed from an industrious man to one who is indifferent and seems to lack spontaneity. There is no evidence of cognitive dysfunction (i.e., Delirium, Dementia, or Amnestic Disorder), Substance Abuse, Major Depression, Anxiety Disorder, or a preinjury Personality Disorder.

CHAPTER 13

SUBSTANCE-RELATED DISORDERS

(59)

(60)

Substances are broadly defined in DSM-IV to include drugs of abuse; the side effects of prescribed or over-the-counter medications; and such toxins as heavy metals, pesticides, and carbon monoxide. Therefore, Substance-Related Disorders encompass the effects of a wide variety of psychoactive chemicals. Disorders in this section are divided into two groups: Substance Use Disorders (Substance Dependence and Abuse) and Substance-Induced Disorders.

The use of certain substances is considered normal in our society. For example, taking prescribed medication to relieve insomnia or pain is a generally accepted practice. The recreational use of alcohol and the consumption of coffee, except among a few groups within our society, are also accepted behaviors. These practices lack the key elements that distinguish the Substance Use Disorders (i.e., Substance Dependence and Abuse). To qualify as a disorder, the maladaptive pattern of substance use must lead to clinically significant impairment or distress.

Substance-Induced Disorders refer to the direct or chronic effects of substances on the central nervous system. Many individuals who regularly ingest substances will have both a Substance Use Disorder and a Substance-Induced Disorder. There are 11 classes of substances discussed in DSM-IV (Table 13.1). Nine classes are associated with both Dependence and Abuse; nicotine is associated with Dependence but not Abuse; and caffeine is not "officially" associated with Dependence or Abuse (DSM-IV Appendix B describes "research criteria" for Caffeine Withdrawal). In this book, Substance Dependence and Substance Abuse (Substance Use Disorders) are defined before specific coded disorders are discussed.

SUBSTANCE USE DISORDERS

Substance Dependence
(significantly modified from DSM-III-R)

(61)

ESSENTIAL FEATURES. As a result of regular substance use, the individual develops impaired control of substance use and continues to use the substance in spite of adverse consequences. Dependence usually, but not always, includes the devel-

TABLE 13.1 DIAGNOSIS ASSOCIATED WITH CLASS OF SUBSTANCES

	Depen-dence	Abuse	Intoxi-cation	With-drawal	Intoxi-cation Delirium	With-drawal Delirium	Dementia	Amnestic Disorder	Psychotic Disorders	Mood Disorders	Anxiety Disorders	Sexual Dysfunctions	Sleep Disorders
Alcohol	X	X	X	X	I	W	P	P	I/W	I/W	I/W	I	I/W
Amphetamines	X	X	X	X	I				I	I/W	I	I	I/W
Caffeine			X								I		I
Cannabis	X	X	X		I				I		I		
Cocaine	X	X	X	X	I				I	I/W	I/W	I	I/W
Hallucinogens	X	X	X		I				I*	I	I		
Inhalants	X	X	X		I		P		I	I	I		
Nicotine	X			X									
Opioids	X	X	X	X	I				I	I		I	I/W
Phencyclidine	X	X	X		I				I	I	I		
Sedatives, hynotics, or anxiolytics	X	X	X	X	I	W	P	P	I/W	I/W	W	I	I/W
Polysubstance	X												
Other	X	X	X	X	I	W	P	P	I/W	I/W	I/W	I	I/W

* Also Hallucinogen Persisting Perception Disorder (flashbacks).

Note: X, I, W, I/W, or P indicates that the category is recognized in DSM-IV. In addition, I indicates that the specifier With Onset During Intoxication may be noted for the category (except for Intoxication Delirium); W indicates that the specifier With Onset During Withdrawal may be noted for the category (except for Withdrawal Delirium); and I/W indicates that either With Onset During Intoxication or With Onset During Withdrawal may be noted for the category. P indicates that the disorder is Persisting. (from DSM-IV, p. 177, copyright 1994, American Psychiatric Association)

opment of tolerance (i.e., one must increase the dose to maintain the same effects), the development of withdrawal symptoms upon discontinuation or dosage reduction, and compulsive drug taking. In order to meet the diagnostic criteria for Substance Dependence, three or more of the cognitive, behavioral, and/or physiological symptoms from use of the chemical must occur over a 12-month period of time.

ASSOCIATED FEATURES. Repeated bouts of Substance-Induced Intoxication are almost always present in the history. Personality and mood disturbances are often present. In chronic Abuse or Dependence, mood lability, suspiciousness, and violent behavior may be seen.

DIFFERENTIAL DIAGNOSIS. An essential feature of a substance-related disorder is clinically significant impairment; therefore, recreational or medically prescribed substance use that does not cause impairment is not considered a disorder. In addition, repeated episodes of Substance Intoxication can occur. A diagnosis of Substance Abuse is made when less severe impairment is present.

DIAGNOSTIC CRITERIA FOR
SUBSTANCE DEPENDENCE
(SEE SPECIFIC SUBSTANCE SECTIONS, FOLLOWING, FOR DSM-IV AND ICD-10 CODES)

A maladaptive pattern of substance use, leading to clinically significant impairment or distress, as manifested by three (or more) of the following, occurring at any time in the same 12-month period:

(1) tolerance, as defined by either of the following:
   (a) a need for markedly increased amounts of the substance to achieve intoxication or desired effect
   (b) markedly diminished effect with continued use of the same amount of the substance
(2) withdrawal, as manifested by either of the following:
   (a) the characteristic withdrawal syndrome for the substance (refer to Criteria A and B of the criteria sets for Withdrawal from the specific substances)
   (b) the same (or a closely related) substance is taken to relieve or avoid withdrawal symptoms
(3) the substance is often taken in larger amounts or over a longer period than was intended
(4) there is a persistent desire or unsuccessful efforts to cut down or control substance use
(5) a great deal of time is spent in activities necessary to obtain the substance (e.g., visiting multiple doctors or driving long distances), use the substance (e.g., chain-smoking), or recover from its effects
(6) important social, occupational, or recreational activities are given up or reduced because of substance use

(7) the substance use is continued despite knowledge of having a persistent or recurrent physical or psychological problem that is likely to have been caused or exacerbated by the substance (e.g., current cocaine use despite recognition of cocaine-induced depression, or continued drinking despite recognition that an ulcer was made worse by alcohol consumption)

Specify if:
With Physiological Dependence: evidence of tolerance or withdrawal (either Item 1 or 2, preceding, is present)

Without Physiological Dependence: no evidence of tolerance or withdrawal (i.e., neither Item 1 nor 2, preceding, is present)

Course specifiers:
Early Full Remission: from 1 to 11 months during which no criteria of Dependence or Abuse are met

(62)

Early Partial Remission: from 1 to 11 months during which one or more Criteria of Dependence or Abuse are met but not the full criteria for Dependence

Sustained Full Remission: for 12 months or more during which no criteria for Dependence or Abuse are met

Sustained Partial Remission: for 12 months or more during which one or more criteria for Dependence or Abuse are met but not the full criteria for Dependence

On Agonist Therapy: taking an agonist, partial agonist, or agonist/antagonist, and no criteria for Dependence or Abuse are met for at least 1 month

In a Controlled Environment: access is restricted by the environment (e.g., locked hospital unit, substance-free jail) for at least the past month

❑ ❑ ❑ ❑

Substance Abuse
(significantly modified from DSM-III-R)

ESSENTIAL FEATURES. This is basically a residual diagnostic category in which the individual has maladaptive behavior as a result of substance use, but does not meet the diagnostic criteria for Substance Dependence—specifically, the history does not include tolerance, withdrawal, or a pattern of compulsiveness. The maladaptive behavior may be either continued substance use despite occupational, psychological, or physical problems, or recurrent use in physically hazardous situations (e.g., operating a punch press while intoxicated).

(63)

ASSOCIATED FEATURES. Repeated bouts of Substance-Induced Intoxication are almost always present in the history. Personality and mood disturbances are often present. In chronic Abuse or Dependence, mood lability, suspiciousness, and violent behavior may be seen.

DIFFERENTIAL DIAGNOSIS. An essential feature of a Substance-Related disorder is clinically significant impairment; therefore, recreational or medically prescribed substance use that does not cause impairment is not considered a disorder. In addition, repeated episodes of Substance Intoxication can occur. A diagnosis of Substance Dependence is made when more severe impairment is present.

DIAGNOSTIC CRITERIA FOR
SUBSTANCE ABUSE
(SEE SPECIFIC SUBSTANCE SECTIONS BELOW
FOR DSM-IV AND ICD-10 CODES)

A. A maladaptive pattern of substance use leading to clinically significant impairment or distress, as manifested by one (or more) of the following, occurring within a 12-month period:
  (1) recurrent substance use resulting in a failure to fulfill major role obligations at work, school, or home (e.g., repeated absences or poor work performance related to substance use; substance-related absences, suspensions, or expulsions from school; neglect of children or household)
  (2) recurrent substance use in situations in which it is physically hazardous (e.g., driving an automobile or operating a machine when impaired by substance use)
  (3) recurrent substance-related legal problems (e.g., arrests for substance-related disorderly conduct)
  (4) continued substance use despite having persistent or recurrent social or interpersonal problems caused or exacerbated by the effects of the substance (e.g., arguments with spouse about consequences of intoxication, physical fights)

B. The symptoms have never met the criteria for Substance Dependence for this class of substance.

☐ ☐ ☐ ☐

SUBSTANCE-INDUCED DISORDERS

Substance Intoxication

ESSENTIAL FEATURES. Intoxication requires recent use or exposure to a substance, development of a reversible specific syndrome known to result from that substance, and the presence of maladaptive behavior or psychological changes.

Note: This definition does not include substance use (e.g., caffeine intake or recreational drugs) unless maladaptive behavior results.

ASSOCIATED FEATURES. Disturbances may occur in perception, attention, wakefulness, clarity of thought, judgment, emotion, and behavior. An individual's particular response to a substance depends on the substance (i.e., type, dose, duration of use), environment, premorbid personality, medical condition, and the individual's expectations.

DIFFERENTIAL DIAGNOSIS. Intoxication is a residual diagnostic category. Therefore, mental disorders due to a medical disorder are considered in the differential diagnosis prior to this diagnosis. For example, neurological diseases can sometimes result in symptoms that resemble an intoxicated state (e.g., a stroke or transient ischemic attack).

DIAGNOSTIC CRITERIA FOR
INTOXICATION
(SEE SPECIFIC SUBSTANCE SECTIONS BELOW
FOR DSM-IV AND ICD-10 CODES)

A. The development of a reversible substance-specific syndrome due to recent ingestion of (or exposure to) a substance.

> **NOTE: Different substances may produce similar or identical syndromes.**

B. Clinically significant maladaptive behavioral or psychological changes that are due to the effect of the substance on the central nervous system (e.g., belligerence, mood lability, cognitive impairment, impaired judgment, impaired social or occupational functioning) and develop during or shortly after use of the substance.

C. The symptoms are not due to a general medical condition and are not better accounted for by another mental disorder.

❑ ❑ ❑ ❑

Substance Withdrawal

ESSENTIAL FEATURES. Withdrawal symptoms develop with recent cessation, or decreased intake, of a substance after prolonged and/or heavy use. Particular withdrawal symptoms are substance specific. For example, symptoms associated with Opioid Withdrawal resemble a viral influenza (e.g., nausea and vomiting, muscle aches, diarrhea, and fever). In order to make this diagnosis, significant distress or impairment in functioning are required.

(65)

DIFFERENTIAL DIAGNOSIS. Withdrawal does not resemble other mental disorders, but can be superimposed on them. An individual in Substance Withdrawal can appear anxious and may be irritable or agitated. When withdrawal symptoms are severe, a delirium is sometimes present. Symptoms of withdrawal can resemble symptoms of a physical disorder (e.g., Opioid Withdrawal can look like influenza).

DIAGNOSTIC CRITERIA FOR
SUBSTANCE WITHDRAWAL
(SEE SPECIFIC SUBSTANCE SECTIONS BELOW
FOR DSM-IV AND ICD-10 CODES)

A. The development of a substance-specific syndrome due to the cessation of (or reduction in) substance use that has been heavy and prolonged.

B. The substance-specific syndrome causes clinically significant distress or impairment in social, occupational, or other important areas of functioning.

C. The symptoms are not due to a general medical condition and are not better accounted for by another mental disorder.

SPECIFIC SUBSTANCES. Except for Intoxication, Dependence, and Withdrawal, most Substance-Induced disorders are described in other Axis I sections (e.g., Psychotic Disorders, Anxiety Disorders, Mood Disorders), as appropriate to their clinical symptoms.

□ □ □ □

....

ALCOHOL-RELATED DISORDERS

Alcohol Use Disorders
Alcohol-Induced Disorders
Alcohol-Related Disorder Not Otherwise Specified (NOS)

Alcohol Use Disorders

303.90 Alcohol Dependence   (ICD-10 code F10.2x)
305.00 Alcohol Abuse   (ICD-10 code F10.1)
(see general criteria for Substance Dependence and
Abuse, preceding)

ASSOCIATED FEATURES AND LABORATORY FINDINGS. Alcohol Dependence and Abuse occur commonly and are often associated with depression, anxiety, insomnia, and abuse of other substances. There is an increased risk of accidents, criminal acts, violence, and suicide. Heavy drinking usually produces an elevation in gamma-glutamyltransferase (GGT), a liver enzyme. The mean corpuscular volume (MCV) of red cells is also sometimes increased. Continued heavy drinking damages almost every organ system.

□ □ □ □

Alcohol-Induced Disorders

303.00 Alcohol Intoxication   (ICD-10 code F10.00)

ASSOCIATED FEATURES. This disorder is sometimes associated with blackouts.

DIAGNOSTIC CRITERIA FOR   (ICD-10 code F10.00)
ALCOHOL INTOXICATION (303.00)

A. Recent ingestion of alcohol.

B. Clinically significant maladaptive behavioral or psychological changes (e.g., inappropriate sexual or aggressive behavior, mood lability, impaired judgment, impaired social or occupational functioning) that developed during, or shortly after, alcohol ingestion.

C. One (or more) of the following signs, developing during, or shortly after, alcohol use:
    (1) slurred speech
    (2) incoordination
    (3) unsteady gait
    (4) nystagmus
    (5) impairment in attention or memory
    (6) stupor or coma

D. The symptoms are not due to a general medical condition and are not better accounted for by another mental disorder.

□ □ □ □

291.8 Alcohol Withdrawal   (ICD-10 code F10.3)
(significantly modified from DSM-III-R)

Withdrawal symptoms begin within a few hours of decreased intake or cessation of alcohol consumption and continue for several days. Less than 5% of individuals, usually those with heavy alcohol intake for a prolonged period, will have severe withdrawal (i.e., Alcohol Withdrawal Delirium). Some individuals will have grand mal seizures.

DIAGNOSTIC CRITERIA FOR   (ICD-10 code F10.3)
ALCOHOL WITHDRAWAL (291.8)

A. Cessation of (or reduction in) alcohol use that has been heavy and prolonged.

B. Two (or more) of the following, developing within several hours to a few days after Criterion A:

(1) autonomic hyperactivity (e.g., sweating or pulse rate greater than 100)
(2) increased hand tremor
(3) insomnia
(4) nausea or vomiting
(5) transient visual, tactile, or auditory hallucinations or illusions
(6) psychomotor agitation
(7) anxiety
(8) grand mal seizures

C. The symptoms in Criterion B cause clinically significant distress or impairment in social, occupational, or other important areas of functioning.

D. The symptoms are not due to a general medical condition and are not better accounted for by another mental disorder.

Specify if:
With Perceptual Disturbances: hallucinations or illusions that are experienced in a context of intact reality testing (i.e., the individual knows they are substance-related and are not real)

CODING NOTE: For hallucinations in the *absence* of appropriate reality testing, consider 291.3 Alcohol-Induced Psychotic Disorder, With Hallucinations, With Onset During Withdrawal, or 291.0 Alcohol Withdrawal Delirium, With Hallucinations.

NOTE: Other Alcohol-Induced Disorders are described in other sections (e.g., Psychotic Disorders, Anxiety Disorders, Mood Disorders), as appropriate to clinical symptoms.

❑ ❑ ❑ ❑

AMPHETAMINE (OR AMPHETAMINE-LIKE)–RELATED DISORDERS

Amphetamine Use Disorders
Amphetamine-Induced Disorders
Amphetamine-Related Disorder Not Otherwise Specified (NOS)

Amphetamine Use Disorders

304.40 Amphetamine Dependence *(ICD-10 code F15.2x)*
305.70 Amphetamine Abuse *(ICD-10 code F15.1)*
(see general criteria for Substance Dependence and Abuse, preceding)

Aggressive, violent, and paranoid behavior may be seen in individuals with Amphetamine Dependence. The symptoms can resemble Schizophrenia, Paranoid Type or Delusional Disorder. Legal problems frequently occur and Sedative

Abuse or Dependence is common to reduce stimulation. Urine screens for amphetamines usually remain positive for 24 to 72 hours after a binge. Two patterns of use are common: daily and episodic (binge) use.

❏ ❏ ❏ ❏

Amphetamine-Induced Disorders
292.89 Amphetamine Intoxication   *(ICD-10 code F15.00)*

DIAGNOSTIC CRITERIA FOR   *(ICD-10 code F15.00)*
AMPHETAMINE INTOXICATION (292.89)

A. Recent use of amphetamine or a related substance (e.g., methylphenidate).

B. Clinically significant maladaptive behavioral or psychological changes (e.g., euphoria or affective blunting; changes in sociability; hypervigilance; interpersonal sensitivity; anxiety, tension, or anger; stereotyped behaviors; impaired judgment; or impaired social or occupational functioning) that developed during, or shortly after, use of amphetamine or a related substance.

C. Two (or more) of the following, developing during, or shortly after, use of amphetamine or a related substance:
   (1) tachycardia or bradycardia
   (2) pupillary dilation
   (3) elevated or lowered blood pressure
   (4) perspiration or chills
   (5) nausea or vomiting
   (6) evidence of weight loss
   (7) psychomotor agitation or retardation
   (8) muscular weakness, respiratory depression, chest pain, or cardiac arrhythmias
   (9) confusion, seizures, dyskinesias, dystonias, or coma

D. The symptoms are not due to a general medical condition and are not better accounted for by another mental disorder.

Specify if:
With Perceptual Disturbances: hallucinations or illusions which are experienced in a context of intact reality testing (the individual knows they are substance induced and are not real) (ICD-10 F15.04)

CODING NOTE: For hallucinations in the absence of appropriate reality testing, consider 292.12 Amphetamine-Induced

Psychotic Disorder, With Hallucinations, or 292.81 Amphetamine Intoxification Delirium, With Hallucinations.

❑ ❑ ❑ ❑

292.0 Amphetamine Withdrawal   (ICD-10 code F15.3)
(significantly modified from DSM-III-R)

ASSOCIATED FEATURES. Weight loss can occur during heavy use; rapid weight gain
can occur during withdrawal.

DIAGNOSTIC CRITERIA FOR   (ICD-10 code F15.3)
AMPHETAMINE WITHDRAWAL (292.0)

A. Cessation of (or reduction in) amphetamine (or a related substance) use that
has been heavy and prolonged.

B. Dysphoric mood and two (or more) of the following physiological changes,
developing within a few hours to several days after Criterion A:
(1) fatigue
(2) vivid, unpleasant dreams
(3) insomnia or hypersomnia
(4) increased appetite
(5) psychomotor retardation or agitation

C. The symptoms in Criterion B cause clinically significant distress or impairment
in social, occupational, or other important areas of functioning.

D. The symptoms are not due to a general medical condition and are not better
accounted for by another mental disorder.

NOTE: Other amphetamine-induced disorders are described in
other DSM-IV sections (e.g., Psychotic Disorders, Anxiety Disorders, Mood Disorders), as appropriate to clinical symptoms.

❑ ❑ ❑ ❑

CAFFEINE-RELATED DISORDERS

305.90 Caffeine Intoxication   (ICD-10 code F15.00)

Heavy use of caffeine can cause anxiety, cardiac arrhythmias, and gastrointestinal and pseudoneurologic symptoms. The differential diagnosis includes Anxiety Disorders, especially Panic Disorder. The differential diagnosis also includes
Amphetamine-Like Drug Intoxication and Substance-Related Withdrawal, as
well as Manic and Hypomanic episode.

DIAGNOSTIC CRITERIA FOR CAFFEINE INTOXICATION (305.9)

(ICD-10 code F15.00)

A. Recent consumption of caffeine, usually in excess of 250 mg (e.g., more than 2–3 cups of brewed coffee).

B. Five (or more) of the following signs, developing during, or shortly after, caffeine use:
- (1) restlessness
- (2) nervousness
- (3) excitement
- (4) insomnia
- (5) flushed face
- (6) diuresis
- (7) gastrointestinal disturbance
- (8) muscle twitching
- (9) rambling flow of thought and speech
- (10) tachycardia or cardiac arrhythmia
- (11) periods of inexhaustibility
- (12) psychomotor agitation

C. The symptoms in Criterion B cause clinically significant distress or impairment in social, occupational, or other important areas of functioning.

D. The symptoms are not due to a general medical condition and are not better accounted for by another mental disorder (e.g., an Anxiety Disorder).

> NOTE: Other Caffeine-Induced Disorders are described in other sections (e.g., Anxiety Disorders), as appropriate to their clinical symptoms.

❑ ❑ ❑ ❑

CANNABIS-RELATED DISORDERS

Cannabis Use Disorders
Cannabis-Induced Disorders
Cannabis-Related Disorder Not Otherwise Specified

Cannabis Use Disorders

304.30 Cannabis Dependence (ICD-10 code F12.2x)
305.20 Cannabis Abuse (ICD-10 code F12.1)
(see general criteria for Substance Dependence and Abuse, preceding)

Cannabis users do not develop physiological dependence and do not consistently experience withdrawal symptoms.

❑ ❑ ❑ ❑

Cannabis-Induced Disorders

292.89 Cannabis Intoxication   (ICD-10 code F12.00)

Individuals who use cannabis typically use other drugs. Mild forms of depression, anxiety, or irritability are very commonly seen in individuals who use cannabis daily. In high doses, the effects are similar to hallucinogens. Urine tests remain positive for many days following use and for weeks following heavy use.

DIAGNOSTIC CRITERIA FOR   (ICD-10 code F12.00)
CANNABIS INTOXICATION (292.89)

A. Recent use of cannabis.

B. Clinically significant maladaptive behavioral or psychological changes (e.g., impaired motor coordination, euphoria, anxiety, sensation of slowed time, impaired judgment, social withdrawal) that developed during, or shortly after, cannabis use.

C. Two (or more) of the following signs, developing within 2 hours of cannabis use:
   (1) conjuctival injection
   (2) increased appetite
   (3) dry mouth
   (4) tachycardia

D. The symptoms are not due to a general medical condition and are not better accounted for by another mental disorder.

Specify if:
With Perceptual Disturbances: hallucinations or illusions that are experienced in a context of intact reality testing (the individual knows they are substance induced and are not real) (ICD-10 F12.04)

CODING NOTE: For hallucinations in the *absence* of appropriate reality testing, consider 292.12 Cannabis-Induced Psychotic Disorder, With Hallucinations, or 292.81 Cannabis Intoxication Delirium, With Hallucinations.

NOTE: Other Cannabis-Induced Disorders are described in other sections (e.g., Psychotic Disorders, Anxiety Disorders, Mood Disorders), as appropriate to their clinical symptoms.

❑ ❑ ❑ ❑

COCAINE-RELATED DISORDERS

Cocaine Use Disorders
Cocaine-Induced Disorders
Cocaine-Related Disorder Not Otherwise Specified (NOS)

Cocaine Use Disorders

304.20 Cocaine Dependence   *(ICD-10 code F14.2x)*
305.60 Cocaine Abuse   *(ICD-10 code F14.1)*
*(see general criteria for Substance Dependence and
Abuse, preceding)*

The euphoria experienced with cocaine is extreme and of brief duration; therefore, individuals develop dependence quickly. Financial problems and criminal activity are common. Conditioned responses to stimuli associated with cocaine are long lasting and can increase the chance of relapse. Urine screen for metabolites of cocaine remains positive for as long as a few days (one-time users) to a week or longer (heavier use and high doses).

"Snorting" (intranasal use) can cause a perforated nasal septum. Dependence is associated with weight loss and malnutrition, myocardial infarction, seizures, stroke, and sudden death. Two patterns of use are commonly seen: daily and episodic ("binge") use.

❑ ❑ ❑ ❑

Cocaine-Induced Disorders

292.89 Cocaine Intoxication   *(ICD-10 code F14.00)*
(significantly modified from DSM-III-R)

DIAGNOSTIC CRITERIA FOR   *(ICD-10 code F14.00)*
COCAINE INTOXICATION (292.89)

A. Recent use of cocaine.

B. Clinically significant maladaptive behavioral or psychological changes (e.g., euphoria or affective blunting; changes in sociability, hypervigilance; interpersonal sensitivity; anxiety, tension, or anger; stereotyped behaviors; impaired judgment; or impaired social or occupational functioning) that developed during, or shortly after, use of cocaine.

C. Two (or more) of the following, developing during, or shortly after, cocaine use:
   (1) tachycardia or bradycardia
   (2) pupillary dilation
   (3) elevated or lowered blood pressure
   (4) perspiration or chills

(5) nausea or vomiting

(6) evidence of weight loss

(7) psychomotor agitation or retardation

(8) muscular weakness, respiratory depression, chest pain, or cardiac arrhythmias

(9) confusion, seizures, dyskinesias, dystonias, or coma

D. The symptoms are not due to a general medical condition and are not better accounted for by another mental disorder.

Specify if:

With Perceptual Disturbances: hallucinations or illusions that are experienced in a context of intact reality testing (the individual knows they are substance induced and are not real) (ICD-10 F14.04)

CODING NOTE: For hallucinations in the *absence* **of appropriate reality testing, consider 292.12 Cocaine-Induced Psychotic Disorder, With Hallucinations,** *or* **292.81 Cocaine Intoxication Delirium, With Hallucinations.**

❑ ❑ ❑ ❑

292.0 Cocaine Withdrawal   (ICD-10 code F14.3)
(significantly modified from DSM-III-R)

DIAGNOSTIC CRITERIA FOR   (ICD-10 code F14.3)
COCAINE WITHDRAWAL (292.0)

A. Cessation of (or reduction in) cocaine use that has been heavy and prolonged.

B. Dysphoric mood and two (or more) of the following physiological changes, developing within a few hours to several days after Criterion A:

(1) fatigue

(2) vivid, unpleasant dreams

(3) insomnia or hypersomnia

(4) increased appetite

(5) psychomotor retardation or agitation

C. The symptoms in Criterion B cause clinically significant distress or impairment in social, occupational, or other important areas of functioning.

D. The symptoms are not due to a general medical condition and are not better accounted for by another mental disorder.

NOTE: Other Cocaine-Induced Disorders are described in other sections (e.g., Psychotic Disorders, Anxiety Disorders, Mood Disorders), as appropriate to clinical symptoms.

❑ ❑ ❑ ❑

HALLUCINOGEN-RELATED DISORDERS

Hallucinogen Use Disorders
Hallucinogen-Induced Disorders
Hallucinogen-Related Disorder Not Otherwise Specified
   (NOS)

Hallucinogen Use Disorders

304.50 Hallucinogen Dependence   *(ICD-10 code F16.2x)*
305.30 Hallucinogen Abuse   *(ICD-10 code F16.1)*

Hallucinogens are a diverse class of substances (e.g., LSD, mescaline, psilocybin, "ecstasy"). Withdrawal from hallucinogens is not always established, but craving is reported. Tolerance develops rapidly, which may explain why daily use is very uncommon.

   While intoxicated, mood lability is often seen, as are fearfulness and intense anxiety. Injuries occur due to impaired judgment. Flashbacks occur and can persist for years.

Hallucinogen-Induced Disorders

292.89 Hallucinogen Intoxication   *(ICD-10 code F16.00)*

DIAGNOSTIC CRITERIA FOR   *(ICD-10 code F16.00)*
HALLUCINOGEN INTOXICATION (292.89)

A. Recent use of a hallucinogen.

B. Clinically significant maladaptive behavioral or psychological changes (e.g., marked anxiety or depression, ideas of reference, fear of losing one's mind, paranoid ideation, impaired judgment, or impaired social or occupational functioning) that developed during, or shortly after, hallucinogen use.

C. Perceptual changes occurring in a state of full wakefulness and alertness (e.g., subjective intensification of perceptions, depersonalization, derealization, illusions, hallucinations, synesthesias) that developed during, or shortly after, hallucinogen use.

D. Two (or more) of the following signs, developing during, or shortly after, hallucinogen use:
   (1) pupillary dilation
   (2) tachycardia
   (3) sweating
   (4) palpitations
   (5) blurring of vision
   (6) tremors
   (7) incoordination

E. The symptoms are not due to a general medical condition and are not better accounted for by another mental disorder.

❑ ❑ ❑ ❑

292.89 Hallucinogen Persisting Perception Disorder (Flashbacks)

(ICD-10 code F16.70)

DIAGNOSTIC CRITERIA FOR HALLUCINOGEN PERSISTING PERCEPTION DISORDER (FLASHBACKS) (292.89)

(ICD-10 code F16.70)

A. The reexperiencing, following cessation of use of a hallucinogen, of one or more of the perceptual symptoms that were experienced while intoxicated with the hallucinogen (e.g., geometric hallucinations, false perceptions of movement in the peripheral visual fields, flashes of color, intensified colors, trails of images of moving objects, positive afterimages, halos around objects, macropsia, and micropsia).

B. The symptoms in Criterion A cause clinically significant distress or impairment in social, occupational, or other important areas of functioning.

C. The symptoms are not due to a general medical condition (e.g., anatomical lesions and infections of the brain, visual epilepsies) and are not better accounted for by another mental disorder (e.g., delirium, dementia, Schizophrenia) or hypnopompic hallucinations.

> NOTE: Other Hallucinogen-Induced Disorders are described in other sections (e.g., Psychotic Disorders, Anxiety Disorders), as appropriate to clinical symptoms.

❑ ❑ ❑ ❑

INHALANT-RELATED DISORDERS

Inhalant Use Disorders
Inhalant-Induced Disorders
Inhalant-Related Disorder Not Otherwise Specified (NOS)

Inhalant Use Disorders

304.60 Inhalant Dependence
305.90 Inhalant Abuse
(see general criteria for Substance Dependence and Abuse, preceding)

(ICD-10 code F18.2x)
(ICD-10 code F18.1)

These are disorders that result from inhalation of hydrocarbons in spray paint, gasoline, glue, paint thinners, and so on. Tolerance is reported, but a withdrawal syndrome is not well described. The odor of the inhalant or residue on clothing may be present at the time of the evaluation. Heavy use can quickly lead to organ damage (kidneys or liver) and significant nervous system injury (peripheral neuropathy, cerebral atrophy, and cerebellar degeneration). Death can occur from cardiovascular dysfunction or respiratory depression.

❏ ❏ ❏ ❏

Inhalant-Induced Disorders

292.89 Inhalant Intoxication   (ICD-10 code F18.00)

DIAGNOSTIC CRITERIA FOR   (ICD-10 code F18.00)
INHALANT INTOXICATION (292.89)

A. Recent intentional use or short-term, high-dose exposure to volatile inhalants (excluding anesthetic gases and short-acting vasodilators).

B. Clinically significant maladaptive behavioral or psychological changes (e.g., belligerence, assaultiveness, apathy, impaired judgment, impaired social or occupational functioning) that developed during, or shortly after, use of or exposure to volatile inhalants.

C. Two (or more) of the following signs, developing during, or shortly after, inhalant use or exposure:
   (1) dizziness
   (2) nystagmus
   (3) incoordination
   (4) slurred speech
   (5) unsteady gait
   (6) lethargy
   (7) depressed reflexes
   (8) psychomotor retardation
   (9) tremor
   (10) generalized muscle weakness
   (11) blurred vision or diplopia
   (12) stupor or coma
   (13) euphoria

D. The symptoms are not due to a general medical condition and are not better accounted for by another mental disorder.

> NOTE: Other Inhalant-Induced Disorders are described in other sections (e.g., Psychotic Disorders, Anxiety Disorders, Mood Disorders), as appropriate to clinical symptoms.

❏ ❏ ❏ ❏

....

NICOTINE-RELATED DISORDERS

305.10 Nicotine Dependence   (ICD-10 code F17.2x)
(see general criteria for Substance Dependence, preceding)

Strong craving during withdrawal may explain the low success rates reported in individuals who attempt to discontinue use. Smoking increases the metabolism of a number of medications.

❑ ❑ ❑ ❑

292.0 Nicotine Withdrawal   (ICD-10 code F17.3)
(significantly modified from DSM-III-R)

DIAGNOSTIC CRITERIA FOR   (ICD-10 code F17.3)
NICOTINE WITHDRAWAL (292.0)

A. Daily use of nicotine for at least several weeks.

B. Abrupt cessation of nicotine use, or reduction in the amount of nicotine used, followed within 24 hours by four (or more) of the following signs:
  (1) dysphoric or depressed mood
  (2) insomnia
  (3) irritability, frustration, or anger
  (4) anxiety
  (5) difficulty concentrating
  (6) restlessness
  (7) decreased heart rate
  (8) increased appetite or weight gain

C. The symptoms in Criterion B cause clinically significant distress or impairment in social, occupational, or other important areas of functioning.

D. The symptoms are not due to a general medical condition and are not better accounted for by another mental disorder.

....

OPIOID-RELATED DISORDERS

Opioid Use Disorders
Opioid-Induced Disorders
Opioid-Related Disorder Not
  Otherwise Specified

Opioid Use Disorders

304.00 Opioid Dependence   *(ICD-10 code F11.2x)*
305.50 Opioid Abuse   *(ICD-10 code F11.1)*
*(see general criteria for Substance Dependence and
Abuse, above)*

Associated criminal activities are common. Urine screens are helpful in diagnosis. The duration of a positive urine after use depends on the biological life of
the drug. Intravenous use causes "tracks" from scarring and damaged veins.
Nationally, upwards of 60% of IV heroin users are HIV positive.

Death rates are as high as 10 per 1,000 per year among individuals with
Opioid Dependence. Babies born to women who are Opioid Dependent develop
withdrawal symptoms that may require medical treatment.

❑ ❑ ❑ ❑

Opioid-Induced Disorders

292.89 Opioid Intoxication   *(ICD-10 code F11.00)*

DIAGNOSTIC CRITERIA FOR   *(ICD-10 code F11.00)*
OPIOID INTOXICATION (292.89)

A. Recent use of an opioid.

B. Clinically significant maladaptive behavioral or psychological changes (e.g.,
initial euphoria followed by apathy, dysphoria, psychomotor agitation or retardation, impaired judgment, or impaired social or occupational functioning)
that developed during, or shortly after, opioid use.

C. Pupillary constriction (or pupillary dilation due to anoxia from severe over-
dose) and one (or more) of the following signs, developing during, or shortly
after, opioid use:
   (1) drowsiness or coma
   (2) slurred speech
   (3) impairment in attention or memory

D. The symptoms are not due to a general medical condition and are not better
accounted for by another mental disorder.

> **Specify if:**
> **With Perceptual Disturbances:** hallucinations or illusions that are
> experienced in a context of intact reality testing (the individual
> knows they are substance induced and are not real) (ICD-10
> F11.04)
>
> **CODING NOTE: For hallucinations in the *absence* of appropriate
> reality testing, consider 292.12 Opioid-Induced Psychotic**

Disorder, With Hallucinations, or 292.81 Opioid-Induced Delirium, With Hallucinations.

▢ ▢ ▢ ▢

292.0 Opioid Withdrawal   (ICD-10 code F11.3)

Time of onset of withdrawal symptoms after the last dose depends on the biological life of the drug. Heroin is short-acting and withdrawal symptoms begin within 6 to 24 hours of last use. Symptoms of withdrawal emerge after 48 to 96 hours of abstinence from longer-acting opioid use, such as methadone or LAAM.

DIAGNOSTIC CRITERIA FOR   (ICD-10 code F11.3)
OPIOID WITHDRAWAL (292.0)

A. Either of the following:
   (1) cessation of (or reduction in) opioid use that has been heavy and prolonged (several weeks or longer)
   (2) administration of an opioid antagonist after a period of opioid use

B. Three (or more) of the following, developing within minutes to several days after Criterion A:
   (1) dysphoric mood
   (2) nausea or vomiting
   (3) muscle aches
   (4) lacrimation or rhinorrhea
   (5) pupillary dilation, piloerection, or sweating
   (6) diarrhea
   (7) yawning
   (8) fever
   (9) insomnia

C. The symptoms in Criterion B cause clinically significant distress or impairment in social, occupational, or other important areas of functioning.

D. The symptoms are not due to a general medical condition and are not better accounted for by another mental disorder.

NOTE: Other Opioid-Induced Disorders are described in other sections (e.g., Psychotic Disorders, Anxiety Disorders, Mood Disorders), as appropriate to clinical symptoms.

▢ ▢ ▢ ▢

PHENCYCLIDINE (OR PHENCYCLIDINE-LIKE)–RELATED DISORDERS

Phencyclidine Use Disorders
Phencyclidine-Induced Disorders
Phencyclidine-Related Disorder Not Otherwise Specified
  (NOS)

Phencyclidine Use Disorders

304.90 Phencyclidine Dependence *(ICD-10 code F19.2x)*
305.90 Phencyclidine Abuse *(ICD-10 code F19.1)*
(see general criteria for Substance Dependence and
Abuse, preceding)

This substance class includes phencyclidine (PCP) and other similarly acting substances, such as ketamine. PCP is a common adulterant of other substances, such as marijuana. Symptoms of PCP withdrawal can occur, but no consistent syndrome is described. Tolerance is not reported in humans.

Phencyclidine-Induced Disorders

292.89 Phencyclidine Intoxication *(ICD-10 code F19.00)*

The effects of intoxication vary widely depending on the dose. Low doses can produce the symptoms listed in Criterion C, below, except for seizures and coma, which occur at high doses.

DIAGNOSTIC CRITERIA FOR *(ICD-10 code F19.00)*
PHENCYCLIDINE INTOXICATION (292.89)

A. Recent use of phencyclidine (or a related substance).

B. Clinically significant maladaptive behavioral changes (e.g., belligerence, as-saultiveness, impulsiveness, unpredictability, psychomotor agitation, impaired judgment, or impaired social or occupational functioning) that developed during, or shortly after, phencyclidine use.

C. Within an hour (less when smoked, "snorted," or used intravenously), two (or more) of the following signs:
  (1) vertical or horizontal nystagmus
  (2) hypertension or tachycardia
  (3) numbness or diminished responsiveness to pain
  (4) ataxia

(5) dysarthria
(6) muscle rigidity
(7) seizures or coma
(8) hyperacusis

D. The symptoms are not due to a general medical condition and are not better accounted for by another mental disorder.

> **Specify if:**
> **With Perceptual Disturbances:** hallucinations or illusions that are experienced in a context of intact reality testing (the individual knows they are substance induced and are not real) (ICD-10 F19.04)
>
> **CODING NOTE:** For hallucinations in the *absence* of appropriate reality testing, consider 292.12 Phencyclidine-Induced Psychotic Disorder, With Hallucinations, or 292.81 Phencyclidine Intoxication Delirium, With Hallucinations.
>
> **NOTE:** Other Phencyclidine-Induced Disorders are described in other sections (e.g., Psychotic Disorders, Anxiety Disorders, Mood Disorders), as appropriate to clinical symptoms.

❏ ❏ ❏ ❏

....

SEDATIVE-, HYPNOTIC-, OR ANXIOLYTIC-RELATED DISORDERS

Sedative, Hypnotic, or Anxiolytic Use Disorders
Sedative-, Hypnotic-, or Anxiolytic-Induced Disorders
Sedative-, Hypnotic-, or Anxiolytic-Related Disorder Not Otherwise Specified (NOS)

Sedative, Hypnotic, or Anxiolytic Use Disorders

304.10 Sedative, Hypnotic, or Anxiolytic Dependence *(ICD-10 code F13.2x)*

305.40 Sedative, Hypnotic, or Anxiolytic Abuse *(ICD-10 code F13.1)*

(see general criteria for Substance Dependence and Abuse, preceding)

This class of substances includes the barbiturates, benzodiazepines, and other substances prescribed for sleeping or anxiety problems (except for buspirone or gepirone). Like alcohol, these medications are central nervous system depressants. The combination of these drugs with alcohol can be fatal in over-dose. Almost all of these substances can be detected in the urine for a significant period of time following ingestion.

□ □ □ □

Sedative-, Hypnotic-, or Anxiolytic-Induced Disorders

292.89 Sedative, Hypnotic, or Anxiolytic Intoxication   (ICD-10 code F13.00)

Taken in excess, these substances produce effects similar to excessive intake of alcohol. The benzodiazepines, taken alone, rarely cause serious respiratory de-pression or death. Barbiturates, however, will cause cessation of respiratory and brain function at higher doses.

DIAGNOSTIC CRITERIA FOR SEDATIVE, HYPNOTIC, OR ANXIOLYTIC INTOXICATION (292.89)   (ICD-10 code F13.00)

A. Recent use of a sedative, hypnotic, or anxiolytic.

B. Clinically significant maladaptive behavioral or psychological changes (e.g., inappropriate sexual or aggressive behavior, mood lability, impaired judg-ment, impaired social or occupational functioning) that developed during, or shortly after, sedative, hypnotic, or anxiolytic use.

C. One (or more) of the following signs, developing during, or shortly after, sed-ative, hypnotic, or anxiolytic use:
   (1) slurred speech
   (2) incoordination
   (3) unsteady gait
   (4) nystagmus
   (5) impairment in attention or memory
   (6) stupor or coma

D. The symptoms are not due to a general medical condition and are not better accounted for by another mental disorder.

□ □ □ □

292.0 Sedative, Hypnotic, or Anxiolytic Withdrawal   (ICD-10 code F13.3)
(significantly modified from DSM-III-R)

Withdrawal from some sedative substances, especially the barbiturates and mep-robamate, can be life threatening. The time of onset of withdrawal symptoms depends on the biological half-life of the abused drug. Short-acting drugs will produce symptoms within a few hours of cessation; long-acting drugs, such as diazepam, may take 1 to 2 weeks.

DIAGNOSTIC CRITERIA FOR SEDATIVE, HYPNOTIC, OR ANXIOLYTIC WITHDRAWAL (292.0)

(ICD-10 F13.3)

A. Cessation of (or reduction in) sedative, hypnotic, or anxiolytic use that has been heavy and prolonged.

B. Two (or more) of the following, developing within several hours to a few days after Criterion A:

(1) autonomic hyperactivity (e.g., sweating or pulse rate greater than 100)
(2) increased hand tremor
(3) insomnia
(4) nausea or vomiting
(5) transient visual, tactile, or auditory hallucinations or illusions
(6) psychomotor agitation
(7) anxiety
(8) grand mal seizures

C. The symptoms in Criterion B cause clinically significant distress or impairment in social, occupational, or other important areas of functioning.

D. The symptoms are not due to a general medical condition and are not better accounted for by another mental disorder.

Specify if:
With Perceptual Disturbances: hallucinations or illusions that are experienced in a context of intact reality testing (the individual knows they are substance induced and are not real)

CODING NOTE: For hallucinations in the *absence* of appropriate reality testing, consider 292.12 Sedative-, Hypnotic-, or Anxiolytic-Induced Psychotic Disorder, With Hallucinations, With Onset During Withdrawal or 292.81 Sedative, Hypnotic, or Anxiolytic Withdrawal Delirium, With Hallucinations.

NOTE: Other Sedative-, Hypnotic-, or Anxiolytic-Induced Disorders are described in other sections (e.g., Psychotic Disorders, Anxiety Disorders, Mood Disorders), as appropriate to clinical symptoms.

□ □ □ □

POLYSUBSTANCE-RELATED DISORDERS

304.80 Polysubstance Dependence   (ICD-10 code F19.2x)

ESSENTIAL FEATURE. An individual is repeatedly using three or more substances from different groups (excluding caffeine and nicotine) during a 12-month period, but no substance predominates. In addition, the Substance Dependence criteria are met when all substances are considered.

❑ ❑ ❑ ❑

OTHER (OR UNKNOWN) SUBSTANCE-RELATED DISORDERS

Other (or Unknown) Substance Use Disorders
Other (or Unknown) Substance-Induced Disorders
Other/Unknown Substance-Related Disorder Not Otherwise
  Specified (NOS)

Diagnosis and coding follow the principles and guidelines for general and specific substances, preceding.

> NOTE: Most Substance-Induced Disorders other than Intoxication, Dependence, and Withdrawal are described in other sections (e.g., Psychotic Disorders, Anxiety Disorders, Mood Disorders), as appropriate to clinical symptoms.

❑ ❑ ❑ ❑

OTHER (OR UNKNOWN) SUBSTANCE DEPENDENCE OR ABUSE
(see general criteria for Substance Dependence
and Abuse, above)

Substances to consider in this category include anabolic steroids, nitrite inhalants, over-the-counter drugs, and prescription drugs not in the other 11 categories (e.g., thyroid extract).

❑ ❑ ❑ ❑

DIFFERENCES BETWEEN DSM-III-R AND DSM-IV SUBSTANCE-RELATED DISORDERS

❑   DSM-IV combines disorders formerly listed in two sections of DSM-III-R (Psychoactive Substance Use Disorders and Psychoactive

Substance-Induced Organic Mental Disorders) into one new section now called **Substance-Related Disorders**.

❑ Many other Substance-Induced Disorders are also listed in sections based on symptom characteristics. They are new disorders in those sections, which include Substance-Induced Mood Disorders (now listed with the Mood Disorders), Substance-Induced Psychotic Disorders (with Schizophrenia and Other Psychotic Disorders), Substance-Induced Anxiety Disorders (in the Anxiety Disorders section), Substance-Induced Sleep Disorder (under Sleep Disorders), and so on.

❑ The number of criteria for **Substance Dependence** has been shortened from nine to seven. Specifically, DSM-III-R's Criterion 4 ("frequent intoxication or withdrawal symptoms when expected to fulfill major role obligation . . .") was moved to DSM-IV's criteria for **Substance Abuse**. DSM-III-R's Criteria 8 and 9, which address withdrawal, were combined into one Substance Dependence criterion in DSM-IV (2a and 2b).

❑ The duration criterion for **Substance Dependence** in DSM-III-R was changed from symptoms persisting for "at least 1 month or have occurred repeatedly over a longer period of time" to three or more criteria "at any time in the same 12-month period" in DSM-IV.

❑ Specifiers (general and course) changed and were expanded in DSM-IV.

❑ DSM-IV maladaptive behavior criteria for **Substance Abuse** were expanded by adding two additional criteria: "recurrent use resulting in failure to fulfill major role obligations" and "recurrent substance-related legal problems."

❑ Substance-specific **intoxication and withdrawal** criteria are changed.

❑ DSM-III-R Alcohol Idiosyncratic Intoxication was eliminated.

❑ All DSM-IV Substance-Related Disorders are categorized in a useful table (Table 1, p. 177, in DSM-IV; Table 13-1, p. 99, in this book.

....

CASE VIGNETTES: SUBSTANCE-RELATED DISORDERS

Case Vignette 1

T.C. is a 20-year-old male who is brought by his wife to the emergency department for evaluation. According to the wife, T.C. has been very agitated for the past few hours. She suspects he is using drugs and reports that he has spent all of their savings. She also states that his behavior has changed over the last 4 months; he is frequently absent from home and has been taking money from her wallet.

T.C.'s vital signs show a tachycardia (rate 120), mild blood pressure elevation (150/95), and a slight fever (100.3° F). On examination, T.C. is quite anxious, has a gross tremor, is pacing the floor and sweating, and complains of severe muscle pain. His pupils are enlarged (mydriasis), and he has rhinorrhea (runny nose). He is anxious to leave and keeps saying, "I'll be O.K. Just let me out of here." He denies regular substance use, but states that he has tried marijuana, cocaine, and heroin. The physical examination reveals recent needle marks on both arms. Toxic screen is positive for opioids.

DIAGNOSIS AND DISCUSSION
Axis I—292.0 Opioid Withdrawal (ICD-10 F11.3)
304.00 Opioid Dependence, With Physiological Dependence (ICD-10 F11.2x)
Axis II—799.9 Diagnosis Deferred (ICD-10 R46.8)

The clinical picture resembles a viral influenza and is typical of Opioid Withdrawal (other symptoms may include lacrimation, diarrhea, yawning, and insomnia.). T.C., as is often the case, did not reveal the reason for his symptoms and only wants to get another "fix" to relieve his intense discomfort. Laboratory tests for drug screening and tests for identification of specific substances are very helpful in the clinical evaluation for possible Substance Abuse and Dependence.

T.C. meets the criteria for Substance Dependence. He has withdrawal symptoms (i.e., muscle aches, pupillary dilation, rhinorrhea, and fever) and no longer spends time with his family. He spends his time in drug-related activities, has spent the family savings, and is taking money from his wife. He exhibits signs and symptoms of physiological dependence; therefore, "With Physiological Dependence" is appropriate. None of the six course specifiers available applies in this particular case. Because insufficient information is available about T.C.'s personality prior to the time of his opioid use, any Axis II diagnosis should be deferred.

Case Vignette 2

C.C. is a 38-year-old self-employed businessman brought for evaluation by his wife, who states, "He is really suspicious and has crazy ideas about our neighbors." She reports that he has had increasing problems over the past 4 months. He has no prior psychiatric history, except for almost daily marijuana (cannabis) use since college. The wife reports that he frequently gets "stoned" at home after work. Additional descriptions by his wife of his recent behavior include "very moody," "very hyper at times, then he will sleep for many hours," "angry and very irritable," and "he is not like the man I married." She reports that his business is failing and their financial problems are severe.

On examination, C.C. appears frightened at times and is quite suspicious at other times. He relates, "I am fine; my neighbor . . . he is trying to steal my money and my home . . . he is part of a criminal cartel." He denies any family history of psychiatric disorders, hallucinations, medical problems, or drug abuse. When asked about his cannabis use, he said angrily, "My wife always exaggerates. I haven't smoked a joint for over a year." He is well-oriented and has good memory function. His toxic screen is positive for cocaine and marijuana.

DIAGNOSIS AND DISCUSSION

Axis 1 292.11 Cocaine-Induced Psychotic Disorder, With Delusions (ICD-10 F14.51), With Onset During Intoxication 304.30 Cannabis Dependence (Provisional) (ICD-10 F12.2x)

Axis II 799.9 Diagnosis deferred on Axis II (ICD-10 R46.8)

Axis III No known medical conditions

Although C.C. denies drug abuse, which is not unusual, his toxic screen and clinical presentation strongly suggest a Cocaine-Induced Psychosis. If the toxic screen had been negative, other diagnoses to consider would have been Bipolar I Disorder and Brief Psychotic Disorder. If the clinician wants to express a slight doubt about the Cocaine-Induced Psychotic Disorder, the word "(probable)" could be added to the diagnosis. Based upon the preliminary history, the wife reports daily cannabis use that, in all likelihood, interferes with family and recreational activities. The word "(provisional)" is added until additional information is obtained.

CHAPTER 14

SCHIZOPHRENIA AND OTHER PSYCHOTIC DISORDERS

Each disorder in this section is characterized by psychosis; however, the term *psychotic* is interpreted in different ways. It is broadest in Schizophrenia, Schizophreniform Disorder, Schizoaffective Disorder, and Brief Psychotic Disorder, in which psychotic refers to delusions, hallucinations, and bizarre or disorganized speech or behavior. In Psychotic Disorder Due to a General Medical Condition and in Substance-Induced Psychotic Disorder, psychotic implies delusions and hallucinations (in the latter diagnosis, only those hallucinations not accompanied by insight). In Delusional Disorder, it refers only to delusions.

GENERAL DIFFERENCES FROM DSM-III-R. Three DSM-III-R sections are combined in this section of DSM-IV: Schizophrenia, Delusional Disorder, and Psychotic Disorders Not Elsewhere Classified. In addition, Psychotic Disorder Due to a General Medical Condition and Substance-Induced Psychotic Disorder (depending on drug/toxin involvement) include syndromes formerly found in DSM-III-R's Organic Delusional Disorder and Organic Hallucinosis. For differences in specific disorders, see below.

SCHIZOPHRENIA
(significantly modified from DSM-III-R)

Paranoid Type
Disorganized Type
Catatonic Type
Undifferentiated Type
Residual Type

ESSENTIAL FEATURES. All of the Schizophrenias exhibit characteristic psychotic symptoms during exacerbations *(active phase)*, as well as functioning below the highest level previously achieved (and/or failure to achieve expected levels of social development). There must be a history of delusions, hallucinations, or characteristic disturbances in affect or form of thought (see following). Psychotic symptoms must have been present for at least 1 month (unless successfully treated before a month has elapsed), and some symptoms or signs must have persisted for at least 6 months. There is often a prodromal phase.

    Positive symptoms can include delusions and hallucinations (the "psychotic" dimension), as well as verbal and behavioral disorganization and catatonia (the "disorganized" dimension). *Negative* symptoms allude to restrictions of affect, thought, verbal productions, and purposeful behavior. *Cognitive* deficits are often seen, although many consider intellectual capacity to be spared.

66

ASSOCIATED FEATURES. Almost any psychiatric symptom may be associated with Schizophrenia. Poor or eccentric grooming, dress, or behavior; psychomotor abnormalities; stereotypic movements; and a perplexed appearance are common, as are concreteness and poverty of speech, ritualistic behavior, magical thinking, various dysphoric moods and feelings, dissociative symptoms, ideas of reference, hypochondriasis and other symptoms of somatization, and illusions. Disturbance of the sensorium is unusual (and mitigates toward other diagnoses), although the patient may be confused or disoriented during acute exacerbation.

    Suicide is not unusual in poorly responsive or inadequately treated patients with Schizophrenia; about 10% die by their own hand. Life expectancy is shortened by other factors as well, including accidents, criminal victimization, and other medical conditions.

ASSOCIATED PHYSICAL AND LABORATORY FINDINGS. Subtle abnormalities in brain anatomy (e.g., ventricular and sulcal size), blood flow, and neurophysiology are often present and may be correlated with severity or chronicity. Neurological findings related to drugs used in treatment may be seen (e.g., extrapyramidal symptoms, Tardive Dyskinesia).

CULTURAL FEATURES. Although Schizophrenia is found in every culture, its presentation—particularly the form and content of psychotic symptoms—varies considerably (e.g., catatonia is relatively uncommon in the United States but is often seen elsewhere). Language and cultural factors should be considered carefully before final diagnosis.

COURSE. The course of Schizophrenia is relevant to the diagnosis. Onset is usually during late adolescence or early adulthood, but it may occur in childhood (in which the criteria are the same but diagnosis is more difficult) or (rarely) after age 45. It may appear to begin suddenly or over a period of months or years. There is usually a *prodromal phase,* which is often noticed only in retrospect. After the *active phase* has remitted somewhat, there is usually a *residual phase.*

67

Return to full premorbid functioning is uncommon, although several factors are associated with better-than-average prognosis (e.g., acute onset, late onset, brief duration of initial exacerbation, and absence of structural brain abnormality). Aggressive treatment of the first psychotic episode may favorably alter the course. The diagnosis should be reconsidered if the patient is able to remain in full remission without treatment.

PREDISPOSING FACTORS. Familial patterns of schizophreniform illness are relatively predisposing, and become much more predictive if the afflicted relative is a parent or sibling. Theories of predisposition related to socioeconomic or parenting factors have not been well supported.

DIFFERENTIAL DIAGNOSIS. General medical conditions, including dementias and deliria, should always be ruled out. Substance-Related Disorders can mimic most or all of the diagnostic criteria. Severe Mood Disorders can produce psychotic symptoms, and mood symptoms are common in Schizophrenia. If the psychotic symptoms are associated solely with mood disturbance, Schizophrenia should not be diagnosed. Schizoaffective Disorder may be difficult to differentiate; DSM-IV suggests that this diagnosis may even alternate with Schizophrenia from one acute episode to another. (One assumes that the disorder is the same, presenting in different ways.) Schizophreniform Disorder should be diagnosed only when the duration of illness is under 6 months, but is otherwise virtually indistinguishable from Schizophrenia. The delusions in Delusional Disorder are not "bizarre"; and hallucinations, disorganization, and negative symptoms are not prominent.

      The criteria for Pervasive Developmental Disorders (e.g., Autism) and other childhood-onset disorders should not be confused with those of Schizophrenia, although the additional diagnosis of Schizophrenia may be made if prominent delusions or hallucinations are present for at least 1 month. Symptoms of Mental Retardation may suggest schizophrenia, but it is easily differentiated.

      Schizoid, Schizotypal and Paranoid Personality Disorders often present with "odd" thinking. Once the "A criteria" (see below) are satisfied, however, Schizophrenia is diagnosed and the Personality Disorder should be described as "premorbid." Transient psychotic symptoms may appear in several other psychiatric disorders, but the patient generally returns to his or her prior level of functioning. Unusual or eccentric religious or cultural beliefs, per se, when shared and accepted by a large group, should not be considered evidence of Schizophrenia.

DIAGNOSTIC CRITERIA FOR ALL SCHIZOPHRENIAS (295.xx) (SEE SUBTYPES, BELOW)

(ICD-10 code F20.xx)

A. *Characteristic symptoms.* Two (or more) of the following, each present for a significant portion of time during a 1-month period (or less if successfully treated):
   (1) delusions
   (2) hallucinations
 –(3) disorganized speech (e.g., frequent derailment or incoherence)
 –(4) grossly disorganized or catatonic behavior
 ?(5) negative symptoms (e.g., affective flattening, alogia, or avolition)

     NOTE: Only one Criterion A symptom is required if delusions are bizarre or hallucinations consist of a voice keeping up a

68

running commentary on the person's behavior or thoughts, or
two or more voices conversing with each other.

B. *Social/occupational dysfunction.* For a significant portion of the time since the
onset of the disturbance, one or more major areas of functioning such as
work, interpersonal relations, or self-care is markedly below the level achieved
prior to onset (or when onset is in childhood or adolescence, failure to
achieve the expected level of interpersonal, academic, or occupational
achievement).

C. *Duration.* Continuous signs of the disturbance persist for at least 6 months.
This 6-month period must include at least 1 month of symptoms (or less if
successfully treated) that meet Criterion A (i.e., active-phase symptoms), and
may include periods of prodromal or residual symptoms. During these prodromal or residual periods, the signs of the disturbance may be manifested by
negative symptoms only or by two or more symptoms from Criterion A present in an attenuated form (e.g., odd beliefs, unusual perceptual experiences).

D. *Schizoaffective and Mood Disorder exclusion.* Schizoaffective Disorder and
Mood Disorder With Psychotic Features have been ruled out because either
(1) no Major Depressive, Manic, or Mixed Episodes have occurred concurrently with the active-phase symptoms, or (2) if mood episodes have occurred
during active-phase symptoms, their total duration has been brief relative to
the duration of the active and residual periods.

E. *Substance/general medical condition exclusion.* The disturbance is not due to
the direct physiological effects of a substance (e.g., a drug of abuse, a medication) or a general medical condition.

F. *Relationship to a Pervasive Developmental Disorder.* If there is a history of Autistic Disorder or another Pervasive Developmental Disorder, the additional diagnosis of Schizophrenia is made only if prominent delusions or hallucinations
are also present for at least a month (less if successfully treated).

Specify:
Classification of longitudinal course. "Episode" refers to exacerbation of prominent psychosis.

Episodic With Interepisode Residual Symptoms (ICD-10 code
F20.x2)
        Specify if: **With Prominent Negative Symptoms**

Episodic With No Interepisode Residual Symptoms (ICD-10
F20.x3)

Continuous (psychotic symptoms are prominent throughout the
period of observation) (ICD-10 F20.x0)
        Specify if: **With Prominent Negative Symptoms**

Single Episode In Partial Remission (ICD-10 F20.x4)
        Specify if: **With Prominent Negative Symptoms**

69

Single Episode In Full Remission (ICD-10 F20.x5)

Other or Unspecified Pattern (ICD-10 F20.x8)

NOTE: Do not classify the course until at least 1 year after initial onset of active-phase symptoms.

CODING NOTE: Course specifiers are no longer given fifth-digit codes in DSM-IV, but ICD-10 does so.

CODING NOTE: Diagnose and code subtypes—Paranoid, Disorganized, Catatonic, Undifferentiated, Residual (see below)— prior to classifying the course (e.g., 295.10 Schizophrenia, Chronic, Disorganized Type, Episodic With Interepisode Residual Symptoms [ICD-10 F20.12]).

....

SUBTYPES OF SCHIZOPHRENIA

The subtypes of Schizophrenia described are defined by the dominant psychotic symptomatology *at the time of the most recent evaluation*. Thus, they may change over time, and the patient may have symptoms of more than one subtype.

NOTE: Other ways of depicting differences among schizophrenic presentations are described in the professional literature. One, which outlines psychotic, disorganized, and negative "dimensions," is described in Appendix B of DSM-IV.

DSM-IV describes an algorhythm for priority of subtype coding: *Catatonic* is assigned whenever catatonic symptoms are prominent. *Disorganized* is diagnosed when its symptoms are prominent and catatonia is not. The next in priority, *Paranoid*, is preempted by conspicuous symptoms of either catatonia or disorganization. *Undifferentiated* implies that positive symptoms are obvious (i.e., there is an active phase), but criteria are not met for any of the preceding subtypes. *Residual* is assigned when there is continuing evidence of Schizophrenia but no prominent positive symptoms to indicate an active phase.

DIAGNOSTIC CRITERIA FOR
SUBTYPES OF SCHIZOPHRENIA

NOTE: All subtypes assume the criteria for Schizophrenia have been met.

295.30 Paranoid Type   (ICD-10 code F20.0x)

A. Preoccupation with one or more delusions or frequent auditory hallucinations.

B. None of the following is prominent: disorganized speech, disorganized or catatonic behavior, or flat or inappropriate affect.

295.10 Disorganized Type   (ICD-10 code F20.1x)

A. All of the following are prominent:
  (1) disorganized speech
  (2) disorganized behavior
  (3) flat or inappropriate affect

B. The criteria are not met for Catatonic Type.

295.20 Catatonic Type   (ICD-10 code F20.2x)

The clinical picture is dominated by at least two of the following:
  (1) motoric immobility as evidenced by catalepsy (including waxy flexibility) or stupor
  (2) excessive motor activity (that is apparently purposeless and not influenced by external stimuli)
  (3) extreme negativism (an apparently motiveless resistance to all instructions or maintenance of a rigid posture against attempts to be moved) or mutism
  (4) peculiarities of voluntary movement as evidenced by posturing (voluntary assumption of inappropriate or bizarre postures), stereotyped movements, prominent mannerisms, or prominent grimacing
  (5) echolalia or echopraxia

295.90 Undifferentiated Type   (ICD-10 code F20.3x)

Symptoms meet Schizophrenia Criterion A (i.e., active phase), but criteria are not met for Catatonic, Disorganized, or Paranoid types.

295.60 Residual Type   (ICD-10 code F20.5x)

A. Absence of prominent delusions, hallucinations, disorganized speech, and grossly disorganized or catatonic behavior (i.e., no longer meets Criterion A).

B. There is continuing evidence of the disturbance, as indicated by the presence of negative symptoms or two or more symptoms listed in schizophrenia Criterion A in an attenuated form (e.g., odd beliefs, unusual perceptual experiences).

❑ ❑ ❑ ❑

295.40 Schizophreniform Disorder   (ICD-10 code F20.8)
(significantly modified from DSM-III-R)

ESSENTIAL FEATURES. Except for duration and Schizophrenia's requirement for impaired functioning (which may occur), the essential features are identical to those of Schizophrenia. If the patient has not recovered at the time of diagnosis, the diagnosis should be qualified as "Provisional" in anticipation of a change to Schizophrenia if the syndrome persists beyond 6 months.

DIFFERENTIAL DIAGNOSIS. The differential diagnosis is similar to that for Schizophrenia.

DIAGNOSTIC CRITERIA FOR
SCHIZOPHRENIFORM DISORDER (295.40)

(ICD-10 code F20.8)

A. Criteria A, D, and E for Schizophrenia are met.

B. An episode of the disorder (including prodromal, active, and residual phases) lasts at least 1 month but less than 6 months. (When the diagnosis must be made without waiting for recovery, it should be qualified as "Provisional.")

Specify if:
Without Good Prognostic Features

With Good Prognostic Features: as evidenced by two (or more) of the following:

(1) onset of prominent psychotic symptoms within 4 weeks of the first noticeable change in usual behavior or functioning
(2) confusion or perplexity at the height of the psychotic episode
(3) good premorbid social and occupational functioning
(4) absence of blunted or flat affect

□ □ □ □

295.70 Schizoaffective Disorder
(significantly modified from DSM-III-R)

(ICD-10 code F25.x)

ESSENTIAL FEATURES. There are symptoms that reflect, at different times during the same period of illness, both schizophrenia-like psychosis and a major mood disturbance (Major Depressive, Manic, or Mixed Episode). If mood symptoms are only briefly present, Schizophrenia should be diagnosed; the definition of brief is a clinical judgment. The diagnosis is based on symptoms *during the most recent episode of illness*, and thus may change to Schizophrenia if future episodes do not meet concurrent mood criteria.

70

ASSOCIATED FEATURES. Associated features are similar to those of Schizophrenia. There may be increased danger of suicide.

DIFFERENTIAL DIAGNOSIS. Schizophrenia and Mood Disorders With Psychotic Features are often difficult to separate from Schizoaffective Disorder. The differential diagnosis is otherwise similar to that of Schizophrenia, preceding.

DIAGNOSTIC CRITERIA FOR   (ICD-10 code F25.x)
SCHIZOAFFECTIVE DISORDER (295.70)

A. An uninterrupted period of illness during which, at some time, there is either a Major Depressive Episode, a Manic Episode, or a Mixed Episode concurrent with symptoms that meet Criterion A for Schizophrenia.

> **NOTE: The Major Depressive Episode must include Criterion A1: depressed mood.**

B. During the same period of illness, there have been delusions or hallucinations for at least 2 weeks in the *absence* of prominent mood symptoms.

C. Symptoms meeting criteria for a mood episode are present for a substantial portion of the total duration of the active and residual periods of the illness.

D. The disturbance is not due to the direct physiological effects of a substance (e.g., a drug of abuse, a medication) or a general medical condition.

> **Specify type:**
> **Bipolar Type:** if the disturbance includes a Manic or a Mixed Manic/Depressive Episode (ICD-10 code F25.0)
>
> **Depressive Type:** if the disturbance only includes Major Depressive Episodes (ICD-10 code F25.1)

◻ ◻ ◻ ◻

297.1 Delusional Disorder   *(ICD-10 code F22.0)*

ESSENTIAL FEATURES. There is a persistent, nonbizarre delusion or system of delusions not due to any other mental disorder, general medical condition, or Substance-Related Disorder. Except when associated with delusions, the behavior is not particularly odd and hallucinations are not prominent. Criterion A for Schizophrenia has never been met. Five delusional themes or "types" may be specified.

In the *Erotomanic Type,* one has a delusion of being loved—usually secretly, romantically, and/or spiritually, and usually by a person of higher status or public prominence. The patient may attempt to monitor or contact the other person. In the *Grandiose Type,* the delusion is one of having great talent, insight, power, or spiritual leadership. In the *Jealous Type,* the person is convinced that his or her spouse or lover is unfaithful, in spite of a lack of any real evidence (although imaginary or trivial "evidence" is often cited by the patient). The *Persecutory Type* contains a delusional theme related to being conspired against, cheated, followed, maligned, or harassed. This is the most common type in many patient populations, and may lead to elaborate, even dangerous behavior by the patient in order to "protect" himself or herself from harm. The *Somatic Type* is manifested by delusions of physical problems, usually very unlikely ones such as foul odors, parasitic infestations, or malfunctioning body parts.

ASSOCIATED AND PREDISPOSING FACTORS. Symptoms of this disorder are disproportionately seen in persons who have emigrated to a new culture (e.g., Asian immigrants in the United States), and sometimes remit upon return to the familiar culture. Deafness or severe stress may predispose one as well, as may certain Personality Disorders (e.g., Paranoid, Schizoid, Avoidant).

DIFFERENTIAL DIAGNOSIS. Any disorder due to a general medical condition (e.g., Alzheimer's dementia) or a substance-related syndrome which can be shown to have initiated and maintained the disturbance preempts a diagnosis of Delusional Disorder. Schizophrenia or Schizophreniform Disorder are also preempting, and have a broader range of symptoms and impairments. Mood Disorders With Psychotic Features may be difficult to differentiate from Delusional Disorder; the clinician should search for an association between the mood disturbance and the appearance of delusions and other psychotic symptoms. Body Dysmorphic Disorder is usually differentiated by the lack of delusional intensity in the somatic preoccupation, although both diagnoses may be made in some patients. Paranoid Personality Disorder does not have persistent delusions.

DIAGNOSTIC CRITERIA FOR (ICD-10 code F22.0)
DELUSIONAL DISORDER (297.1)

A. Nonbizarre delusions (i.e., involving situations that might occur in real life, such as being followed, poisoned, infected, loved at a distance, deceived by one's spouse or lover, or having a disease) of at least 1 month's duration.

B. Criterion A for Schizophrenia has never been met.

> NOTE: Tactile and olfactory hallucinations may be present in Delusional Disorder if they are related to the delusional theme.

C. Apart from the impact of the delusion(s) or its ramifications, functioning is not markedly impaired and behavior is not obviously odd or bizarre.

D. If DSM-IV-described mood episodes have occurred concurrently with delusions, their total duration has been brief relative to the duration of the delusional periods.

E. The disturbance is not due to the direct physiological effects of a substance (e.g., a drug of abuse, a medication) or a general medical condition.

> **Specify type** (based on the predominant delusional theme):
> **Erotomanic Type:** delusions that another person, usually of higher status, is in love with the individual
>
> **Grandiose Type:** delusions of inflated worth, power, knowledge, identity, or special relationship to a deity or famous person
>
> **Jealous Type:** delusions that one's sexual partner is unfaithful

71

Persecutory Type: delusions that one (or someone to whom he/she is close) is being malevolently treated in some way

Somatic Type: delusions that one has some physical defect or general medical condition

Mixed Type: delusions characteristic of more than one of the above types, but no one theme predominates

Unspecified Type: no clearly predominant type of delusion, or the predominant type is not listed above

□ □ □ □

298.8 Brief Psychotic Disorder　　　　　　(ICD-10 code F23.xx)
(similar to Brief Reactive Psychosis in DSM-III-R)
(significantly modified from DSM-III-R)

ESSENTIAL FEATURES. There is a sudden onset of psychotic features lasting from 1 day to 1 month, with eventual full return to the premorbid functioning level. The disorder includes psychosis due to the psychological—but not the physiological—effects of a general medical condition.

PREDISPOSING FACTORS. Preexisting psychopathology, especially Personality Disorders, predispose the patient to Brief Psychotic Disorder, although one should not automatically infer the preexistence of a Personality Disorder.

DIFFERENTIAL DIAGNOSIS. Disorders due to a general medical condition and Substance-Related Disorders must be ruled out. Schizophreniform Disorder and Mood Disorders With Psychotic Features that persist longer than 1 month (but may remit sooner with successful treatment) should be considered, as should Delusional Disorder, Factitious Disorder With Psychological Symptoms, and Malingering (when primary gain is suggested). All of the above preempt Brief Psychotic Disorder. Transient psychoses associated with primitive Personality Disorders usually do not merit a separate diagnosis, but Brief Psychotic Disorder may be appropriate if the symptoms last more than a day.

DIAGNOSTIC CRITERIA FOR　　　　　　(ICD-10 code F23.xx)
BRIEF PSYCHOTIC DISORDER (298.8)

A. Presence of one (or more) of the following symptoms:
   (1) delusions
   (2) hallucinations
   (3) disorganized speech (e.g., frequent derailment or incoherence)
   (4) grossly disorganized or catatonic behavior

   NOTE: Do not include a symptom that is a culturally sanctioned response pattern.

B. The duration of an episode of the disturbance is at least 1 day but less than 1 month, with eventual full return to premorbid level of functioning.

C. The disturbance is not better accounted for by a Mood Disorder With Psychotic Features, Schizoaffective Disorder, or Schizophrenia, and is not due to the direct physiological effects of a substance (e.g., a drug of abuse, a medication) or a general medical condition.

> **Specify if:**
> **With Marked Stressor(s) (brief reactive psychosis):** if symptoms occur shortly after, and apparently in response to, events that, singly or together, would be markedly stressful to almost anyone in similar circumstances in the person's culture (ICD-10 code F23.81)
>
> **Without Marked Stressor(s):** if psychotic symptoms do *not* occur shortly after, or are not apparently in response to, events that, singly or together, would be markedly stressful to almost anyone in similar circumstances in the person's culture (ICD-10 code F23.80)
>
> **With Postpartum Onset:** if onset is within 4 weeks postpartum

❑ ❑ ❑ ❑

297.3 Shared Psychotic Disorder (Folie à Deux) (ICD-10 code F24)
(Induced Psychotic Disorder in DSM-III-R)

ESSENTIAL FEATURES. There is a delusional system that develops as a result of a close relationship with a (typically) dominant psychotic person ("inducer," "primary case"). The delusions are at least partly shared by both persons, are not usually bizarre, and often are specific to the two people. Larger families or groups are occasionally involved.

ASSOCIATED FEATURES. Interruption of the relationship with the "primary case" person usually decreases the delusional beliefs in the second person.

DIFFERENTIAL DIAGNOSIS. Delusional Disorder, Schizophrenia, and Schizoaffective Disorder, in which either the requisite close relationship with a dominant psychotic person is missing or the psychosis preceded any shared delusions, are considered in the differential diagnosis. If the delusions do not fade on separation from the primary case, consider another diagnosis.

DIAGNOSTIC CRITERIA FOR   (ICD-10 code F24)
SHARED PSYCHOTIC DISORDER (297.3)

A. A delusion develops in an individual in the context of a close relationship with another person(s), who has an already established delusion.

B. The delusion is similar in content to that of the person who already has the established delusion.

C. The disturbance is not better accounted for by another Psychotic Disorder (e.g., Schizophrenia) or a Mood Disorder With Psychotic Features, and is not due to the direct physiological effects of a substance (e.g., a drug of abuse, a medication) or a general medical condition.

❑ ❑ ❑ ❑

293.xx Psychotic Disorder Due to a General Medical Condition

(ICD-10 code F06.x)

(includes DSM-III-R's non-substance-related Organic Delusional Disorder and Organic Hallucinosis)
(new in DSM-IV)

.81 With Delusions (ICD-10 code F06.2)
.82 With Hallucinations (ICD-10 code F06.0)

NOTE: See special coding procedures following Diagnostic Criteria.

ESSENTIAL FEATURES. There are prominent delusions or hallucinations directly caused by the physiological effects of a general medical condition (but not exclusively expressed during Delirium, Alzheimer's, or Vascular Dementia). Hallucinations may be in any sensory form. Full criteria for a particular Psychotic Disorder need not be met.

ASSOCIATED FEATURES AND PHYSICAL AND LABORATORY FINDINGS. Associated features and findings are those of the underlying general medical condition.

DIFFERENTIAL DIAGNOSIS. The symptoms are not merely psychological reactions to the general medical condition but are caused by its physiological effects. Symptoms seen exclusively during Delirium are coded elsewhere. Hallucinations related to Sleep Disorders preempt this diagnosis. Other Psychotic Disorders and Substance-Induced Psychotic Disorder should be ruled out. If one is uncertain whether or not the symptoms are due to a general medical condition, Psychotic Disorder NOS should be considered.

DIAGNOSTIC CRITERIA FOR PSYCHOTIC DISORDER DUE TO . . . (SPECIFY GENERAL MEDICAL CONDITION) (293.81 OR 293.82)

(ICD-10 code F06.2 or F06.0)

A. Prominent hallucinations or delusions.

B. There is evidence from the history, physical examination, or laboratory findings that the disturbance is a direct physiological consequence of a general medical condition.

C. The disturbance is not better accounted for by another mental disorder.

D. The disturbance does not occur exclusively during the course of a delirium.

> **Code:**
> **293.81 With Delusions:** if delusions are the predominant symptom (ICD-10 F06.2)
>
> **293.82 With Hallucinations:** if hallucinations are the predominant symptom (ICD-10 F06.0)
>
> **CODING NOTE: Include the name of the general medical condition in the Axis I diagnosis (e.g., 293.81, Psychotic Disorder Due to Malignant Lung Neoplasm, With Delusions), and *also* code the general medical condition on Axis III. (See DSM-IV Appendix G for ICD-9-CM disease and E codes.)**
>
> **CODING NOTE: If delusions are part of a preexisting dementia, indicate them by coding the Dementia subtype, if available (e.g., 290.20 Dementia of the Alzheimer's Type, With Late Onset, With Delusions).**

❏ ❏ ❏ ❏

29x.xx Substance-Induced Psychotic Disorder (includes DSM-III-R substance-related Organic Delusional Disorder and Organic Hallucinosis) (new in DSM-IV)

(ICD-10 codes refer to substance codes)

> NOTE: See special coding procedures following Diagnostic Criteria.

ESSENTIAL FEATURES. There are prominent hallucinations or delusions directly caused by the physiological effects of a substance, including the effects of prescription use, poisoning, intoxication, or withdrawal. If hallucinations are the prominent feature, the patient does not appreciate the fact that they are substance induced. Hallucinations may be in any sensory form. Full criteria for a particular Psychotic Disorder need not be met.

ASSOCIATED FEATURES AND PHYSICAL AND LABORATORY FINDINGS. Associated features and findings are those of the underlying substance, intoxication, or withdrawal syndrome.

DIFFERENTIAL DIAGNOSIS. The symptoms clearly exceed those usually associated with intoxication or withdrawal. They are not merely psychological reactions but are caused by physiological effects of the substance. Other Psychotic Disorders and Psychotic Disorder Due to a General Medical Condition should be ruled out. If uncertain whether or not symptoms are substance induced, consider Psychotic Disorder NOS.

DIAGNOSTIC CRITERIA FOR
SUBSTANCE-INDUCED PSYCHOTIC DISORDER
(291.3, 291.5, 292.11, 292.12)

(ICD-10 codes refer to substance codes)

A. Prominent hallucinations or delusions.

> NOTE: Do not include hallucinations if the person has insight that they are substance induced.

B. There is evidence from the history, physical examination, or laboratory findings of either (1) or (2):
 (1) the symptoms in Criterion A developed during, or within a month of, Substance Intoxication or Withdrawal
 (2) medication use is etiologically related to the disturbance

> NOTE: Symptoms must be in excess of those usually associated with Substance Intoxication or Withdrawal *and* must be sufficiently severe to warrant clinical attention independent of the intoxication or withdrawal.

C. The disturbance is not better accounted for by a Psychotic Disorder that is not substance induced (e.g., the symptoms precede the onset of the substance abuse or dependence, persist for a substantial period of time [e.g., over a month] after the cessation of acute withdrawal or severe intoxication, or are substantially in excess of what would be expected given the character, duration, or amount of the substance used; *or* there is other evidence that suggests the existence of an independent non-substance-induced disorder [e.g., a history of recurrent non-substance-related episodes]).

D. The disturbance does not occur exclusively during the course of delirium.

Specify subtype:
With Delusions: delusions are the predominant symptom

With Hallucinations: hallucinations are the predominant symptom

Specify if:
With Onset During Intoxication: if the DSM-IV criteria are met for Intoxication and the symptoms develop during intoxication

With Onset During Withdrawal: if the DSM-IV criteria are met for Withdrawal from the substance and the symptoms develop during, or shortly after, a withdrawal syndrome

(See Table 13.1, p. 99, for applicability by substance.)

CODING NOTE: Code the (Specific Substance)-Induced Psychotic Disorder as follows: 291.5 Alcohol, With Delusions (ICD-10 F10.51)

291.3 Alcohol, With Hallucinations (ICD-10 F10.52)
292.11 Amphetamine (or Related Substance), With Delusions (ICD-10 F15.51)
292.12 Amphetamine (or Related Substance), With Hallucinations (ICD-10 F15.52)
292.11 Cannabis, With Delusions (ICD-10 F12.51)
292.12 Cannabis, With Hallucinations (ICD-10 F12.52)
292.11 Cocaine, With Delusions (ICD-10 F14.51)
292.12 Cocaine, With Hallucinations (ICD-10 F14.52)
292.11 Hallucinogen, With Delusions (ICD-10 F16.51)
292.12 Hallucinogen, With Hallucinations (ICD-10 F16.52)
292.11 Inhalant, With Delusions (ICD-10 F18.51)
292.12 Inhalant, With Hallucinations (ICD-10 F18.52)
292.11 Opioid, With Delusions (ICD-10 F11.51)
292.12 Opioid, With Hallucinations (ICD-10 F11.52)
292.11 Phencyclidine (or Similar Substance), With Delusions (ICD-10 F19.51)
292.12 Phencyclidine (or Similar Substance), With Hallucinations (ICD-10 F19.52)
292.11 Sedative/Hypnotic/Anxiolytic, With Delusions (ICD-10 F13.51)
292.12 Sedative/Hypnotic/Anxiolytic, With Hallucinations (ICD-10 F13.52)
292.11 Other (or Unknown) Substance, With Delusions (ICD-10 F19.51)
292.12 Other (or Unknown) Substance, With Hallucinations (ICD-10 F19.52)

Example: 292.11 Amphetamine-Induced Psychotic Disorder, With Delusions, With Onset During Intoxication (ICD-10 code F15-51)

CODING NOTE: Also code Substance-Specific Intoxication or Withdrawal if criteria are met.

□ □ □ □

298.9 Psychotic Disorder Not Otherwise Specified (NOS)　　　　(ICD-10 code F29)

ESSENTIAL FEATURES. Psychotic symptoms that do not meet criteria for any other Psychotic Disorder, or for which there is inadequate information about the symptoms and features to make a specific diagnosis, for example:

□ Postpartum Psychosis that does not meet the criteria for another Psychotic Disorder or Mood Disorder With Psychotic Features.

□ Persistent auditory hallucinations in the absence of any other features.

□ Situations in which the clinician has concluded that a Psychotic Disorder is present, but the clinician is unable to determine whether it is primary, due to a general medical condition, or substance induced.

□ □ □ □

DIFFERENCES BETWEEN DSM-III-R AND DSM-IV PSYCHOTIC DISORDERS

❑ DSM-III-R sections for Schizophrenia, Delusional Disorder, and Psychotic Disorders Not Elsewhere Classified were combined into DSM-IV's **Schizophrenia and Other Psychotic Disorders** section.

❑ Criterion list "A" for **Schizophrenia** is simplified and includes negative symptoms, alogia, and avolition. Duration criteria for the active phase is lengthened from 1 week to 1 month. Specific *Prodromal* and *Residual* symptoms were eliminated. Longitudinal course specifiers were changed to conform to ICD-10 and are not associated with fifth-digit number codes.

❑ For **Schizophrenia Subtypes,** DSM-IV deleted the "stable" form of Paranoid Schizophrenia. Catatonic Type now requires two of five criteria. Disorganized Type requires both disorganized speech and disorganized behavior.

❑ **Schizophreniform Disorder** has a minimum symptom duration of 1 month.

❑ In **Schizoaffective Disorder,** the criteria now focus on the uninterrupted episode of illness rather than the lifelong pattern.

❑ **Delusional Disorder** added a new Mixed Type.

❑ **Brief Psychotic Disorder** (similar to DSM-III-R's Brief Reactive Psychosis) criteria are generally broadened. A marked stressor is not required. Minimum duration is now 1 day. Three new specifiers (presence or absence of stressors, postpartum onset) may be used.

❑ **Psychotic Disorder Due to a General Medical Condition** is new, and includes disorders diagnosed in DSM-III-R as non-substance-related Organic Delusional Disorder and Organic Hallucinosis.

❑ **Substance-Induced Psychotic Disorder** is new, and combines DSM-III-R's substance-related Organic Delusional Disorder and Organic Hallucinosis. The subtypes are also new.

CASE VIGNETTES: SCHIZOPHRENIA AND OTHER PSYCHOTIC DISORDERS

Case Vignette 1

D.E., a 46-year-old man, has a long history of psychiatric and social problems. He enlisted in the army at age 20, after dropping out of college. He scored very well on military intelligence tests but was unable to complete basic training because of apparent confusion under stress and difficulty concentrating on training tasks. After an early discharge, D.E. tried to return to school and was referred to the mental health center after he was found wandering around campus in a heavy trenchcoat on a hot day.

A few weeks later D.E. was committed to a state mental hospital after starting a fire in his dormitory room "to help me stay warm so I can study." He was found to have delusions that he was unable to control his body temperature and would freeze to death if he weren't careful. He responded to treatment with neuroleptic medication, but he discontinued taking it after discharge from the hospital. Over the next 25 years D.E. was hospitalized on many occasions, each time with delusions of body deterioration of some sort, or of persecution by vaguely described "dark angels." The delusions were often accompanied by the voices of the dark angels, or of reassuring white angels. He did not adapt well socially, never married, has not been able to work, and has never had serious problems with the law.

At this time, D.E. is living semiautonomously in a boarding home, where he spends his days watching television or walking about a nearby park. He expresses few emotions and has little motivation. He scrupulously avoids illicit drugs and alcohol, although he smokes 20–30 hand-rolled cigarettes a day. He takes antipsychotic medication daily. He has not been completely free of his symptoms since they first appeared, although they don't trouble him very much.

DIAGNOSIS AND DISCUSSION
Axis I—295.30 Schizophrenia, Chronic, Paranoid Type, Episodic With Interepisode Residual Symptoms, With Prominent Negative Symptoms (ICD-10 F20.02)
Axis II—V71.09 No Diagnosis or Condition on Axis II (ICD-10 Z03.2)

D.E. meets the criteria for Schizophrenia, with no indication that his symptoms have been caused by a substance, general medical condition, or Mood Disorder. He meets the duration criteria for chronicity, and continues to have residual symptoms. His schizophrenic symptoms are characterized by systematized delusions with accompanying hallucinations related to the delusional theme. The prominence of the hallucinations is one factor differentiating his diagnosis from Delusional Disorder. There is no mention of incoherence, catatonia, or gross disorganization in any of the exacerbations (active phases) of his illness. Negative symptoms are prominent.

Case Vignette 2

C.R., a 44-year-old woman, was arrested after harassing a local television newscaster with telephone calls and letters asserting that he had fathered, then absconded with, her child. She denied any wish to harm him but steadfastly pursued him with demands that he give her "visitation rights" to "their" child. She said she understood that he would be unable to marry her, or even to outwardly acknowledge his love for her, because of his delicate public position.

There was no indication that the newscaster had ever had a relationship with C.R., although evidence from his files and from her apartment indicated that her fantasied relationship with him had existed for several years. There was no indication of hallucinations, disturbance of affect, significant Mood Disorder, or organic illness, and the woman had never been treated for a psychiatric disorder.

DIAGNOSIS AND DISCUSSION

Axis I—297.1 Delusional Disorder, Erotomanic Type (ICD-10 F22.0)
Axis II—799.9 Diagnosis Deferred on Axis II (ICD-10 R46.8)

The disorder appears limited to delusions, which meet criteria for Erotomanic Type. There is no mention of organic or affective symptoms, and no indication that Criterion A for Schizophrenia has ever been met. The delusions eliminate a diagnosis of Paranoid Personality Disorder, and there is no mention of any other symptoms of premorbid Personality Disorder.

Case Vignette 3

V.V., a 20-year-old apprentice electrician, was hospitalized 6 weeks ago with acute confusion and psychosis, including looseness of associations and statements that God had spoken to him and given him great powers. He showed no severe blunting of affect. He was doing well, in his training and socially, until about 3 months ago, when he began to show deterioration in productivity and ability to concentrate. V.V. drinks socially and has used marijuana occasionally, but there is no evidence of continuous abuse or other drug use.

The patient has not recently been physically ill, is taking no prescribed medications, has a normal physical exam, and apparently has not been exposed to industrial or environmental toxins. At present, V.V. has responded to hospitalization and medication but is still delusional.

DIAGNOSIS AND DISCUSSION

Axis I—295.40 Schizophreniform Disorder, Provisional, With Good Prognostic Features (ICD-10 F20.8)
Axis II—799.9 Diagnosis Deferred on Axis II (ICD-10 R46.8)

V.V. meets Criteria A and C for Schizophrenia but does not meet the duration criterion for either Schizophrenia or Brief Psychotic Disorder. Although his grandiosity may suggest a Manic or Hypomanic Episode, there is no mention of other criteria for any Mood Disorder. Environmental (e.g., industrial) toxins and Substance Abuse have both been considered as sources of the psychosis, but they are not apparently a part of the clinical picture. The patient has not recovered fully, mandating a "Provisional" notation until recovery occurs, duration and other criteria for Schizophrenia are met, or other diagnostic information comes to light. His good premorbid functioning, confusion during psychosis, and absence of blunt or flattened affect are "good prognostic features."

CHAPTER 15

MOOD DISORDERS

Mood describes a prolonged, pervasive affective state, such as a depression or elation, that colors an individual's perception of the world. The Mood Disorders have in common a disturbance of mood and psychiatric symptoms, such as those of a hypomanic, manic, or depressive syndrome. Mood Disorders are divided into Depressive Disorders, Bipolar Disorders, Substance-Induced Mood Disorder, and Mood Disorder Due to a General Medical Condition.

Before the coded disorders and specifiers in this diagnostic category are discussed, the reader must understand the definitions of **Major Depressive Episode, Manic Episode, Mixed Episode,** and **Hypomanic Episode**. These syndromes, which are not separately coded, are described separately in DSM-IV because they are building blocks for the disorders.

MAJOR DEPRESSIVE EPISODE
(significantly modified from DSM-III-R)

ESSENTIAL FEATURES. The person must have, for at least a 2-week period, either a pervasive depressed mood (in children or adolescents the mood may be irritable) or loss of pleasure or interest in almost all activities (referred to as anhedonia). In addition, at least four other depressive symptoms are present. The Major Depressive Episode cannot be due to a general medical condition or a substance, or secondary to Bereavement.

ASSOCIATED FEATURES. Accompanying clinical features may include tearfulness, anxiety, obsessive ruminations, Panic Attacks, phobias, and excessive health concerns. In children, separation anxiety may be prominent. When delusions and hallucinations occur, they are usually mood congruent. For example, the individual may believe that his bowels are rotting in spite of receiving normal medical evaluations. The most serious associated features are suicide and suicide attempts.

DIFFERENTIAL DIAGNOSIS. When an individual has symptoms that meet the diagnostic criteria for a Major Depressive Episode (MDE), the clinician must look

75

76

77

145

for potential causes. A Mood Disorder is often caused directly by something other than a Depressive or Bipolar Disorder (and is then referred to as a secondary Mood Disorder). For example, MDE is sometimes caused by a medical illness or a substance, and the related disorder diagnosed as a Mood Disorder Due to a General Medical Condition, With Major Depressive-like Features or a Substance-Induced Mood Disorder, With Depressive Features.

Other entities and diagnoses to consider are Mixed Episode, in which depressive and manic symptoms are combined; Dementia, in which symptoms of brain disease produce apathy and severe lack of motivation that may be mistaken for depression; and Manic Episode With Irritable Mood, in which the absence of euphoria and the presence of irritability are misclassified as a Major Depressive Episode With Agitation.

Some depressive symptoms occur normally during Bereavement, others do not. DSM-IV's Major Depressive Episode Criterion E identifies the usual time course for Bereavement (2 months) and specifies symptoms that suggest a diagnosis of Major Depression (e.g., suicidal ideation, psychomotor retardation, and marked disability). The behavior associated with Attention-Deficit/Hyperactivity Disorder can also give the appearance of an individual who has an agitated-anxious depression. When depressive symptoms are a response to a stressor and are not as severe as a Major Depressive Episode, consider Adjustment Disorder With Depressed Mood.

DIAGNOSTIC CRITERIA FOR
MAJOR DEPRESSIVE EPISODE

A. Five (or more) of the following symptoms have been present during the same 2–week period and represent a change from previous functioning; at least one of the symptoms is either (1) depressed mood or (2) loss of interest or pleasure.

> **NOTE: Do not include symptoms that are clearly due to a general medical condition, or mood-incongruent delusions or hallucinations.**

   (1) depressed mood most of the day, nearly every day, as indicated by either subjective report (e.g., feels sad or empty) or observation made by others (e.g., appears tearful)

   NOTE: In children and adolescents, can be irritable mood.

   (2) markedly diminished interest or pleasure in all, or almost all, activities most of the day, nearly every day (as indicated by either subjective account or observation made by others)

   (3) significant weight loss when not dieting or weight gain (e.g., a change of more than 5% of body weight in a month), or decrease or increase in appetite nearly every day

   NOTE: In children, consider failure to make expected weight gains.

(4) insomnia or hypersomnia nearly every day

(5) psychomotor agitation or retardation nearly every day (observable by others; not merely subjective feelings of restlessness or being slowed down)

(6) fatigue or loss of energy nearly every day

(7) feelings of worthlessness or excessive or inappropriate guilt (which may be delusional) nearly every day (not merely self-reproach or guilt about being sick)

(8) diminished ability to think or concentrate, or indecisiveness, nearly every day (either by subjective account or as observed by others)

(9) recurrent thoughts of death (not just fear of dying), recurrent suicidal ideation without a specific plan, or a suicide attempt or a specific plan for committing suicide

B. The symptoms do not meet criteria for a Mixed Episode (see p. 149).

C. The symptoms cause clinically significant distress or impairment in social, occupational, or other important areas of functioning.

D. The symptoms are not due to the direct physiological effects of a substance (e.g., a drug of abuse, a medication) or a general medical condition (e.g., hypothyroidism).

E. The symptoms are not better accounted for by Bereavement (i.e., after the loss of a loved one, the symptoms persist for longer than 2 months or are characterized by marked functional impairment, morbid preoccupation with worthlessness, suicidal ideation, psychotic symptoms, or psychomotor retardation).

□ □ □ □

MANIC EPISODE
(significantly modified from DSM-III-R)

ESSENTIAL FEATURES. The individual experiences a distinct period of elated, expansive, or irritable mood lasting at least 1 week (or any duration if hospitalization is required). In addition, symptoms such as grandiosity, decreased need for sleep, talkativeness, flight of ideas, distractibility, increase in activity, and involvement in risky activity are present. This disturbance must result in marked dysfunction on the job or in school, in social activities, or in relationships with others. In addition, the condition is not due to a general medical condition or is not substance induced.

ASSOCIATED FEATURES. An individual with Manic Episodes frequently resists treatment. Clinical features include mood lability (e.g., rapid shifts from anger to depression) and depressive symptoms may last moments, minutes, or, more rarely, days. When delusions and hallucination occur, they are usually mood congruent. For example, the individual with an elated mood may believe he is endowed with special powers. Catatonic symptoms may also be seen.

DIFFERENTIAL DIAGNOSIS. Virtually every biologic treatment for depression (e.g., antidepressants, electroconvulsive therapy, light therapy) can precipitate a Manic Episode in certain individuals. When a substance causes a Manic Episode, the diagnosis is Substance-Induced Mood Disorder With Manic Features, rather than Bipolar I Disorder. Other diagnoses to rule out are Hypomanic Episode (i.e., patient is not psychotic, not severely ill enough to warrant hospitalization, or does not have marked functional impairment), or a Mood Disorder Due to a General Medical Condition, With Manic Features (e.g., hyperthyroidism). One should look for a combination of depressive and manic symptoms (a Mixed Episode). Individuals who have severe Attention-Deficit/Hyperactivity Disorder can appear hyperactive and inattentive. Age of onset can usually differentiate AD/HD from a Manic Episode. Psychotic Disorders, such as Schizophrenia, are sometimes confused with mania, especially when the person is acutely agitated and psychotic.

DIAGNOSTIC CRITERIA FOR
MANIC EPISODE

A. A distinct period of abnormally and persistently elevated, expansive, or irritable mood, lasting at least 1 week (or any duration if hospitalization is necessary).

B. During the period of mood disturbance, three (or more) of the following symptoms have persisted (four if the mood is only irritable) and have been present to a significant degree:
  (1) inflated self-esteem or grandiosity
  (2) decreased need for sleep (e.g., feels rested after only 3 hours of sleep)
  (3) more talkative than usual or pressured to keep talking
  (4) flight of ideas or subjective experience that thoughts are racing
  (5) distractibility (i.e., attention too easily drawn to unimportant or irrelevant external stimuli)
  (6) increase in goal-directed activity (either socially, at work or school, or sexually) or psychomotor agitation
  (7) excessive involvement in pleasurable activities that have a high potential for painful consequences (e.g., engaging in unrestrained buying sprees, sexual indiscretions, or foolish business investments)

C. The symptoms do not meet criteria for a Mixed Episode (see p. 149).

D. The mood disturbance is sufficiently severe to cause marked impairment in occupational functioning or in usual social activities or relationships with others, or to necessitate hospitalization to prevent harm to self or others; or there are psychotic features.

E. The symptoms are not due to the direct physiological effects of a substance (e.g., a drug of abuse, a medication, or other treatment) or a general medical condition (e.g., hyperthyroidism).

> NOTE: Manic-like episodes that are clearly caused by somatic antidepressant treatment (e.g., medication, electroconvulsive therapy, light therapy) should not count toward a diagnosis of Bipolar I Disorder.

❑ ❑ ❑ ❑

MIXED EPISODE
(significantly modified from DSM-III-R)

ESSENTIAL FEATURES. There is a rapidly alternating mood state (e.g., sad, euphoric, irritable) with symptoms severe enough to meet all the diagnostic criteria—except duration—of a Manic Episode and a Major Depressive Episode nearly every day during at least a 1-week period. The mood disorder is not caused by a substance or a general medical condition. Psychosis and suicidal ideation are frequently present.

DIFFERENTIAL DIAGNOSIS. Certain substances, for example high doses of steroids, can cause marked mood instability. When this occurs, the diagnosis is Substance-Induced Mood Disorder, specifically Steroid-Induced Mood Disorder, With Mixed Features. Medical illnesses, such as Cushing's Syndrome or severe thyroid dysfunction, can also cause mood instability. In these cases, the diagnosis of Mood Disorder Due to a General Medical Condition, With Mixed Features, is given. Other diagnoses to consider are Manic Episode (especially when an irritable mood is present), or Major Depressive Episode (especially if the individual is anxious and dysphoric). Attention-Deficit/Hyperactivity Disorder is considered in the differential diagnosis because hyperactivity, impulsivity, and poor judgment are associated with both disorders; the age of onset for AD/HD, before age 7, helps the clinician discriminate between them.

DIAGNOSTIC CRITERIA FOR
MIXED EPISODE

A. The criteria (except for duration) are met both for a Manic Episode (see p. 148) and for a Major Depressive Episode (see p. 146) (except for duration) nearly every day during at least a 1-week period.

B. The mood disturbance is sufficiently severe to cause marked impairment in occupational functioning or in usual social activities or relationships with others, or to necessitate hospitalization to prevent harm to self or others; or there are psychotic features.

C. The symptoms are not due to the direct physiological effects of a substance (e.g., a drug of abuse, a medication, or other treatment) or a general medical condition (e.g., hyperthyroidism).

> **NOTE: Mixed-like episodes that are clearly caused by somatic antidepressant treatment (e.g., medication, electroconvulsive therapy, light therapy) should not count toward a diagnosis of Bipolar I Disorder.**

◻ ◻ ◻ ◻

HYPOMANIC EPISODE
(criteria new in DSM-IV)

ESSENTIAL FEATURES. As in a Manic Episode, the predominant mood is either elevated, expansive, or irritable, and there are similar associated symptoms. The mood must last at least 4 days. However, the disturbance is not severe enough to cause marked impairment (in job, social activities, or relationships) or require hospitalization. Delusions or hallucinations are never present. The episode is not caused by a substance or a general medical condition (e.g., hyperthyroidism).

DIFFERENTIAL DIAGNOSIS. Remember, the distinction between a Manic and a Hypomanic Episode is based upon the degree of impairment and severity of symptoms. In a Manic Episode, the impairment is marked, hospitalization is usually required, and psychosis is typically present. Just as medical conditions and substances can cause mania, they can also cause hypomania. When this occurs, the diagnosis is Mood Disorder Due to a General Medical Condition, With Manic Features, or a Substance-Induced Mood Disorder, With Manic Features. Attention-Deficit/Hyperactivity Disorder, because symptoms include impulsivity and hyperactivity, is also considered in the differential diagnosis. Finally, the clinician must decide whether the individual's mood is "normal" ("euthymic"); the DSM-IV requirement that manic/hypomanic symptoms last throughout 4 days helps to discriminate normal from abnormally elevated mood.

DIAGNOSTIC CRITERIA FOR
HYPOMANIC EPISODE

A. A distinct period of persistently elevated, expansive, or irritable mood, lasting throughout at least 4 days, that is clearly different from the usual non-depressed mood.

B. During the period of mood disturbance, three (or more) of the following symptoms have persisted (four if the mood is only irritable) and have been present to a significant degree:
   (1) inflated self-esteem or grandiosity
   (2) decreased need for sleep (e.g., feels rested after only 3 hours of sleep)

(3) more talkative than usual or pressure to keep talking

(4) flight of ideas or subjective experience that thoughts are racing

(5) distractibility (i.e., attention too easily drawn to unimportant or irrelevant external stimuli)

(6) increase in goal-directed activity (either socially, at work or school, or sexually) or psychomotor agitation

(7) excessive involvement in pleasurable activities that have a high potential for painful consequences (e.g., the person engages in unrestrained buying sprees, sexual indiscretions, or foolish business investments)

C. The episode is associated with an unequivocal change in functioning that is uncharacteristic of the person when not symptomatic.

D. The disturbance in mood and the change in functioning are observable by others.

E. The episode is not severe enough to cause marked impairment in social or occupational functioning, or to necessitate hospitalization, and there are no psychotic features.

F. The symptoms are not due to the direct physiological effects of a substance (e.g., a drug of abuse, a medication) or a general medical condition (e.g., hyperthyroidism).

> NOTE: Hypomanic-like episodes that are clearly caused by somatic antidepressant treatment (e.g., medication, electroconvulsive therapy, light therapy) should not count toward a diagnosis of Bipolar II Disorder.

❑ ❑ ❑ ❑

SPECIFIERS
(new and significantly modified from DSM-III-R)

The Mood Disorders have a large number of potential specifiers. The specifiers vary from one diagnosis to another; some specifiers are associated with codes and some are not. This is sometimes confusing. This section lists the criteria and definitions for all specifiers used with Mood Disorders.

Severity/Psychotic/Remission Specifiers for Major Depressive Episode
(several new in DSM-IV)

DIAGNOSTIC CRITERIA FOR SEVERITY/PSYCHOTIC/REMISSION SPECIFIERS FOR CURRENT/MOST RECENT MAJOR DEPRESSIVE EPISODE

> CODING NOTE: Code in fifth digit. Can be applied to the most recent Major Depressive Episode in Major Depressive Disorder

and to a Major Depressive Episode in Bipolar I or II Disorder only if it is the most recent type of mood episode.

.xl Mild: Few, if any, symptoms in excess of those required to make the diagnosis and symptoms result in only minor impairment in occupational functioning or in usual social activities or relationships with others.

.x2 Moderate: Symptoms or functional impairment between "mild" and "severe."

.x3 Severe Without Psychotic Features: Several symptoms in excess of those required to make the diagnosis, **and** symptoms markedly interfere with occupational functioning or with usual social activities or relationships with others.

.x4 Severe With Psychotic Features: Delusions or hallucinations. If possible, specify whether the psychotic features are mood-congruent or mood-incongruent:

> **Mood-Congruent Psychotic Features:** Delusions or hallucinations whose content is entirely consistent with the typical depressive themes of personal inadequacy, guilt, disease, death, nihilism, or deserved punishment.

> **Mood-Incongruent Psychotic Features:** Delusions or hallucinations whose content does not involve typical depressive themes of personal inadequacy, guilt, disease, death, nihilism, or deserved punishment. Included are such symptoms as persecutory delusions (not directly related to depressive themes), thought insertion, thought broadcasting, and delusions of control.

.x5 In Partial Remission: Symptoms of a Major Depressive Episode are present but full criteria are not met, or there is a period without any significant symptoms of a Major Depressive Episode lasting less than 2 months following the end of the Major Depressive Episode. (If the Major Depressive Episode was superimposed on Dysthymic Disorder, the diagnosis of Dysthymic Disorder alone is given once the full criteria for a Major Depressive Episode are no longer met.)

.x6 In Full Remission: During the past 2 months, no significant signs or symptoms of the disturbance were present.

.x0 Unspecified.

□ □ □ □

Severity/Psychotic/Remission Specifiers for Manic Episode

DIAGNOSTIC CRITERIA FOR
SEVERITY/PSYCHOTIC/REMISSION SPECIFIERS
FOR CURRENT/MOST RECENT MANIC EPISODE

CODING NOTE: Code in fifth digit. These can be applied to a Manic Episode in Bipolar I Disorder only if it is the most recent type of mood episode.

.xl Mild: Minimum symptom criteria are met for a Manic Episode.
.x2 Moderate: Extreme increase in activity or impairment in judgment, but not to the extent of being "severe."

.x3 Severe Without Psychotic Features: Almost continual supervision is required to prevent physical harm to self or others.

.x4 Severe With Psychotic Features: Delusions or hallucinations. If possible, specify whether the psychotic features are mood-congruent or mood-incongruent:

> **Mood-Congruent Psychotic Features:** Exhibits delusions or hallucinations whose content is entirely consistent with the typical manic themes of inflated worth, power, knowledge, identity, or special relationship to a deity or famous person.
>
> **Mood-Incongruent Psychotic Features:** Delusions or hallucinations whose content does not involve typical manic themes of inflated worth, power, knowledge, identity, or special relationship to a deity or famous person. Included are such symptoms as persecutory delusions (not directly related to grandiose ideas or themes), thought insertion, and delusions of being controlled.

.x5 In Partial Remission: Symptoms of a Manic Episode are present but full criteria are not met, or there is a period without any significant symptoms of a Manic Episode lasting less than 2 months following the end of the Manic Episode.

.x6 In Full Remission: During the past 2 months no significant signs or symptoms of the disturbance were present.

.x0 Unspecified.

□ □ □ □

Severity/Psychotic/Remission Specifiers for Mixed Episode

DIAGNOSTIC CRITERIA FOR
SEVERITY/PSYCHOTIC/REMISSION SPECIFIERS
FOR CURRENT/MOST RECENT MIXED EPISODE

> **CODING NOTE: Code in fifth digit.** These can be applied to a Mixed Episode in Bipolar I Disorder only if it is the most recent type of mood episode.

.x1 Mild: No more than minimum symptom criteria are met for both a Manic Episode and a Major Depressive Episode.

.x2 Moderate: Symptoms or functional impairment are between "mild" and "severe."

.x3 Severe Without Psychotic Features: Almost continual supervision is required to prevent physical harm to self or others.

.x4 Severe With Psychotic Features: Exhibits delusions or hallucinations. If possible, specify whether the psychotic features are mood-congruent or mood-incongruent:

> **Mood-Congruent Psychotic Features:** Delusions or hallucinations whose content is entirely consistent with the typical manic or depressive themes.
>
> **Mood-Incongruent Psychotic Features:** Delusions or hallucinations whose content does not involve typical manic or depressive themes. Included are such symptoms as persecutory delusions (not directly related to grandiose or de-

pressive themes), thought insertion, and delusions of being controlled.

.x5 In Partial Remission: Symptoms of a Mixed Episode are present but full criteria are not met, or there is a period without any significant symptoms of a Mixed Episode lasting less than 2 months following the end of the Mixed Episode.

x6 In Full Remission: During the past 2 months, no significant signs of symptoms of the disturbance were present.

.x0 Unspecified.

▢ ▢ ▢ ▢

"Chronic" Specifier

"Chronic" can be applied to the current or most recent Major Depressive Episode in Major Depressive Disorder and to a Major Depressive Episode in Bipolar I or II Disorder (if it is the most recent type of mood episode).

DIAGNOSTIC CRITERION FOR
CHRONIC SPECIFIER

Full criteria for a Major Depressive Episode have been met continuously for at least the past 2 years.

▢ ▢ ▢ ▢

"Catatonic Features" Specifier
(new in DSM-IV)

"With Catatonic Features" can be applied to the current or most recent Major Depressive Episode, Manic Episode, or Mixed Episode in Major Depressive Disorder, Bipolar I Disorder, or Bipolar II Disorder.

DIAGNOSTIC CRITERIA FOR
WITH CATATONIC FEATURES SPECIFIER

The clinical picture is dominated by at least two of the following:

(1) motoric immobility as evidenced by catalepsy (including waxy flexibility) or stupor

(2) excessive motor activity that is apparently purposeless and not influenced by external stimuli

(3) extreme negativism (an apparently motiveless resistance to all instructions or maintenance of a rigid posture against attempts to be moved) or mutism

(4) peculiarities of voluntary movement as evidenced by posturing (volun-

tary assumption of inappropriate or bizarre postures), stereotyped
movements, prominent mannerisms, or prominent grimacing
(5) echolalia or echopraxia

□ □ □ □

"Melancholic Features" Specifier

"With Melancholic Features" can be applied to the current or most recent Major
Depressive Episode in Major Depressive Disorder and to a Major Depressive
Episode in Bipolar I or Bipolar II Disorder (if it is the most recent type of mood
episode).

DIAGNOSTIC CRITERIA FOR
WITH MELANCHOLIC FEATURES SPECIFIER

A. Either of the following, occurring during the most severe period of the current
episode:
(1) loss of pleasure in all, or almost all, activities
(2) lack of reactivity to usually pleasurable stimuli (does not feel much better, even temporarily, when something good happens)

B. Three (or more) of the following:
(1) distinct quality of depressed mood (i.e., the depressed mood is experienced as distinctly different from the kind of feeling experienced after
the death of a loved one)
(2) depression regularly worse in the morning
(3) early morning awakening (at least 2 hours before usual time of
awakening)
(4) marked psychomotor retardation or agitation
(5) significant anorexia or weight loss
(6) excessive or inappropriate guilt

□ □ □ □

"Atypical Features" Specifier
(new in DSM-IV)

"With Atypical Features" can be applied when the following features predominate during the most recent 2 weeks of a Major Depressive Episode in Major
Depressive Disorder or in Bipolar I or Bipolar II Disorder when the Major Depressive Episode is the most recent type of mood episode, or when these features
predominate during the most recent 2 years of Dysthymic Disorder.

DIAGNOSTIC CRITERIA FOR
WITH ATYPICAL FEATURES SPECIFIER

A. Mood reactivity (i.e., mood brightens in response to actual or potential positive events).

B. Two (or more) of the following features:
  (1) significant weight gain or increase in appetite
  (2) hypersomnia
  (3) leaden paralysis (i.e., heavy, leaden feelings in arms or legs)
  (4) long-standing pattern of interpersonal rejection sensitivity (not limited to episodes of mood disturbance) that results in significant social or occupational impairment

C. Criteria are not met for With Melancholic Features or With Catatonic Features during the episode being considered.

82

❑ ❑ ❑ ❑

"Postpartum Onset" Specifier
(new in DSM-IV)

"With Postpartum Onset" can be applied to the current or most recent Major Depressive, Manic, or Mixed Episode in Major Depressive Disorder, Bipolar I Disorder, or Bipolar II Disorder; or to Brief Psychotic Disorder

DIAGNOSTIC CRITERION FOR
POSTPARTUM ONSET SPECIFIER

Onset of the episode is within 4 weeks postpartum

❑ ❑ ❑ ❑

Longitudinal Course Specifiers
(With and Without Full Interepisode Recovery)

83

These specifiers can be applied to Recurrent Major Depressive Disorder or Bipolar I or II Disorder.

DIAGNOSTIC CRITERIA FOR
LONGITUDINAL COURSE SPECIFIERS
(new in DSM-IV)

With Full Interepisode Recovery: if full remission is attained between the two most recent Mood Episodes

Without Full Interepisode Recovery: if full remission is not attained between the two most recent Mood Episodes

❏ ❏ ❏ ❏

"Seasonal Pattern" Specifier

"With Seasonal Pattern" can be applied to the pattern of Major Depressive Episodes in Bipolar I Disorder, Bipolar II Disorder, or Major Depressive Disorder, Recurrent.

DIAGNOSTIC CRITERIA FOR
SEASONAL PATTERN SPECIFIER

A. There has been a regular temporal relationship between the onset of Major Depressive Episodes in Bipolar I or Bipolar II Disorder or Major Depressive Disorder, Recurrent, and a particular time of the year (e.g., regular appearance of the Major Depressive Episode in the fall or winter).

> **NOTE: Do not include cases in which there is an obvious effect of seasonal-related psychosocial stressors (e.g., regularly being unemployed every winter).**

B. Full remissions (or a change from depression to mania or hypomania) also occur at a characteristic time of the year (e.g., depression disappears in the spring).

C. In the last 2 years, two Major Depressive Episodes have occurred that demonstrate the temporal seasonal relationships defined in Criteria A and B, and no nonseasonal Major Depressive Episodes have occurred during that same period.

D. Seasonal Major Depressive Episodes (as described above) substantially outnumber the nonseasonal Major Depressive Episodes that may have occurred over the individual's lifetime.

❏ ❏ ❏ ❏

"Rapid-Cycling" Specifier
(new in DSM-IV)
"With Rapid Cycling" can be applied to Bipolar I Disorder or Bipolar II Disorder.

DIAGNOSTIC CRITERIA FOR
RAPID-CYCLING SPECIFIER

At least four episodes of a mood disturbance in the previous 12 months that meet criteria for a Major Depressive, Manic, Mixed, or Hypomanic Episode.

84

NOTE: Episodes are demarcated either by partial or full remission for at least 2 months *or* a switch to an episode of opposite polarity (e.g., Major Depressive Episode to Manic Episode).

▫ ▫ ▫ ▫

DEPRESSIVE DISORDERS

Major Depressive Disorder, Single Episode
Major Depressive Disorder, Recurrent
Dysthymic Disorder
Depressive Disorder Not Otherwise Specified (NOS)

296.xx Major Depressive Disorder
(Single or Recurrent; see specific criteria following)

(ICD-10 codes
F32.x, F33.x)

ESSENTIAL FEATURES. The individual has had one or more Major Depressive Episodes without a Manic, Mixed or Hypomanic Episode. The Major Depressive Episode is not caused by a substance or a general medical condition, and cannot be better accounted for by one of the Psychotic Disorders.

ASSOCIATED FEATURES. If untreated, a significant number of individuals will follow a chronic course with considerable residual symptoms and impairment. Some persons who are diagnosed with Dysthymic Disorder will experience a superimposed Major Depressive Episode (so-called double-depression).

Major Depression is twice as common in adult women as men. Presence of Major Depression in first-degree relatives increases the risk of developing the disorder up to threefold. Five to 10% of individuals with Major Depressive Episodes will eventually develop Bipolar I Disorder. Severe psychosocial stressors often precipitate an episode. In addition, up to 25% of individuals with significant general medical conditions will develop a Major Depressive Episode.

DIFFERENTIAL DIAGNOSIS. When an individual has symptoms that meet the diagnostic criteria for a Major Depressive Episode (MDE), the clinician must look for potential causes. A Mood Disorder is often caused directly by something other than Major Depressive Disorder, such as medical illness or substance use. This is referred to as a Secondary Mood Disorder. For example, MDE is sometimes caused by a medical illness or a substance. These are diagnosed as a Mood Disorder Due to a General Medical Condition, With Major Depressive-like Features or a Substance-Induced Mood Disorder, With Depressive Features.

When diagnosing Major Depressive Episode, one should rule out Mixed Episode, in which depressive and manic symptoms are combined; Dementia can produce apathy and severe lack of motivation that is sometimes mistaken for depression; and Manic Episode With an Irritable Mood, in which the absence of euphoria and the presence of irritability are mistakenly classified as a Major Depressive Episode With Agitation. Individuals with Cyclothymic Disorder also have mood swings, although the depressive and manic symptoms are not sufficiently severe to meet the criteria for a Major Depressive or Manic Episode.

Some depressive symptoms occur normally during Bereavement, while others do not. DSM-IV's Major Depressive Episode Criterion E identifies a usual time course for improvement in Bereavement (2 months) and symptoms that suggest Major Depression (e.g., marked impairment, suicidal ideation, psychomotor retardation). The behavior associated with Attention-Deficit/Hyperactivity Disorder can also give the appearance of an individual with an agitated-anxious depression. Major Depressive Episodes occur commonly with other mental disorders as well, especially Substance-Related Disorders, Anxiety Disorders, Eating Disorders, and Borderline Personality Disorder.

When depressive symptoms are in response to a stressor and are not severe enough to meet the criteria for a Major Depressive Episode, consider a diagnosis of Adjustment Disorder With Depressed Mood. When a Major Depression has psychotic features, it must be distinguished from Schizoaffective Disorder and Schizophrenia. A Schizoaffective Disorder diagnosis requires 2 weeks of delusions or hallucinations in the absence of a prominent mood disturbance. A depressed mood often occurs in individuals with Schizophrenia or other Psychotic Disorders. When the criteria for a Major Depressive Episode are met in addition to the criteria for a Psychotic Disorder, a diagnosis of Depressive Disorder Not Otherwise Specified is made, in addition to the diagnosis of the specific Psychotic Disorder (e.g., Delusional Disorder).

DIAGNOSTIC CRITERIA FOR MAJOR DEPRESSIVE DISORDER, SINGLE EPISODE (296.2X)

(ICD-10 code F32.x)

A. Presence of a single Major Depressive Episode (p. 146).

B. The Major Depressive Episode is not better accounted for by Schizoaffective Disorder and is not superimposed on Schizophrenia, Schizophreniform Disorder, Delusional Disorder, or Psychotic Disorder Not Otherwise Specified.

C. There has never been a Manic Episode (p. 148), a Mixed Episode (p. 149), or a Hypomanic Episode (p. 150).

> NOTE: This exclusion does not apply if all of the manic-like, mixed-like, or hypomanic-like episodes are substance or treatment induced or are due to the direct physiological effects of a general medical condition.

> **Specify (for current or most recent episode):**
> Severity/Psychotic/Remission Specifiers (p. 151)

> Chronicity (p. 154)

> With Catatonic Features (p. 154)

With Melancholic Features (p. 155)

With Atypical Features (p. 156)

With Postpartum Onset (p. 156)

❑ ❑ ❑ ❑

DIAGNOSTIC CRITERIA FOR MAJOR DEPRESSIVE DISORDER, RECURRENT (296.3X)

(ICD-10 code F33.x)

A. Presence of two or more Major Depressive Episodes (p. 146).

> NOTE: To be considered separate episodes, there must be an interval of at least 2 consecutive months in which criteria are not met for a Major Depressive Episode.

B. The Major Depressive Episodes are not better accounted for by Schizoaffective Disorder and are not superimposed on Schizophrenia, Schizophreniform Disorder, Delusional Disorder, or Psychotic Disorder Not Otherwise Specified.

C. There has never been a Manic Episode (p. 148), a Mixed Episode (p. 149), or a Hypomanic Episode (p. 150).

> NOTE: This exclusion does not apply if all of the manic-like, mixed-like, or hypomanic-like episodes are substance or treatment induced or are due to the direct physiological effects of a general medical condition.

Specify (for current or most recent episode):
Severity/Psychotic/Remission Specifiers (p. 151)

Chronicity (p. 154)

With Catatonic Features (p. 154)

With Melancholic Features (p. 155)

With Atypical Features (p. 155)

With Postpartum Onset (p. 156)

Specify:
Longitudinal Course Specifiers (With and Without Interepisode Recovery) (p. 156)

With Seasonal Pattern (p. 157)

❑ ❑ ❑ ❑

300.4 Dysthymic Disorder   (ICD-10 code F34.1)
(significantly modified from DSM-III-R)

ESSENTIAL FEATURES. Dysthymia is a chronic mood disturbance involving frequent periods of depressive mood and a few depressive symptoms. Specifically, during a 2-year period (1) depressive mood is present "for most of the day, for more days than not"; (2) depressive symptoms are never absent for more than 2 months; and (3) no Major Depressive Episode occurs during the first two years of the disorder. The diagnosis is not made if the disturbance is superimposed on a Psychotic Disorder, or if the disturbance is caused by a substance or a general medical disorder. There is no history of a Manic, Mixed, or Hypomanic Episode, or of Cyclothymic Disorder.

ASSOCIATED FEATURES. There are no delusions or hallucinations. Individuals with Dysthymic Disorder often also have an Axis II Personality Disorder. Major Depressive Episodes may be superimposed on this disorder (double-depression, see Criterion D, following). In fact, 10% of individuals with Dysthymic Disorder will develop a Major Depressive Episode in any one year. Depressed children and adolescents often show deterioration in school performance and behavior, and are often irritable.

   A dysthymic-like disorder can result from chronic Axis I disorders (especially Substance-Related Disorders) and/or Axis III medical disorders. In children and adolescents, Attention-Deficit/Hyperactivity Disorder, Conduct Disorder, Mental Retardation, or a chaotic environment may predispose one to Dysthymic Disorder.

DIFFERENTIAL DIAGNOSIS. Because the criteria for Dysthymic Disorder require depressive symptoms for "at least 2 years," or 1 year in adolescents, it is usually easy to differentiate Dysthmic Disorder from normal fluctuations in mood or Adjustment Disorder With Depressed Mood. Major Depressive Disorder usually consists of several distinct episodes, whereas the depressive symptoms associated with Dysthymic Disorder last for many years and are less severe.

   Substance-Induced Mood Disorder, With Depressive Features, is diagnosed when the symptoms are a direct result of a substance. Chronic Psychotic Disorders, such as Schizophrenia, Delusional Disorder, and Schizoaffective Disorder, are commonly associated with depressive symptoms, so a separate diagnosis of Dysthmic Disorder is not warranted. Mood Disorder Due to a General Medical Condition, With Depressive Features, is diagnosed when the depressive symptoms are a direct consequence of a medical disorder (e.g., Parkinson's Disease). The diagnosis of Cyclothymic Disorder is considered in the differential diagnosis of Dysthymic Disorder. Episodes of hypomanic symptoms during the 2-year period differentiates the two.

DIAGNOSTIC CRITERIA FOR   (ICD-10 code F34.1)
DYSTHYMIC DISORDER (300.4)

A. Depressed mood for most of the day, for more days than not, as indicated either by subjective account or observation by others, for at least 2 years.

NOTE: In children and adolescents, mood can be irritable and duration must be at least 1 year.

B. Presence, while depressed, of two (or more) of the following:
(1) poor appetite or overeating
(2) insomnia or hypersomnia
(3) low energy or fatigue
(4) low self-esteem
(5) poor concentration or difficulty making decisions
(6) feelings of hopelessness

C. During the 2-year period (1 year for children or adolescents) of the disturbance, the person has never been without the symptoms in Criteria A and B for more than 2 months at a time.

D. No Major Depressive Episode (p. 146) has been present during the first 2 years of the disturbance (1 year for children and adolescents); i.e., the disturbance is not better accounted for by chronic Major Depressive Disorder, or Major Depressive Disorder, In Partial Remission.

NOTE: There may have been a previous Major Depressive Episode provided there was a full remission (no significant signs or symptoms for 2 months) before development of the Dysthymic Disorder. In addition, after the initial 2 years (1 year in children or adolescents) of Dysthymic Disorder, there may be superimposed episodes of Major Depressive Disorder, in which case both diagnoses may be given when the criteria are met for a Major Depressive Episode.

E. There has never been a Manic Episode (p. 148), a Mixed Episode (p. 149), or a Hypomanic Episode (p. 150), and criteria have never been met for Cyclothymic Disorder.

F. The disturbance does not occur exclusively during the course of a chronic Psychotic Disorder, such as Schizophrenia or Delusional Disorder.

G. The symptoms are not due to the direct physiological effects of a substance (e.g., a drug of abuse, a medication) or a general medical condition (e.g., hypothyroidism).

H. The symptoms cause clinically significant distress or impairment in social, occupational, or other important areas of functioning.

Specify if:
Early Onset: if onset is before age 21 years

Late Onset: if onset is age 21 years or older

Specify if, for most recent 2 years of Dysthymic Disorder:
With Atypical Features (p. 155)

❑ ❑ ❑ ❑

311 Depressive Disorder Not Otherwise Specified

(ICD-10 code F32.9)

ESSENTIAL FEATURES. A disorder with depressive features that does not meet the criteria for one of the Mood Disorders, Adjustment Disorder With Depressed Mood, or Adjustment Disorder With Anxiety and Depressed Mood.

❏ ❏ ❏ ❏

BIPOLAR DISORDERS

Bipolar I Disorders
Bipolar II Disorder
Cyclothymic Disorder
Bipolar Disorder Not Otherwise Specified (NOS)

Bipolar I Disorders

296.0x Bipolar I Disorder, Single Manic Episode (new in DSM-IV)	*(ICD-10 code F30.x)*
296.40 Bipolar I Disorder, Most Recent Episode Hypomanic (new in DSM-IV)	*(ICD-10 code F31.0)*
296.4x Bipolar I Disorder, Most Recent Episode Manic	*(ICD-10 code F31.x)*
296.6x Bipolar I Disorder, Most Recent Episode Mixed	*(ICD-10 code F31.6)*
296.5x Bipolar I Disorder, Most Recent Episode Depressed	*(ICD-10 code F31.x)*
296.7 Bipolar I Disorder, Most Recent Episode Unspecified (new in DSM-IV)	*(ICD-10 code F31.9)*

In Bipolar Disorders, one or more Manic (Bipolar I Disorder) or Hypomanic Episodes (Bipolar II Disorder) are associated with one or more Major Depressive Episodes. Bipolar Disorders are diagnosed according to the clinical features of the current or most recent episode.

> NOTE: Numerous specifiers for Bipolar Disorders were added in DSM-IV. They vary by diagnosis and are described in this chapter.

ESSENTIAL FEATURES. Bipolar I Disorder is characterized by one or more Manic *or* Mixed Episodes. Most individuals also have Major Depressive Episodes over the course of illness. Manic or Mixed Episodes caused by either substances or a general medical condition do *not* qualify for this diagnosis. The clinician must also ensure that the episode is not better accounted for by a Psychotic Disorder. Diagnostic classification in this category is somewhat complicated. The clinician must first decide if the Manic Episode is single or recurrent. Recurrence is uniquely defined as a shift in polarity (i.e., Manic Episode to Major Depressive Episode or vice versa), or a manic-symptom-free interval of at least 2 months before manic symptoms return. Single episode is defined as one Manic Episode, or any confluence of Hypomanic-Manic-Mixed Symptoms. If the disorder is considered recurrent, the disorder is diagnosed according to the nature of the current or most recent episode. Specifiers are selected to describe the current episode and the pattern of episodes.

DIFFERENTIAL DIAGNOSIS. In order to make a diagnosis of Bipolar I Disorder, the clinician must confirm that an individual has had at least one Manic Episode, or at least one Manic Episode plus a Mixed or Major Depressive Episode. If the individual has had a Hypomanic Episode and a Major Depressive Episode, the correct diagnosis is Bipolar II Disorder. If the depressive and manic symptoms are of at least 2 years duration and do not meet criteria for a Major Depressive or a Manic Episode, the diagnosis is Cyclothymic Disorder. When symptoms of mania, depression, mixed mood, or hypomania are caused directly by a medical disorder, such as thyroid disease or a stroke, the correct diagnosis is Mood Disorder Due to a General Medical Condition. If a substance causes mania, even if the substance is an antidepressant or ECT, the diagnosis is Substance-Induced Mood Disorder, With Manic Features.

The history helps to differentiate Major Depressive Disorder or Dysthymic Disorder from Bipolar I Disorder, because an individual with the latter diagnosis will have had one or more Manic and/or Mixed Episodes. Individuals with Bipolar I Disorder or one of the Psychotic Disorders (i.e., Schizophrenia, Schizoaffective Disorder, or Delusional Disorder) can exhibit similar symptoms; however, the individual with a Psychotic Disorder will have psychosis in the absence of mood symptoms, but the patient with Bipolar I will not. If an individual has mood cycles that occur too rapidly to meet the diagnostic criteria for a Major Depressive or Manic Episode, the diagnosis is Bipolar Disorder Not Otherwise Specified.

DIAGNOSTIC CRITERIA FOR   (ICD-10 code F30.x)
BIPOLAR I DISORDER, SINGLE MANIC EPISODE (296.0X)

A. Presence of only one Manic Episode (p. 148) and no past Major Depressive Episodes.

> NOTE: Recurrence is defined as either a change in polarity from depression or an interval of at least 2 months without manic symptoms.

B. The Manic Episode is not better accounted for by Schizoaffective Disorder and is not superimposed on Schizophrenia, Schizophreniform Disorder, Delusional Disorder, or Psychotic Disorder Not Otherwise Specified.

Specify if:
Mixed: if symptoms meet criteria for a Mixed Episode (p. 149)

Specify (for current or most recent episode):
Severity/Psychotic/Remission Specifiers (p. 152)

With Catatonic Features (p. 154)

With Postpartum Onset (p. 156)

❑ ❑ ❑ ❑

DIAGNOSTIC CRITERIA FOR
(ICD-10 code F31.0)
BIPOLAR I DISORDER, MOST RECENT EPISODE
HYPOMANIC (296.40)

A. Currently (or most recently) in a Hypomanic Episode (p. 150).

B. There has previously been at least one Manic Episode (p. 148) or Mixed Epi-- sode (p. 149).

C. The mood symptoms cause clinically significant distress or impairment in so- cial, occupational, or other important areas of functioning.

D. The mood episodes in Criteria A and B are not better accounted for by Schizoaffective Disorder and are not superimposed on Schizophrenia, Schizo- phreniform Disorder, Delusional Disorder, or Psychotic Disorder Not Other- wise Specified.

> **Specify:**
> **Longitudinal Course Specifiers (With and Without Interepisode Recovery)** (p. 156)
>
> **With Seasonal Pattern** (applies only to the pattern of Major De- pressive Episodes) (p. 157)
>
> **With Rapid Cycling** (p. 157)

❑ ❑ ❑ ❑

DIAGNOSTIC CRITERIA FOR
(ICD-10 code F31.x)
BIPOLAR I DISORDER, MOST RECENT EPISODE
MANIC (296.4X)

A. Currently (or most recently) in a Manic Episode (p. 148).

B. There has previously been at least one Major Depressive Episode (p. 146), Manic Episode (p. 148), or Mixed Episode (p. 149).

C. The mood episodes in Criteria A and B are not better accounted for by Schizoaffective Disorder and are not superimposed on Schizophrenia, Schizophreniform Disorder, Delusional Disorder, or Psychotic Disorder Not Otherwise Specified.

> **Specify (for current or most recent episode):**
> Severity/Psychotic/Remission Specifiers (p. 152)
>
> **With Catatonic Features** (p. 154)
>
> **With Postpartum Onset** (p. 156)
>
> **Specify:**
> Longitudinal Course Specifiers (With and Without Interepisode Recovery) (p. 156)
>
> **With Seasonal Pattern** (applies only to the pattern of Major Depressive Episodes) (p. 157)
>
> **With Rapid Cycling** (p. 157)

❏ ❏ ❏ ❏

DIAGNOSTIC CRITERIA FOR   (ICD-10 code F31.6)
BIPOLAR I DISORDER, MOST RECENT EPISODE MIXED (296.6X)

A. Currently (or most recently) in a Mixed Episode (p. 149).

B. There has previously been at least one Major Depressive Episode (p. 146), Manic Episode (p. 148), or Mixed Episode (p. 149).

C. The mood episodes in Criteria A and B are not better accounted for by Schizoaffective Disorder and are not superimposed on Schizophrenia, Schizophreniform Disorder, Delusional Disorder, or Psychotic Disorder Not Otherwise Specified.

> **Specify (for current or most recent episode):**
> Severity/Psychotic/Remission Specifiers (p. 153)
>
> **With Catatonic Features** (p. 154)
>
> **With Postpartum Onset** (p. 156)
>
> **Specify:**
> Longitudinal Course Specifiers (With and Without Interepisode Recovery) (p. 156)

With Seasonal Pattern (applies only to the pattern of Major Depressive Episodes) (p. 157)

With Rapid Cycling (p. 157)

❏ ❏ ❏ ❏

DIAGNOSTIC CRITERIA FOR BIPOLAR I DISORDER, MOST RECENT EPISODE DEPRESSED (296.5X)

(ICD-10 code F31.x)

A. Currently (or most recently) in a Major Depressive Episode (p. 146).

B. There has previously been at least one Manic Episode (p. 148) or Mixed Episode (p. 149).

C. The mood episodes in Criteria A and B are not better accounted for by Schizoaffective Disorder and are not superimposed on Schizophrenia, Schizophreniform Disorder, Delusional Disorder, or Psychotic Disorder Not Otherwise Specified.

Specify (for current or most recent episode):
Severity/Psychotic/Remission Specifiers (p. 151)

Chronic (p. 154)

With Catatonic Features (p. 154)

With Melancholic Features (p. 155)

With Atypical Features (p. 155)

With Postpartum Onset (p. 156)

Specify:
Longitudinal Course Specifiers (With and Without Interepisode Recovery) (p. 156)

With Seasonal Pattern (applies only to the pattern of Major Depressive Episodes) (p. 157)

With Rapid Cycling (p. 157)

❏ ❏ ❏ ❏

DIAGNOSTIC CRITERIA FOR BIPOLAR I DISORDER, MOST RECENT EPISODE UNSPECIFIED (296.7)

(ICD-10 code F31.9)

A. Criteria, except for duration, are currently (or most recently) met for a Manic (p. 148), a Hypomanic (p. 150), a Mixed (p. 149), or a Major Depressive Episode (p. 146).

B. There has previously been at least one Manic Episode (p. 148) or Mixed Episode (p. 149).

C. The mood symptoms cause clinically significant distress or impairment in social, occupational, or other important areas of functioning.

D. The mood symptoms in Criteria A and B are not better accounted for by Schizoaffective Disorder and are not superimposed on Schizophrenia, Schizophreniform Disorder, Delusional Disorder, or Psychotic Disorder Not Otherwise Specified.

E. The mood symptoms in Criteria A and B are not due to the direct physiological effects of a substance (e.g., a drug of abuse, a medication, or other treatment) or a general medical condition (e.g., hyperthyroidism).

> **Specify:**
> **Longitudinal Course Specifiers (With and Without Interepisode Recovery)** (p. 156)
>
> **With Seasonal Pattern** (applies only to the pattern of Major Depressive Episodes) (p. 157)
>
> **With Rapid Cycling** (p. 157)

❑ ❑ ❑ ❑

296.89 Bipolar II Disorder
(new in DSM-IV)

(ICD-10 code F31.8)

ESSENTIAL FEATURES. Bipolar II Disorder is characterized as one or more Major Depressive Episodes associated with one or more Hypomanic Episodes. Previous Manic or Mixed Episodes preclude this diagnosis—Bipolar I Disorder is the appropriate diagnosis.

> **NOTE: Some patients immediately following a Major Depressive Episode can appear hypomanic because they are happy the depression is over.**

ASSOCIATED FEATURES. The majority of Hypomanic Episodes occur immediately before or after a Major Depressive Episode. Recurrence of mood symptoms over the individual's lifetime is common. Psychotic symptoms do not occur during Hypomanic Episodes but can occur as part of a Major Depressive Episode.

DIFFERENTIAL DIAGNOSIS. In Bipolar I Disorder, an individual has had at least one Manic Episode, or at least one Manic Episode plus a Mixed or Major Depressive Episode. If the individual has had a Hypomanic Episode and a Major Depressive Episode, the diagnosis is Bipolar II Disorder. If the depressive and manic symptoms are of at least 2 years duration and do not meet criteria for a Major Depressive or a Manic Episode, the diagnosis is Cyclothymic Disorder. When symptoms of mania, depression, mixed mood, or hypomania are directly caused by a medical disorder, such as thyroid disease or a stroke, the correct diagnosis is Mood Disorder Due to a General Medical Condition. If a substance causes hypomania, even if the substance is an antidepressant or ECT, the diagnosis is Substance-Induced Mood Disorder, With Manic Features.

The history helps to differentiate major Depressive Disorder or Dysthymic Disorder from Bipolar II Disorder, because an individual with the latter diagnosis will have had one or more Hypomanic Episodes. Individuals with Psychotic Disorders (i.e., Schizophrenia, Schizoaffective Disorder, or Delusional Disorder) will have psychosis in the absence of mood symptoms. If an individual has mood cycles that occur too rapidly to meet the diagnostic criteria for a Major Depressive, Hypomanic or Manic Episode, the diagnosis is Bipolar Disorder Not Otherwise Specified.

DIAGNOSTIC CRITERIA FOR BIPOLAR II DISORDER (296.89)

(ICD-10 code F31.8)

A. Presence (or history) of one or more Major Depressive Episodes (p. 146).

B. Presence (or history) of at least one Hypomanic Episode (p. 150).

C. There has never been a Manic Episode (p. 148) or a Mixed Episode (p. 149).

D. The mood symptoms in Criteria A and B are not better accounted for by Schizoaffective Disorder and are not superimposed on Schizophrenia, Schizophreniform Disorder, Delusional Disorder, or Psychotic Disorder Not Otherwise Specified.

E. The symptoms cause clinically significant distress or impairment in social, occupational, or other important areas of functioning.

Specify for current or most recent episode:
Hypomanic: if currently (or most recently) in a Hypomanic Episode (p. 150)

Depressed: if currently (or most recently) in a Major Depressive Episode (p. 146)

Specify for current Major Depressive Episode (or most recent episode if it is the most recent type of mood episode)

NOTE: Fifth-digit numeric codes specified on p. 151 cannot be used here because the code for Bipolar II Disorder already uses the fifth digit.

Chronic (p. 154)

With Catatonic Features (p. 154)

With Melancholic Features (p. 155)

With Atypical Features (p. 155)

With Postpartum Onset (p. 156)

Specify:
Longitudinal Course Specifiers (With and Without Interepisode Recovery) (p. 156)

With Seasonal Pattern: (applies only to the pattern of Major Depressive Episodes) (p. 157)

With Rapid Cycling (p. 157)

❑ ❑ ❑ ❑

301.13 Cyclothymic Disorder   (ICD-10 code F34.0)

ESSENTIAL FEATURES. Cyclothymic Disorder is a chronic mood disturbance involving frequent hypomanic symptoms and frequent periods of depressive mood or anhedonia that do not meet criteria for a Major Depressive Episode. During the first 2 years of the disturbance (1 year for children and adolescents), there is neither a Manic Episode nor a Major Depressive Episode and the individual has not been symptom free for more than 2 months at a time. The diagnosis is not made if the disturbance is superimposed on a Psychotic Disorder, or if the disturbance is substance induced or caused by a general medical condition.

ASSOCIATED FEATURES. There may be social, academic, interpersonal, or occupational difficulties caused by recurrent mood swings. Substance-Related and Sleep Disorders are common.

DIFFERENTIAL DIAGNOSIS. The individual with Cyclothymic Disorder has clinically significant, sometimes rapid, mood shifts; however, the mood symptoms do not meet the criteria for a Major Depressive, Mixed, or Manic Episode (i.e., not Bipolar I Disorder With Rapid Cycling or Bipolar II Disorder With Rapid Cycling). When a mood disturbance is directly caused by a substance, the diagnosis is Substance-Induced Mood Disorder. If the Mood Disorder is the direct result of a medical illness, such as Multiple Sclerosis, a diagnosis of Mood Disorder Due to a General Medical Condition is made. Individuals with Borderline Personality Disorder typically have marked mood shifts. Both diagnoses are made if the criteria for both are met.

DIAGNOSTIC CRITERIA FOR CYCLOTHYMIC DISORDER (301.13)

(ICD-10 code F34.0)

A. For at least 2 years, the presence of numerous periods with hypomanic symptoms (p. 150) and numerous periods with depressive symptoms that do not meet criteria for a Major Depressive Episode.

> **NOTE: In children and adolescents, the duration must be at least 1 year.**

B. During the above 2-year period (1 year in children and adolescents), the person has not been without the symptoms in Criterion A for more than 2 months at a time.

C. No Major Depressive Episode (p. 146), Manic Episode (p. 148), or Mixed Episode (p. 149) has been present during the first 2 years of the disturbance.

> **NOTE: After the initial 2 years (1 year in children and adolescents) of Cyclothymic Disorder, there may be superimposed Manic or Mixed Episodes (in which case both Bipolar I Disorder and Cyclothymic Disorder may be diagnosed) or Major Depressive Episodes (in which case both Bipolar II Disorder and Cyclothymic Disorder may be diagnosed).**

D. The symptoms in Criterion A are not better accounted for by Schizoaffective Disorder and are not superimposed on Schizophrenia, Schizophreniform Disorder, Delusional Disorder, or Psychotic Disorder Not Otherwise Specified.

E. The symptoms are not due to the direct physiological effects of a substance (e.g., a drug of abuse, a medication) or a general medical condition (e.g., hyperthyroidism).

F. The symptoms cause clinically significant distress or impairment in social, occupational, or other important areas of functioning.

❑ ❑ ❑ ❑

296.80 Bipolar Disorder Not Otherwise Specified (NOS)

(ICD-10 code F31.9)

ESSENTIAL FEATURES. A disorder in which manic or hypomanic features exist but the disturbance does not meet the criteria for any other Bipolar Disorders. An example would be a patient who has mania symptoms and depressive symptoms that alternate so that the duration criteria are not met for either disorder.

❑ ❑ ❑ ❑

OTHER MOOD DISORDERS

293.83 Mood Disorder Due to a General Medical Condition (significantly modified from DSM-III-R)

(ICD-10 code F06.xx)

ESSENTIAL FEATURES. This diagnosis is given when a general medical condition directly causes a significant mood disturbance (e.g., depressed, elevated, or irritable mood). The clinician needs to rule out other mental disorders and Delirium prior to making this diagnosis. There is equal distribution by sex and an increased risk of suicide.

DIFFERENTIAL DIAGNOSIS. Depression frequently accompanies Dementia, especially Vascular Dementia. When a Major Depressive Episode occurs during the course of either Vascular Dementia or Dementia of the Alzheimer's Type, the subtype "With Depressed Mood" is used. In Delirium, mood symptoms are sometimes seen; however, the rapid onset and dramatic fluctuations in mental status seen with Delirium rarely cause diagnostic confusion. Occasionally, an individual with a quiet Delirium, such as that which occurs with hepatic encephalopathy, is mistakenly diagnosed as depressed. Substance-Induced Mood Disorders are common. The clinician must look for evidence that the Mood Disorder is the direct result of a substance (i.e., review medications and drugs of abuse, check blood and urine for substances).

Other diagnoses to consider are Major Depressive Disorder and Bipolar I or II Disorder. In these disorders, there is no causal link between the medical illness and Mood Disorder. If the individual has a maladaptive response to the medical illness, a diagnosis of Adjustment Disorder with Depressed Mood is appropriate. When the clinician cannot determine whether the Mood Disorder is primary (i.e., Mood Disorder is not directly caused by a medical illness or substance) or secondary (i.e., caused by a substance or medical condition), a diagnosis of Mood Disorder Not Otherwise Specified is used.

DIAGNOSTIC CRITERIA FOR MOOD DISORDER DUE TO . . . [INDICATE GENERAL MEDICAL CONDITION] (293.83)

(ICD-10 code F06.xx)

A. A prominent and persistent disturbance in mood predominates in the clinical picture and is characterized by either (or both) of the following:
   (1) depressed mood or markedly diminished interest or pleasure in all, or almost all, activities
   (2) elevated, expansive, or irritable mood

B. There is evidence from the history, physical examination, or laboratory findings that the disturbance is the direct physiological consequence of a general medical condition.

C. The disturbance is not better accounted for by another mental disorder (e.g., Adjustment Disorder With Depressed Mood in response to the stress of having a general medical condition).

D. The disturbance does not occur exclusively during the course of a delirium.

E. The symptoms cause clinically significant distress or impairment in social, occupational, or other important areas of functioning.

> **Specify type:**
> **With Depressive Features:** if the predominant mood is depressed but the full criteria are not met for a Major Depressive Episode
>
> **With Major Depressive-Like Episode:** if the full criteria are met (except Criterion D) for a Major Depressive Episode (p. 146)
>
> **With Manic Features:** if the predominant mood is elevated, euphoric, or irritable
>
> **With Mixed Features:** if the symptoms of both mania and depression are present but neither predominates
>
> **CODING NOTE: Include the name of the general medical condition on Axis I (e.g., 293.83 Mood Disorder Due to Hypothyroidism, With Depressive Features); also code the general medical condition on Axis III (see Appendix G for codes).**
>
> **CODING NOTE: If depressive symptoms occur as part of a preexisting dementia, indicate the depressive symptoms by coding the appropriate subtype of the dementia if one is available (e.g., 290.21 Dementia of the Alzheimer's Type, With Late Onset, With Depressed Mood).**

❑ ❑ ❑ ❑

---.---* Substance-Induced Mood Disorder (ICD-10 code F--.--)
(significantly modified from DSM-III-R)
(see Substance-Related Disorders for specific codes)

ESSENTIAL FEATURES. This diagnosis is given when a substance, which is broadly defined in DSM-IV as drugs of abuse, prescribed medications, other treatment for depression (e.g., ECT), and toxic exposure, directly cause a significant mood disturbance (e.g., depressed, elevated, or irritable mood). The clinician needs to rule out other mental disorders and Delirium prior to using this diagnosis. There is an increased risk of suicide. Mood Disorders are sometimes associated with intoxication (e.g., alcohol) and withdrawal (e.g., cocaine).

DIFFERENTIAL DIAGNOSIS. Mood symptoms occur commonly during Substance Intoxication and Substance Withdrawal. Only if the mood symptoms are greater than normally expected does the clinician make the diagnosis of a Substance-Induced Mood Disorder. Mood symptoms are also common during Delirium and are not diagnosed as a Mood Disorder. The clinician must also rule out primary Mood Disorders (e.g., Major Depressive Disorder, Bipolar I or II Disorder) and Mood Disorder Due to a General Medical Condition. The latter diagnosis is, at times, difficult to distinguish from a Substance-Induced Mood Disorder, because some patients both have medical illnesses and are taking numerous medications. The history can sometimes clarify the cause of the mood disturbance or, when possible, one might discontinue a potentially offending medication and observe for improvement.

DIAGNOSTIC CRITERIA FOR
SUBSTANCE-INDUCED MOOD DISORDER
(SEE SPECIFIC CODES FOLLOWING)

A. A prominent and persistent disturbance in mood predominates in the clinical picture and is characterized by either (or both) of the following:
  (1) depressed mood or markedly diminished interest or pleasure in all, or almost all, activities
  (2) elevated, expansive, or irritable mood
B. There is evidence from the history, physical examination, or laboratory findings of either (1) or (2):
  (1) the symptoms in Criterion A developed during, or within a month of, Substance Intoxication or Withdrawal
  (2) medication use is etiologically related to the disturbance
C. The disturbance is not better accounted for by a Mood Disorder that is not substance induced. Evidence that the symptoms are better accounted for by a Mood Disorder that is not substance induced might include the following: the symptoms precede the onset of the substance use (or medication use); the symptoms persist for a substantial period of time (e.g., about a month) after the cessation of acute withdrawal or severe intoxication or are substantially in excess of what would be expected given the type or amount of the substance used or the duration of use; or there is other evidence that suggests the existence of an independent non-substance-induced Mood Disorder (e.g., a history of recurrent Major Depressive Episodes).

D. The disturbance does not occur exclusively during the course of a delirium.

E. The symptoms cause clinically significant distress or impairment in social, occupational, or other important areas of functioning.

> NOTE: This diagnosis should be made instead of a diagnosis of Substance Intoxication or Substance Withdrawal only when the mood symptoms are in excess of those usually associated with

the intoxication or withdrawal syndrome and when the symptoms are sufficiently severe to warrant independent clinical
attention.

Code (Specific Substance)-Induced Mood Disorder:
291.8 Alcohol (ICD-10 F10.8); **292.84 Amphetamine (or Amphetamine-Like Substance)** (ICD-10 F15.8); **292.84 Cocaine** (ICD-
10 F14.8); **292.84 Hallucinogen** (ICD-10 F16.8); **292.84 Inhalant**
(ICD-10 F18.8); **292.84 Opioid** (ICD-10 F11.8); **292.84
Phencyclidine (or Phencyclidine-Like Substance)** (ICD-10 F19.8);
292.84 Sedative, Hypnotic, or Anxiolytic (ICD-10 F13.8); **292.84
Other (or Unknown) Substance** (ICD-10 F19.8)

Specify type:
With Depressive Features: if the predominant mood is depressed

With Manic Features: if the predominant mood is elevated, euphoric, or irritable

With Mixed Features: if symptoms of both mania and depression
are present and neither predominates

Specify if (see Table 13.1 on p. 99 for applicability by substance):
With Onset During Intoxication: if the criteria are met for Intoxication with the substance and the symptoms develop during the
intoxication syndrome

With Onset During Withdrawal: if criteria are met for Withdrawal
from the substance and the symptoms develop during, or shortly
after, a withdrawal syndrome

❑ ❑ ❑ ❑

DIFFERENCES BETWEEN DSM-III-R AND DSM-IV MOOD DISORDERS

❑ Mood Disorders were significantly modified in DSM-IV. This section
   is now divided into six parts: Mood Episodes, Depressive Disorders,
   Bipolar Disorders, Other Mood Disorders, Specifiers Describing Most
   Recent Episode, and Course of Recurrent Episodes. This section grew
   from 20 pages in DSM-III-R to 74 pages in DSM-IV.

❑ DSM-IV added separate diagnostic criteria for **Mixed Episode** and **Hypomanic Episode**.

❑ The diagnostic criteria for **Major Depressive Episode** were modified to include the requirement that symptoms must "cause clinically significant distress or impairment." Specific guidelines to separate a Major Depressive Episode from normal Bereavement are also provided (Criterion E).

❑ The diagnostic criteria for **Manic Episode** were revised to include the requirement that a mood disturbance last at least 1 week. Also, Substance-Induced Mania no longer qualifies toward a diagnosis of Bipolar Disorder; it is now diagnosed as a **Substance-Induced Mood Episode, with Manic Features**.

❑ The requirement that a Manic Episode not be superimposed on Schizophrenia or other Psychotic Disorders was eliminated from diagnostic criteria.

❑ For all Mood Disorders, the number of specifiers was greatly expanded.

❑ DSM-III-R's Organic Mood Disorders were replaced with **Mood Disorder Due to a General Medical Condition** and **Substance-Induced Mood Disorder**.

❑ New **Specifiers** include **With Catatonic Features, With Atypical Features, With Postpartum Onset, With Rapid Cycling**, and **Longitudinal Course Specifiers**.

❑ With the exception of **In Partial Remission** (for which DSM-IV adds a time criterion of less than 2 months without significant symptoms) and **In Full Remission** (for which DSM-IV requires 2 months without symptoms, rather than the 6 months required in DSM-III-R), Severity Criteria are almost identical for Manic and Depressive Episodes.

❑ DSM-III-R's Dysthymia is now called **Dysthymic Disorder**. Criterion H was added, which requires that "symptoms cause clinically significant distress or impairment." In addition, Dysthymic Disorder cannot be caused by a substance or a general medical condition (DSM-III-R classified these as "secondary type"). DSM-III-R's primary and secondary specifiers are eliminated.

❑ **Depressive Disorder Not Otherwise Specified** no longer has a seasonal pattern specifier.

❑ **Bipolar Disorders** are divided into six **Bipolar I** Disorders, which are classified according to whether the episode is single or recurrent and according to the characteristics of the most recent or current episode, and **Bipolar II** Disorder.

❑ DSM-III-R's Cyclothymia is now called **Cyclothymic Disorder** and a criterion was added that requires that symptoms cause clinically significant distress or impairment.

....

CASE VIGNETTES: MOOD DISORDERS

Case Vignette 1

C.J. is a 34-year-old bank executive who is brought for evaluation by her husband. According to the husband, C.J. was in excellent health until 2 weeks ago, when she began staying up later and later at night. He was initially not too concerned, until she began awakening him to talk about the "revolutionary" new ideas she had about creating an international bank cartel. He notes she was "full of energy" and talked rapidly about the many ideas that she had. He became quite concerned when at 3 A.M. C.J. telephoned the president of the bank where she works to discuss her ideas. She then began telephoning European banks in an attempt to find partners for her business venture. When her husband confronted her about the inappropriateness of her phone calls, she became enraged and accused him of purposefully attempting to sabotage her venture. She was brought to the emergency room by the husband and two friends.

On examination, C.J.'s speech is quite rapid and she jumps quickly from one subject to another. She states that she is about to revolutionize banking and control the world currency market. When questioned about the likelihood of achieving this goal, she becomes irritable and threatens to leave. She admits to auditory hallucinations that are telling her how to corner the market on gold and other precious metals. The patient is on no medications, has no prior psychiatric history (including no prior depressive episodes), and denies drug abuse. Family history is positive for Mood Disorders. Her younger brother had a severe depression 2 years ago that required hospitalization, and her mother was diagnosed as Manic-Depressive many years ago. Her physical examination and laboratory valves are normal, and a toxic screen for drugs is negative.

DIAGNOSIS AND DISCUSSION

Axis I—296.04 Bipolar I Disorder, Single Manic Episode, Severe, With Psychotic Features (Mood-Congruent), (ICD-10 F30.2)
Axis II—V71.09 No diagnosis or 799.9 Diagnosis Deferred (ICD-10 Z03.2, R46.8)
Axis III—No known medical condition

C.J.'s symptoms and behavior are typical of a Manic Episode. Her mood is expansive. She is grandiose, talkative, has flight of ideas, and is having mood-congruent hallucinations. She also has a markedly decreased need for sleep. Her impairment is severe. There is no evidence of a Substance-Induced Mood Disorder or a Mood Disorder Due to a General Medical Condition. There is no evidence of any preexisting Psychotic Disorder or a Major Depressive Episode, and C.J.'s hallucinations appeared concurrently with the Mood Disorder.

Case Vignette 2

T.F. is a 28-year-old government employee referred by his family physician for evaluation. He reports a 3-month history of worsening anxiety that is especially bad early in the morning. "I wake up at 3 in the morning and I can't get back to sleep. My thoughts torment me." He also reports decreased energy, inability to concentrate at his job, decreased appetite with a 10-pound weight loss, and suicidal ideation. "I feel so hopeless that suicide seems like an option." He also states, "There is nothing in my life that I enjoy."

T.F. is tearful during evaluation. He lacks animation and has few body movements during the session. His mood is quite depressed. He denies prior hypomanic or manic episodes. Mental status exam reveals slowed thinking and no evidence of psychosis. He does report two previous depressive periods, one in late adolescence and another during his senior year in college. During the latter episode, his symptoms were severe enough that he was unable to attend classes. "I almost failed that semester." Both depressive episodes remitted in a few months without treatment; he "felt like normal" during remission. He denies drug abuse or use and has no medical problems. The family history is positive for depression in a paternal grandfather, and in his father, and he reports that a depressed uncle committed suicide about 10 years ago.

DIAGNOSIS AND DISCUSSION

Axis I—296.33 Major Depressive Disorder, Recurrent, Severe Without Psychotic Features, With Melancholic Features, With Full Interepisode Recovery (ICD-10 F33.2)
Axis II—V71.09 No diagnosis or 799.9 Diagnosis Deferred (ICD-10 Z03.2, R46.8)
Axis III—No known medical condition

T.F. presents with signs and symptoms of a severe Major Depressive Episode. According to the history, he has had two previous depressive episodes, and no reported history of mania, hypomanic, drug abuse, or medical illness. There is no evidence of psychosis. Therefore, T.F. has a Major Depressive Disorder that is recurrent and severe without psychotic features. Concerning the specifiers for this diagnosis (see p. 354 of DSM-IV), the disorder is not chronic (i.e., is not 2 years in duration) but does have Melancholic Features. Specifically, T.F. lacks pleasure in all activities and has early morning awakening, depression regularly worse in the morning, psychomotor retardation, significant weight loss, and excessive guilt. The Longitudinal Course Specifier that describes this case is "With Full Interepisode Recovery" (i.e., he recovers completely between depressive episodes). Additional inquiry is needed to see if a seasonal pattern exists in T.F.'s case.

CHAPTER 16

ANXIETY DISORDERS

CODING NOTE: Posttraumatic Stress Disorder is now coded 309.81. Code Substance-Induced Anxiety Disorders according to the substance involved.

NOTE: Some Anxiety Disorders are not classified here (e.g., Separation Anxiety Disorder listed under Disorders Usually First Evident in Infancy, Childhood, or Adolescence; Sexual Aversion Disorder listed under Sexual Disorders).

ESSENTIAL FEATURES. The characteristic features of the Anxiety Disorders are clinically significant anxiety and, for some, avoidance behavior.

PANIC ATTACK AND AGORAPHOBIA

These syndromes, which are not separately coded, are described separately in DSM-IV because of frequent references to them in the various disorders.

Panic Attack

ESSENTIAL FEATURES. The primary features are sudden, acute, intense fear or discomfort, accompanied by somatic and/or cognitive symptoms. The context in which the Panic Attack occurs is often characteristic of the disorder in which it is found. **Unexpected (uncued)** Panic Attacks, required for any Panic Disorder diagnosis, are spontaneous (i.e., not associated with a situational trigger). **Situationally bound (cued)** Panic Attacks, in which an attack almost invariably occurs upon exposure to, or in anticipation of, a situational trigger ("cue"), are characteristic of phobias. **Situationally predisposed** Panic Attacks are associated with a situational trigger but do not always occur (or may develop some time after exposure). Any form of Panic Attack may appear in any Anxiety Disorder.

Diagnostic Criteria
FOR PANIC ATTACK
(NOT A CODABLE DISORDER)

(86)

A discrete period of intense fear or discomfort, in which four (or more) of the following symptoms develop abruptly and reach a peak within 10 minutes:

    (1) palpitations, pounding heart, or accelerated heart rate
    (2) sweating
    (3) trembling or shaking
    (4) sensations of shortness of breath or smothering
    (5) feeling of choking
    (6) chest pain or discomfort
    (7) nausea or abdominal distress
    (8) feeling dizzy, unsteady, lightheaded, or faint
    (9) derealization (feelings of unreality) or depersonalization (being detached from oneself)
 (10) fear of losing control or going crazy
 (11) fear of dying
 (12) paresthesias (numbness or tingling sensations)
 (13) chills or hot flushes

Specify type:
Unexpected (uncued)

Situationally bound (cued)

Situationally predisposed

NOTE: A "limited-symptom attack" is an episode meeting fewer than four criteria but otherwise identical to a Panic Attack.

□ □ □ □

Agoraphobia

ESSENTIAL FEATURES. There is intense fear of, or discomfort in, settings from which escape is difficult or embarrassing, or in which help (e.g., to alleviate a panic attack) is not available.

Diagnostic Criteria
FOR AGORAPHOBIA
(NOT A CODABLE DISORDER)

(87)

A. Anxiety about being in places or situations from which escape might be difficult (or embarrassing) or in which help might not be available in the event of having an unexpected or situationally predisposed Panic Attack or panic-like symptoms. Agoraphobic fears typically involve characteristic clusters of situations that include being outside the home alone, being in a crowd or standing in line, being on a bridge, and traveling in a bus, train, or automobile.

> NOTE: Consider a diagnosis of Specific Phobia if the avoidance is limited to one or only a few specific situations, or Social Phobia if the avoidance is limited to social situations.

B. The situations are avoided (e.g., travel is restricted), or else are endured with marked distress or with anxiety about having a Panic Attack or panic-like symptoms, or require the presence of a companion.

C. The anxiety or phobic avoidance is not better accounted for by another mental disorder, such as Social Phobia (e.g., avoidance limited to social situations because of fear of embarrassment), Specific Phobia (e.g., avoidance limited to one type of situation), Obsessive-Compulsive Disorder (e.g., avoidance of dirt in someone with an obsession about contamination), Posttraumatic Stress Disorder (e.g., avoidance of stimuli associated with a severe stressor), or Separation Anxiety Disorder (e.g., avoidance of leaving home or relatives).

❑ ❑ ❑ ❑

Panic Disorder
(significantly modified from DSM-III-R)

300.01 Panic Disorder Without Agoraphobia	(ICD-10 code F41.0)
300.21 Panic Disorder With Agoraphobia	(ICD-10 code F40.01)

ESSENTIAL FEATURES. There are recurrent, *unexpected* Panic Attacks followed by at least 1 month of persistent concern about further attacks, their meaning, or some change in behavior related to them. Agoraphobia is present or absent, depending on the type of Panic Disorder. (See criteria for Panic Attack and Agoraphobia.) Frequency and severity of attacks varies a great deal, and "limited-symptom attacks" (in which panic is felt but not all criteria for Panic Attack are met) may occur. The agoraphobic type is very common.

ASSOCIATED FEATURES. Patients are often apprehensive between attacks, usually in fear of another attack or some life-threatening condition (e.g., terminal illness). Mood disturbance, including Major Depressive Disorder, is common. Self-medication with legal or illegal substances is common and should be separately diagnosed. Onset is typically in adolescence or early adulthood.

PHYSICAL AND LABORATORY FINDINGS. Except for occasional respiratory alkalosis, routine laboratory tests are usually normal. Panic response to sodium lactate infusion may be greater than in other Anxiety Disorders. Inconsistent association with mitral valve prolapse and thyroid disease has been reported.

PREDISPOSING FACTORS. In susceptible individuals, the predisposing factors include Separation Anxiety Disorder, sudden loss of social support, and disruption of important interpersonal relationships.

DIFFERENTIAL DIAGNOSIS. Anxiety or panic related to organic factors, including medications, Substance Abuse, Substance Withdrawal (including caffeine), and any of a large number of physical disorders preempt the diagnosis (see disorders below). Major Depressive Episode and Somatization Disorder should be differentiated from Panic Disorder, although each can coexist with it. Other Anxiety Disorders may coexist with Panic Disorder unless specifically preempted; however, care should be taken to be sure the symptoms of Panic Attack are not better accounted for by one of the other disorders (see below). An additional diagnosis of Generalized Anxiety Disorder should not be made if the patient's anxiety between Panic Attacks is focused on the fear of having another.

Differentiating Panic Disorder With Agoraphobia from Specific Phobia, Situational Type or Social Phobia is often difficult, and may rest with a determination of when and where the first Panic Attack occurred. If it occurred in a setting which then became phobic, and Panic Attacks do not occur in other settings, consider Specific Phobia. If unexpected Panic Attacks occur in separate settings, without phobic dread, consider Panic Disorder Without Agoraphobia.

DIAGNOSTIC CRITERIA FOR
PANIC DISORDER WITHOUT AGORAPHOBIA
(300.01) OR WITH AGORAPHOBIA (300.21)

(ICD-10 codes F41.0
or F40.01)

A. Both (1) and (2), below:
  (1) There are recurrent, unexpected Panic Attacks (see definition/criteria, above).
  (2) At least one of the attacks has been followed by 1 month (or more) of one (or more) of the following:
    (a) persistent concern about having additional attacks
    (b) worry about the implications of the attack or its consequences (e.g., losing control, having a heart attack, "going crazy")
    (c) a significant change in behavior related to the attacks

B. Absence or presence of Agoraphobia (specify Without Agoraphobia, 300.01 or With Agoraphobia, 300.21, respectively; see definition/criteria for Agoraphobia, above).

C. The panic attacks are not due to the direct physiological effects of a substance (e.g., a drug of abuse, a medication) or a general medical condition (e.g., hyperthyroidism).

D. The panic attacks are not better accounted for by another mental disorder, such as Social Phobia (e.g., occurring on exposure to feared social situations), Specific Phobia (e.g., on exposure to a specific phobic situation), Obsessive-Compulsive Disorder (e.g., on exposure to dirt in someone with an obsession about contamination), Posttraumatic Stress Disorder (e.g., in response tostimuli associated with a severe stressor), or Separation Anxiety Disorder (e.g., in response to being away from home or close relatives).

☐ ☐ ☐ ☐

300.22 Agoraphobia Without History of Panic Disorder

(ICD-10 code F40.00)

ESSENTIAL FEATURES. There is Agoraphobia with no known history of panic disorder. The person may be afraid of having a Panic Attack or fear an embarrassing or incapacitating event (such as becoming dizzy, falling, or enuretic). Limited-symptom attacks (see criteria for Panic Attack, above) and panic-like symptoms may occur. Fears of embarrassment or incapacitation must be clinically significant and clearly exceed realistic expectations (e.g., fear of diarrhea in a person with ulcerative colitis, fear of getting lost or confused in an unfamiliar environment).

COMPLICATIONS. Some patients subsequently develop Panic Disorder.

DIFFERENTIAL DIAGNOSIS. Avoidant behavior may be seen in some Psychotic or Delusional Disorders with persecutory features, and in Major Depressive Episodes. Social Phobia and Specific Phobias may be associated with similar avoidance patterns; the former is differentiated by its focus on the fear of what one will do, rather than fear of the setting itself. Panic Disorder With Agoraphobia, which preempts this diagnosis, is differentiated by its history of Panic Attacks. Concerns about genuinely incapacitating or embarrassing situations must reach excessive proportions before Agoraphobia may be diagnosed.

DIAGNOSTIC CRITERIA FOR AGORAPHOBIA WITHOUT HISTORY OF PANIC DISORDER (300.22)

(ICD-10 code F40.00)

A. The presence of Agoraphobia (see criteria above) related to fear of developing panic-like symptoms (e.g., dizziness or diarrhea).

B. Criteria have never been met for Panic Disorder (see preceding).

C. The disturbance is not due to the direct physiological effects of a substance (e.g., a drug of abuse, a medication) or a general medical condition.

D. If an associated general medical condition is present, the fear described in Criterion A is clearly in excess of that usually associated with the condition.

NOTE: The anxiety or phobic avoidance should not be better accounted for by another mental disorder, such as Specific Pho-

bia, Separation Anxiety Disorder, Obsessive-Compulsive Disorder, Posttraumatic Stress Disorder, or Social Phobia.

❑ ❑ ❑ ❑

300.29 Specific Phobia   (ICD-10 code F40.2)
(Simple Phobia in DSM-III-R)
(significantly modified from DSM-III-R)

ESSENTIAL FEATURES. This disorder is characterized by a persistent and excessive
or unreasonable fear of a clearly definable object or situation *other than* fear of a
Panic Attack or social situation. During some phase of the disturbance, exposure
to the phobic stimulus almost invariably provokes immediate anxiety, and
marked anticipatory anxiety occurs if exposure is imminent. The diagnosis is
made only if the fear or avoidance interferes with the person's normal routine,
social activities, or relationships, or if there is marked distress about having the
fear; *and* it is clearly excessive given its context.

ASSOCIATED FEATURES. Associated features include restrictions of occupation,
school, and/or lifestyle. Other, unrelated Anxiety Disorders are often present.

CULTURAL AND AGE-RELATED FEATURES. Adolescents and adults recognize the fear
as unreasonable. Children, however, are often unaware that their phobias are
excessive or unusual and may thus not display distress about them. Cultural
sanction for some unusual fears (e.g., fears of magic or spirits) should be considered, and may preclude the diagnosis in certain groups.

DIFFERENTIAL DIAGNOSIS. Other Phobic and Anxiety Disorders can be distinguished by the clear focus of the unreasonable fear and by the lack of pervasive
anxiety in Specific Phobia. In Posttraumatic Stress Disorder, the phobic stimulus
is associated, in reality or symbolically, with the trauma. Anxiety about dirt or
contamination in Obsessive-Compulsive Disorder should not be confused with
a Specific Phobia. Persons with Schizophrenia or other Psychotic Disorders usually do not recognize their phobic symptoms as excessive or unreasonable. Hypochondriasis involves the feeling that one *has* a disease rather than a fear of
contracting it. Eating Disorders may involve avoidance of food and related cues
but should be easily distinguished from Specific Phobia.

DIAGNOSTIC CRITERIA FOR   (ICD-10 code F40.2)
SPECIFIC PHOBIA (300.29)

A. Marked and persistent fear that is excessive or unreasonable, cued by the
   presence or anticipation of a specific object or situation (e.g., flying, heights,
   animals, receiving an injection, seeing blood).

B. Exposure to the phobic stimulus almost invariably provokes an immediate anxiety response, which may take the form of a situationally bound or situationally predisposed Panic Attack.

> **NOTE: In children, the anxiety may be expressed by crying, tantrums, freezing, or clinging.**

C. The person recognizes that the fear is excessive or unreasonable.

> **NOTE: In children, this feature may be absent.**

D. The phobic situation(s) is avoided or else is endured with intense anxiety or distress.

E. Avoidance, anxious anticipation, or distress in the feared situation interferes significantly with the person's normal routine, occupational (or academic) functioning, or social activities or relationships; *or* there is marked distress about having the phobia.

F. In individuals under age 18 years, the duration is at least 6 months.

G. The anxiety, Panic Attacks, or phobic avoidance associated with the specific object or situation are not better accounted for by another mental disorder, such as Obsessive-Compulsive Disorder (e.g., fear of dirt in someone with an obsession about contamination), Posttraumatic Stress Disorder (e.g., avoidance of stimuli associated with a severe stressor), Separation Anxiety Disorder (e.g., avoidance of school), Social Phobia (e.g., avoidance of social situations because of fear of embarrassment), Panic Disorder With Agoraphobia, or Agoraphobia Without History of Panic Disorder.

> **Specify type:**
> **Animal Type** (e.g., dogs, snakes)
>
> **Natural Environment Type** (e.g., heights, storms, water)
>
> **Blood-Injection-Injury Type** (e.g., venipuncture, bleeding cuts)
>
> **Situational Type** (e.g., planes, elevators, or enclosed places)
>
> **Other Type** (e.g., phobic avoidance of situations that may lead to choking, vomiting, or contracting an illness; or, in children, avoidance of loud sounds or costumed characters)

❑ ❑ ❑ ❑

300.23 Social Phobia (Social Anxiety Disorder)   *(ICD-10 code F40.1)*
(Now includes DSM-III-R Avoidant Disorder of
Childhood, formerly 313.21)

ESSENTIAL FEATURES. There is an excessive and persistent fear of situations in which the patient is exposed to possible scrutiny by others, and a fear that he or she may act in a way that will be humiliating or embarrassing. The Social Phobia may be general or circumscribed. It must be unrelated to fears of Panic Attack (although situational Panic Attacks are common), Stuttering, trembling, or symptoms of other Axis I or Axis III disorders. Marked anticipatory anxiety is the rule. The diagnosis should be made only if avoidant behavior interferes with social or vocational functioning, or if the patient has marked distress about the fear.

ASSOCIATED FEATURES. Restrictions of occupation, school, and/or lifestyle are seen. Other, unrelated Anxiety Disorders are often present.

CULTURAL AND AGE-RELATED FEATURES. Adolescents and adults recognize that their anxiety is unreasonable. Children are often unaware that the fear is unusual and thus may not display distress about it. Culturally expected social avoidance behaviors do not imply this disorder; however, extreme and excessive concerns characteristic of patients in some cultures (e.g., about offending others with body odor) should be given the diagnosis.

DIFFERENTIAL DIAGNOSIS. Simple avoidance of social situations that commonly are a source of some distress (e.g., reasonable fear of public speaking or performing) should be considered. Avoidant Personality Disorder may coexist with the disorder. Pervasive Developmental Disorder and Schizoid Personality Disorder are differentiated from Social Phobia by their lack of interest in and capacity for social situations. Other Anxiety Disorders and Other Axis I disorders (e.g., Mood Disorders) should be diagnosed instead if they better explain the symptoms; they may be comorbid if the criteria are separate and distinct.

DIAGNOSTIC CRITERIA FOR (ICD-10 code F40.1)
SOCIAL PHOBIA (300.23)

A. A marked and persistent fear of one or more social or performance situations in which the person is exposed to unfamiliar people or to possible scrutiny by others. The individual fears that he or she will act in a way (or show anxiety symptoms) that will be humiliating or embarrassing.

> NOTE: In children, there must be evidence of the capacity for age-appropriate social relationships with familiar people and the anxiety must occur in peer settings, not just in interactions with adults.

B. Exposure to the feared social situation almost invariably provokes anxiety, which may take the form of a situationally bound or situationally predisposed Panic Attack.

> NOTE: In children, the anxiety may be expressed by crying, tantrums, freezing, or shrinking from social situations with unfamiliar people.

C. The person recognizes that the fear is excessive or unreasonable.

> NOTE: In children, this feature may be absent.

D. The feared social or performance situations are avoided or else endured with intense anxiety or distress.

E. The avoidance, anxious anticipation, or distress in the feared social or performance situation(s) interferes significantly with the person's normal routine, occupational (academic) functioning, or social activities or relationships; *or* there is marked distress about having the phobia.

F. In individuals under age 18 years, the duration is at least 6 months.

G. The fear or avoidance is not due to the direct physiological effects of a substance (e.g., a drug of abuse, a medication) or a general medical condition, and is not better accounted for by another mental disorder (e.g., Panic Disorder With or Without Agoraphobia, Separation Anxiety Disorder, Body Dysmorphic Disorder, a Pervasive Developmental Disorder or Schizoid Personality Disorder).

H. If a general medical condition or another mental disorder is present, the fear in Criterion A is unrelated to it (e.g., the fear is not of Stuttering, trembling in Parkinson's disease, or exhibiting abnormal eating behavior in Anorexia Nervosa or Bulimia Nervosa).

Specify if:
Generalized: if the fears include most social situations (also consider the additional diagnosis of Avoidant Personality Disorder)

□ □ □ □

300.3 Obsessive-Compulsive Disorder   (ICD-10 code F42.8)

ESSENTIAL FEATURES. The essential feature of this disorder is recurrent obsessions or compulsions sufficiently severe to cause marked distress, consume considerable time, and/or significantly interfere with the patient's normal routine and/or occupational, social, or interpersonal functioning. The obsessions (or at least the energy consumed by them) are dysphoric. Attempts to resist the compulsions lead to a sense of mounting tension that can be immediately relieved by yielding to them.

ASSOCIATED FEATURES. Depression, anxiety, and phobic avoidance of situations related to obsessions (e.g., dirt, contamination) are commonly seen. The compulsions and/or phobic avoidance may markedly restrict social, occupational, or academic activities.

CULTURAL AND AGE-FELATED FEATURES. Children with this disorder may not be distressed by it. When help is sought, it is usually at the request of a parent.

DIFFERENTIAL DIAGNOSIS. Some ordinary behaviors (such as "checking") are common in the general population but do not reach the level of impairment or distress required for Obsessive-Compulsive Disorder. Many potentially injurious activities in which patients engage excessively, such as those associated with Eating Disorders, Paraphilias, Gambling, or Substance Abuse, may be confused with compulsions; however, true compulsions and the activity they generate is not usually pleasurable and the wish to resist is not based in concern about detrimental consequences.

Depressive Disorders are frequently associated with obsessive guilt or rumination; however, the obsessions are usually mood congruent and are rarely associated with compulsions. Obsessions and compulsions associated with Psychotic Disorders are usually ego-syntonic and not recognized as unrealistic. Symptoms of Obsessive-Compulsive Disorder can reach psychotic proportions, in which case an additional diagnosis (e.g., Delusional Disorder, Psychotic Disorder NOS) should be considered.

The disorder should be differentiated from the stereotypic behavior of Tourette's Disorder and Stereotypic Movement Disorder, although it may co-exist with them. Symptoms directly related to general medical conditions or Substance Abuse are not diagnosed here, nor is any disorder in which the obsessions or compulsions are related solely to another mental disorder. Thus Body Dysmorphic Disorder, Trichotillomania, and phobias preempt the diagnosis.

Obsessive-Compulsive Disorder is quite distinct from the Axis II Obsessive-Compulsive Personality Disorder, which is not characterized by obsessions or compulsions and involves a pervasive and lifelong character style rather than a set of symptoms.

DIAGNOSTIC CRITERIA FOR OBSESSIVE-COMPULSIVE DISORDER (300.3)

(ICD-10 code F42.8)

A. Either obsessions or compulsions:

Obsessions as defined by (1), (2), (3), and (4):

(1) recurrent and persistent thoughts, impulses, or images that are experienced, at some time during the disturbance, as intrusive and inappropriate, and cause marked anxiety or distress

(2) the thoughts, impulses, or images are not simply excessive worries about real-life problems

(3) the person attempts to ignore or suppress the thoughts, impulses, or images, or to neutralize them with another thought or action

(4) the person recognizes that the obsessional thoughts, impulses, or images are from his or her own mind (not imposed from without as in thought insertion)

Compulsions as defined by (1) and (2):

(1) repetitive behaviors (e.g., hand washing, ordering, checking) or mental acts (e.g., praying, counting, repeating words silently) the person feels driven to perform in response to an obsession, or according to rules that must be rigidly applied

(2) the behaviors or mental acts are aimed at preventing or reducing distress or preventing some dreaded event or situation; however, these be-

haviors or mental acts either are not connected in a realistic way with what they are designed to neutralize or prevent, or are clearly excessive

B. At some point during the course of the disorder, the person has recognized that the obsessions or compulsions are excessive or unreasonable.

> **NOTE: This does not apply to children.**

C. The obsessions or compulsions cause marked distress, are time consuming (take more than 1 hour a day), or significantly interfere with the person's normal routine, occupational (or academic) functioning, or usual social activities or relationships.

D. If another Axis I disorder is present, the content of the obsessions or compulsions is not restricted to it (e.g., preoccupation with food in the presence of an Eating Disorder; hair pulling in the presence of Trichotillomania; concern with appearance in the presence of Body Dysmorphic Disorder; preoccupation with drugs in the presence of a Substance Use Disorder; preoccupation with having a serious illness in the presence of Hypochondriasis; preoccupation with sexual urges or fantasies in the presence of a paraphilia; or guilty ruminations in the presence of Major Depressive Disorder).

E. The disturbance is not due to the direct physiological effects of a substance (e.g., a drug of abuse, a medication) or a general medical condition.

> **Specify if:**
> **With Poor Insight:** if for most of the time during the current episode, the person does not recognize that the obsessions and compulsions are excessive or unreasonable.

❑ ❑ ❑ ❑

309.81 Posttraumatic Stress Disorder (PTSD) (ICD-10 code F43.1)
(309.89 in DSM-III-R)
(significantly modified from DSM-III-R)

ESSENTIAL FEATURES. One sees characteristic symptoms following an event that is extremely traumatic and experienced with intense fear, terror, and/or helplessness. The event must be directly experienced, observed, or related to a family member or other "close associate." Death, serious injury, or threat to physical integrity is required. Symptoms include persistent re-experiencing, persistent avoidance, or persistently increased arousal. The precipitating stressor is not generally one which is usually well tolerated by most other members of the cultural group (e.g., death of a loved one, ordinary traffic accident). The stressor may arise from natural, accidental, or purposeful events, and usually develops within the first 3 months (see Acute Stress Disorder 308.3, following). The disorder does not develop in every victim; when it does, it is often preceded by Acute Stress Disorder.

ASSOCIATED FEATURES. Depression and anxiety, which may be separately diagnosed, are commonly seen. Compulsive behavior or changes of routine or lifestyle may occur. "Pseudo-organic" symptoms, such as memory problems, difficulty concentrating, or emotional lability may occur, and may be confused with Somatoform Disorders. "Survivor's guilt" may be seen, particularly if others were killed in the traumatic event. Impairment may be mild or severe, and may affect almost any aspect of life. Phobic avoidance of real or symbolic reminders of the trauma may occur.

AGE-SPECIFIC FEATURES. PTSD may present differently in children (see below).

DIFFERENTIAL DIAGNOSIS. Adjustment Disorder implies less-than-extreme trauma, and may or may not include all of the criteria below. Symptoms that predate the trauma should not be used to support a diagnosis of PTSD. PTSD is preempted if the symptoms, even if related to extreme trauma, are better accounted for by other mental disorders (e.g., Anxiety Disorders, Depressive Disorders, Conversion Disorder, Brief Psychotic Disorder). In other cases, comorbidity is permitted. Symptom exaggeration or malingering should be carefully considered in cases that involve financial gain, other benefits, or litigation.

DIAGNOSTIC CRITERIA FOR POSTTRAUMATIC STRESS DISORDER (309.81)   (ICD-10 code F43.1)

A. The person has been exposed to a traumatic event in which both of the following were present:

(1) the person experienced, witnessed, or was confronted with an event or events that involved actual or threatened death or serious injury, or a threat to the physical integrity of self or others

(2) the person's response involved intense fear, helplessness, or horror

NOTE: In children, this may be expressed instead by disorganized or agitated behavior.

B. The traumatic event is persistently reexperienced in one (or more) of the following ways:

(1) recurrent and intrusive distressing recollections of the event, including images, thoughts, or perceptions

NOTE: In young children, repetitive play may occur in which themes or aspects of the trauma are expressed.

(2) recurrent distressing dreams of the event

NOTE: In children, there may be frightening dreams without recognizable content.

(3) acting or feeling as if the traumatic event were recurring (includes a sense of reliving the experience, illusions, hallucinations, and dissociative

flashback episodes, including those that occur on awakening or when intoxicated)

NOTE: Young children may reenact the trauma.

    (4) intense psychological distress at exposure to internal or external cues that symbolize or resemble an aspect of the traumatic event

    (5) physiological reactivity upon exposure to internal or external cues that symbolize or resemble an aspect of the traumatic event

C. Persistent avoidance of stimuli associated with the trauma and numbing of general responsiveness (not present before the trauma), as indicated by three (or more) of the following:

    (1) efforts to avoid thoughts, feelings, or conversations associated with the trauma

    (2) efforts to avoid activities, places, or people that arouse recollections of the trauma

    (3) inability to recall an important aspect of the trauma

    (4) markedly diminished interest or participation in significant activities

    (5) feeling of detachment or estrangement from others

    (6) restricted range of affect (e.g., unable to have loving feelings)

    (7) sense of a foreshortened future (e.g., does not expect to have a career, marriage, children, or a normal life span)

D. Persistent symptoms of increased arousal (not present before the trauma), as indicated by two (or more) of the following:

    (1) difficulty falling or staying asleep

    (2) irritability or outbursts of anger

    (3) difficulty concentrating

    (4) hypervigilance

    (5) exaggerated startle response

E. Duration of the disturbance (symptoms in Criteria B, C, and D) is more than 1 month.

F. The disturbance causes clinically significant distress or impairment in social, occupational, or other important areas of functioning.

Specify if:
Acute: if duration of symptoms is less than 3 months

NOTE: Do not confuse PTSD, Acute, with Acute Stress Disorder [p. 192].

Chronic: if duration of symptoms is 3 months or more

Specify if:
With Delayed Onset: if onset of symptoms is at least 6 months after the stressor

❑ ❑ ❑ ❑

308.3 Acute Stress Disorder
(new in DSM-IV)

(ICD-10 code F43.0)

ESSENTIAL FEATURES: One sees characteristic symptoms caused by, and occurring within 1 month after, exposure to an extremely traumatic event. Individuals who develop this disorder are at high risk for PTSD.

ASSOCIATED FEATURES. See PTSD, as clinically appropriate.

DIFFERENTIAL DIAGNOSIS. See PTSD, which has similar symptoms but different duration and time of onset. Symptoms seen immediately after a trauma must be differentiated from preempting general medical conditions and Substance-Induced Disorders.

DIAGNOSTIC CRITERIA FOR ACUTE STRESS DISORDER (308.3)

(ICD-10 code 43.0)

A. The person has been exposed to a traumatic event in which both of the following were present:
  (1) the person experienced, witnessed, or was confronted with an event or events that involved actual or threatened death or serious injury, or a threat to the physical integrity of oneself or others
  (2) the person's response involved intense fear, helplessness, or horror

B. Either while experiencing or after experiencing the distressing event, the individual has three (or more) of the following dissociative symptoms:
  (1) a subjective sense of numbing, detachment, or absence of emotional responsiveness
  (2) a reduction in awareness of one's surroundings (e.g., "being in a daze")
  (3) derealization
  (4) depersonalization
  (5) dissociative amnesia (i.e., inability to recall an important aspect of the trauma)

C. The traumatic event is persistently reexperienced in at least one of the following ways: recurrent images, thoughts, dreams, illusions, flashbacks, or a sense of reliving the experience; or distress on exposure to reminders of the trauma.

D. Marked avoidance of stimuli that arouse recollections of the trauma (e.g., thoughts, feelings, conversations, activities, places, people).

E. Marked symptoms of anxiety or increased arousal (e.g., difficulty sleeping, irritability, poor concentration, hypervigilance, exaggerated startle response, motor restlessness).

F. The disturbance causes clinically significant distress or impairment in social, occupational, or other important areas of functioning, or impairs the individual's ability to pursue some necessary task, such as obtaining necessary assistance or mobilizing personal resources by telling family members about the traumatic experience.

G. The disturbance lasts for a minimum of 2 days and a maximum of 4 weeks, and occurs within 4 weeks of the traumatic event.

H. The disturbance is not due to the direct physiological effects of a substance (e.g., a drug of abuse, a medication) or a general medical condition, is not better accounted for by Brief Psychotic Disorder, and is not merely an exacerbation of a preexisting Axis I or Axis II disorder.

❑❑❑❑

300.02 Generalized Anxiety Disorder (GAD)　　(ICD-10 code F41.1)
(significantly modified from DSM-III-R; now includes Overanxious Disorder of Childhood [formerly 313.00])

ESSENTIAL FEATURES. There is excessive anxiety and worry which are pervasive, chronic, and not solely associated with features of another Axis I disorder (e.g., panic, public embarrassment, obsessions or compulsions).

ASSOCIATED FEATURES. Somatic symptoms of anxiety are common, as are depressive symptoms, unrelated Panic Disorder, Substance Abuse, or somatic symptoms (any of which may be comorbid).

DIFFERENTIAL DIAGNOSIS. Anxiety that is substance-induced or due to a general medical condition (including Substance Withdrawal, covert or overt physical illness, or caffeine intoxication) is preempting. When the worry is focused on a particular subject, as in some other Anxiety Disorders, the diagnosis should not be made. Generalized anxiety occurring during the course of other disorders (e.g., Mood Disorder, Psychotic Disorder) should not be used to support this diagnosis. Adjustment Disorder With Anxiety rarely meets the criteria of Generalized Anxiety Disorder, and a psychosocial stressor is present.

DIAGNOSTIC CRITERIA FOR　　(ICD-10 code F41.1)
GENERALIZED ANXIETY DISORDER (300.02)

A. Excessive anxiety and worry (apprehensive expectation), occurring more days than not for at least 6 months, about a number of events or activities (such as work or school performance).

B. The person finds it difficult to control the worry.

C. The anxiety and worry are associated with three (or more) of the following, with at least some symptoms present more days than not for the past 6 months:

>   NOTE: Only one item is required in children.

>   (1) restlessness or feeling "keyed up" or "on edge"
>   (2) being easily fatigued
>   (3) difficulty concentrating or "mind going blank"

(4) irritability

(5) muscle tension

(6) sleep disturbance (difficulty falling or staying asleep, or restless, unsatisfying sleep)

D. The focus of the anxiety and worry is not confined to features of an Axis I
disorder. For example, the anxiety or worry is not about having a Panic Attack
(as in Panic Disorder), being embarrassed in public (as in Social Phobia), being contaminated (as in Obsessive-Compulsive Disorder), being away from
home or close relatives (as in Separation Anxiety Disorder), gaining weight (as
in Anorexia Nervosa), having multiple physical complaints (as in Somatization
Disorder), or having a serious illness (as in Hypochondriasis), and the anxiety
and worry do not occur exclusively during Posttraumatic Stress Disorder.

E. The anxiety, worry, or physical symptoms cause clinically significant distress
or impairment in social, occupational, or other important areas of
functioning.

F. The disturbance is not due to the direct physiological effects of a substance
(e.g., a drug of abuse, a medication) or a general medical condition (e.g., hyperthyroidism), and does not occur exclusively during a Mood Disorder, Psychotic Disorder, or Pervasive Developmental Disorder.

▫ ▫ ▫ ▫

293.89 Anxiety Disorder Due to a General Medical Condition

(ICD-10 code F06.4)

*(includes non-substance-related Organic Anxiety
Disorder/Syndrome, formerly 294.80 in DSM-III-R)*
(new in DSM-IV)

NOTE: See special coding procedures under Diagnostic Criteria.

ESSENTIAL FEATURES. There is clinically significant anxiety directly caused by the
physiological effects of a general medical condition (but not exclusively expressed during a Delirium). The symptoms may be those of any of the Anxiety
Disorders discussed in this section, but full criteria for a particular disorder need
not be met.

ASSOCIATED FEATURES AND PHYSICAL AND LABORATORY FINDINGS. Associated features and findings are those of the underlying general medical condition.

DIFFERENTIAL DIAGNOSIS. The symptoms are not merely psychological reactions
to the general medical condition but are caused by its physiological effects.
Symptoms seen exclusively during Delirium are coded elsewhere. Other Anxiety
Disorders and Adjustment Disorders should be ruled out. If one is uncertain
whether or not the symptoms are due to a general medical condition, Anxiety
Disorder NOS should be considered.

DIAGNOSTIC CRITERIA FOR ANXIETY DISORDER DUE TO . . . (SPECIFY GENERAL MEDICAL CONDITION) (293.89)

(ICD-10 code F06.4)

A. Prominent anxiety, Panic Attacks, or obsessions or compulsions dominate the clinical picture.

B. There is evidence from the history, physical examination, or laboratory findings that the disturbance is a direct physiological consequence of a general medical condition.

C. The disturbance is not better accounted for by another mental disorder (e.g., Adjustment Disorder With Anxiety in which the stressor is a serious medical condition).

D. The disturbance does not occur exclusively during the course of a delirium.

E. The disturbance causes clinically significant distress or impairment in social, occupational, or other important areas of functioning.

Specify if:
(depending on symptoms dominating the clinical presentation)
With Generalized Anxiety

With Panic Attacks

With Obsessive-Compulsive Symptoms

CODING NOTE: Include the name of the general medical condition in the Axis I diagnosis (e.g., 293.89, Anxiety Disorder Due to Pheochromocytoma, With Generalized Anxiety) and *also* code the general medical condition on Axis III. (See DSM-IV Appendix G for ICD-9-CM disease and E codes.)

❑ ❑ ❑ ❑

291.8, 292.89 Substance-Induced Anxiety Disorder
(includes substance-related Organic Anxiety Disorder, formerly 294.80 in DSM-III-R)
(new in DSM-IV)

(ICD-10 codes refer to substance codes)

NOTE: See special coding procedures under Diagnostic Criteria.

ESSENTIAL FEATURES. There is clinically significant anxiety directly caused by the physiological effects of a substance (e.g., drug of abuse or medication), including prescription use, poisoning, intoxication, or withdrawal. The symptoms may be those of any of the Anxiety Disorders already discussed, but full criteria for a particular disorder need not be met.

ASSOCIATED FEATURES AND PHYSICAL AND LABORATORY FINDINGS. Associated features and findings are those of the underlying substance, intoxication, or withdrawal syndrome.

DIFFERENTIAL DIAGNOSIS. The symptoms clearly exceed those usually associated with intoxication or withdrawal. They are not merely psychological reactions but are caused by physiological effects of the substance. If the patient is taking medication for a general medical condition, the clinician should be certain that condition is not the source of the anxiety. Other Anxiety Disorders and Adjustment Disorders should be ruled out. If one is uncertain whether or not the symptoms are substance induced, consider Anxiety Disorder NOS.

DIAGNOSTIC CRITERIA FOR SUBSTANCE-INDUCED ANXIETY DISORDER (291.8 or 292.89)

(ICD-10 codes refer to specific substance codes)

A. Prominent anxiety, Panic Attacks, or obsessions or compulsions dominate the clinical picture.

B. There is evidence from the history, physical examination, or laboratory findings of either (1) or (2):

(1) the symptoms in Criterion A developed during, or within 1 month of, Substance Intoxication or Withdrawal

(2) medication use is etiologically related to the disturbance

C. The disturbance is not better accounted for by an Anxiety Disorder that is not substance induced. Evidence that the symptoms are better accounted for by an Anxiety Disorder that is not substance induced might include the following: The symptoms precede the onset of the substance use (or medication use); the symptoms persist for a substantial period of time (e.g., about a month) after the cessation of acute withdrawal or severe intoxication or are substantially in excess of what would be expected given the type or amount of the substance used or the duration of use; or there is other evidence suggesting the existence of an independent non-substance-induced Anxiety Disorder (e.g., a history of recurrent non-substance-related episodes).

D. The disturbance does not occur exclusively during the course of a delirium.

E. The disturbance causes clinically significant distress or impairment in social, occupational, or other important areas of functioning.

> **Specify if:** (based on symptoms dominating the clinical presentation)
> With Generalized Anxiety
>
> With Panic Attacks
>
> With Obsessive-Compulsive Symptoms
>
> With Phobic Symptoms

Specify if:
With Onset During Intoxication: DSM-IV criteria are met for In-toxication and the anxiety symptoms develop during the intoxica-tion syndrome

With Onset During Withdrawal: DSM-IV criteria are met for With-drawal from the substance and the anxiety symptoms develop dur-ing, or shortly after, a withdrawal syndrome

(See table in DSM-IV, p.177, for applicability by substance.)

CODING NOTE: Code the (Specific Substance)-Induced Anxiety Disorder as follows: 291.8 Alcohol (ICD-10 F10.8); 292.89 Am-phetamine (or Related Substance) (ICD-10 F15.8), Caffeine (ICD-10 F15.8), Cannabis (ICD-10 F12.8), Cocaine (ICD-10 F14.8), Hallucinogen (ICD-10 F16.8), Inhalant (ICD-10 F18.8), Phencyclidine (or Related Substance) (ICD-10 F19.8), Sedative/Hypnotic/Anxiolytic, or Other or Unknown Substance (ICD-10 F15.8).

CODING NOTE: Also code Substance-Specific Intoxication or Withdrawal if criteria are met.

❑ ❑ ❑ ❑

300.00 Anxiety Disorder Not Otherwise Specified (NOS)
(ICD-10 code F41.9)

This category includes disorders with prominent, clinically significant anxiety or phobic avoidance that do not meet criteria for any specific Anxiety Disorder, Adjustment Disorder With Anxiety, or Adjustment Disorder With Mixed Anx-iety and Depressed Mood.

❑ ❑ ❑ ❑

DIFFERENCES BETWEEN DSM-III-R AND DSM-IV ANXIETY DISORDERS

❑ **Acute Stress Disorder** (308.3) is new in DSM-IV, as are diagnoses for **Substance-Induced Anxiety Disorder** and **Anxiety Disorder Due to a General Medical Condition.**

❑ **Agoraphobia** is similar but more specifically defined.

❑ **Panic Disorder Without Agoraphobia** is reorganized and more spe-cific, but generally similar. Severity of agoraphobic avoidance and Panic Attacks is no longer specified.

❑ In DSM-IV, DSM-III-R's simple phobia was renamed Specific Phobias. Types have been added, as have special considerations and duration criteria for children.

❑ **Social Phobia** incorporates DSM-III-R's Avoidant Disorder of Child-hood (formerly 313.21) by adding special considerations and duration criteria for children.

❑ **Obsessive-Compulsive Disorder** now has a specifier (With Poor In-sight). Definitions of obsession and compulsion are clearer but generally similar. One can now have a mental compulsion.

❑ **In Posttraumatic Stress Disorder,** the stressor is now defined in terms of the person's response to it and is no longer required to be "outside the range of normal human experience" (although it must be "extreme" and involve actual or threatened death, severe injury, or threat to physical integrity). Clinically significant distress or impairment is now required. Acute and chronic specifiers were added. **Note that PTSD is now coded 309.81.**

❑ In **Generalized Anxiety Disorder,** the symptom set (Criterion C) was simplified and is probably more reliable. The diagnosis now requires "excessive" anxiety and worry, no longer mentioning "unrealistic." Dif-ficulty controlling the worry must be present. DSM-III-R's Overanxious Disorder of Childhood (formerly 313.00) is now included under GAD, and special consideration has been added for children.

❑ **Anxiety Disorder Due to a General Medical Condition** is new in DSM-IV. Differences from DSM-III-R's non-substance-related Or-ganic Anxiety Disorder/syndrome (formerly 294.80) include the speci-fiers **With Generalized Anxiety, With Panic Attacks,** and **With Obsessive-Compulsive Symptoms** (based on symptoms dominating the clinical presentation).

❑ **Substance-Induced Anxiety Disorder** is new in DSM-IV. Differ-ences from DSM-III-R's substance/medication-related Organic Anxiety Disorder/syndrome (formerly 294.80) include the specifiers **With On-set During Intoxication** and **With Onset During Withdrawal,** as well as specifiers listed for Anxiety Disorder Due to a General Medical Condition (listed above).

CASE VIGNETTES: ANXIETY DISORDERS

Case Vignette 1

F.S. presents with extraordinary concern about the safety of his wife and young daughter. He rarely leaves them alone; when away (e.g., at work), he telephones home every hour. He has lost one job because of this, and his wife has threatened to leave him if he does not seek psychiatric help. Six months ago, the symptoms, which have been present for years, became worse after his wife had a serious automobile accident.

F.S. describes recurrent, unbidden thoughts in which dangerous events befall his family and he is not there to save them. He knows the thoughts are "silly" and that they come from his own mind rather than any real danger, but he cannot resist contacting his wife or daughter in some way to be certain they are safe. His wife has arranged to lift the telephone receiver briefly, then hang up, which is usually sufficient to allay his fears for an hour or so.

There is no history of significant medical illness or Substance Abuse. The patient completed 2 years of college and has a responsible job. He performs well, and is not particularly perfectionistic, overly conscientious (except with regard to his family's safety), rigid, or preoccupied with details.

DIAGNOSIS AND DISCUSSION

Axis I—300.3 Obsessive-Compulsive Disorder (ICD-10 code F42.8)
Axis II—V71.09 No Diagnosis or Condition on Axis II (ICD-10 code Z03.2)

F.S. has obsessive-compulsive symptoms, with superficial insight about them. There is no indication of Obsessive-Compulsive Personality Disorder, which is quite distinct from Axis I Obsessive-Compulsive Disorder. Criteria are not met for Posttraumatic Stress Disorder or any other Anxiety Disorder.

Case Vignette 2

For the past 6 months, H.P., a 35-year-old woman, has had increasing anxiety and occasional panic attacks. Although the anxiety and panic were initially not associated with any particular situation they are now associated with her work as a personnel director for a large corporation. When she goes to work, she often—sometimes more than once a week—has sudden attacks of nausea, perspiring, a feeling of unreality and impending doom, trembling, and dyspnea. These symptoms become quite intense within a few minutes and last less than half an hour. H.P. dreads the episodes, which are so uncomfortable that she occasionally prevents them by staying home rather than going to the office.

She has noticed that the episodes, which initially came randomly and unexpectedly, have recently become more specifically associated with certain responsibilities, such as board meetings and presentations to her superiors. H.P. denies any discomfort from the meetings and presentations themselves, saying that she enjoys her position, handles it well, and feels very comfortable as a member of the management team. She is not affected in ordinary social situations or while working with people in other settings. The patient has never had other psychiatric symptoms, enjoys a normal family life, and is in good health. She takes no medications, has a low caffeine intake, and denies drug or alcohol abuse. Physical examination, with thyroid tests and echocardiogram, is normal.

DIAGNOSIS AND DISCUSSION

Axis I—300.01 Panic Disorder Without Agoraphobia (ICD-10 code F41.0)
Axis II—V71.09 No Diagnosis or Condition on Axis II (ICD-10 code Z03.2)

H.P. has some agoraphobic symptoms, but there is really only one setting that precipitates the attacks. Her attacks meet the criteria for Panic Disorder, having at one time been unexpected (although they later became associated with specific work settings). They do not meet criteria for Social Phobia, Specific Phobia, or Generalized Anxiety Disorder because her fear is of the Panic Attacks, not (consciously) of a social or work situation itself. There is no mention of any precipitating psychosocial stressor. The fulfilled criteria for Panic Disorder preempt a diagnosis of Adjustment Disorder. Important organic considerations have been ruled out. She lacks chronic or pervasive symptoms of Personality Disorder.

CHAPTER 17

SOMATOFORM DISORDERS

Individuals with Somatoform Disorders report physical symptoms that suggest a general medical condition. However, thorough evaluation of the patient's complaint does not reveal a medical condition, Substance-Related Disorder, or another mental disorder that explains the individual's complaint, *or* any pathology found cannot explain the degree of impairment present. There is usually strong evidence, or a strong presumption, that the physical symptoms are connected to psychological factors or conflicts. The symptom production in Somatoform Disorders is not intentional (or conscious), unlike the symptoms reported in Malingering or Factitious Disorder.

300.81 Somatization Disorder (Briquet's Syndrome) (significantly modified from DSM-III-R)

(ICD-10 code F45.0)

ESSENTIAL FEATURES. There is a long-standing pattern of multiple, recurrent medical complaints without an apparent physical disorder or, if a general medical condition is present, complaints are in excess of what is expected. Complaints are often presented in a dramatic fashion, the medical history is complicated, and the complaint results in medical treatment or causes impairment. In the past, many medical diagnoses have been considered. This disorder begins before age 30, is quite rare in men, and has a chronic, fluctuating course. In order to make the diagnosis, there must be a history of pain reported from four different sites or functions (e.g., sexual intercourse). In addition to pain complaints, there must be a history of two gastrointestinal symptoms, one sexual symptom, and one pseudoneurological symptom.

ASSOCIATED FEATURES. The language used by these individuals is very graphic and exaggerated. For example, when asked about a relatively small cut that required a few stitches, the individual might say, "The doctor almost fainted when he saw so much bleeding!" These individuals see numerous doctors and often obtain consultations from well-known clinics. Anxious and depressed mood are frequent. Antisocial behavior, as well as occupational, interpersonal, and marital difficulties, is common. Nonbizarre hallucinations are sometimes reported, such as hearing one's name called. Personality Disorders (e.g., Antisocial, Borderline,

201

and Histrionic), Major Depressive Disorder, and Substance-Related Disorder are also frequently associated. There may be male first-degree relatives with Antisocial Personality Disorder or Substance-Related Disorders, and female relatives with Somatization Disorder.

DIFFERENTIAL DIAGNOSIS. The clinician must always be concerned about the possibility that an individual has an undiagnosed medical condition. After a medical disorder is eliminated as an explanation for physical complaints, rule out Anxiety Disorders, especially Panic Disorder, because anxiety frequently manifests itself through somatic symptoms (e.g., palpitations, sweating, shortness of breath, dizziness, etc.). Another diagnostic consideration is Schizophrenia, in which the somatic delusions are usually bizarre and alert the clinician to the more serious diagnosis.

Patients with Somatization Disorder have conversion symptoms; however, a person with Conversion Disorder does not have the other diffuse, multisystem medical complaints that are diagnostic of Somatization Disorder. Individuals with Mood Disorders, especially Major Depressive Disorders, frequently have somatic symptoms and exaggerated concerns about their bodies. One should also consider Factitious Disorder with Predominantly Physical Signs and Symptoms (i.e., the manufacturing of physical signs and symptoms in order to become a medical patient) and Malingering (i.e., lying about physical symptoms to obtain a particular goal, such as compensation).

DIAGNOSTIC CRITERIA FOR (ICD-10 code F45.0)
SOMATIZATION DISORDER (300.81)

A. A history of many physical complaints beginning before age 30 years that occur over a period of several years and result in treatment being sought or significant impairment in social, occupational, or other important areas of functioning.

B. Each of the following criteria must have been met, with individual symptoms occurring at any time during the course of the disturbance:

    (1) *four pain symptoms:* a history of pain related to at least four different sites or functions (e.g., head, abdomen, back, joints, extremities, chest, rectum, during menstruation, during sexual intercourse, or during urination)

    (2) *two gastrointestinal symptoms:* a history of at least two gastrointestinal symptoms other than pain (e.g., nausea, bloating, vomiting other than during pregnancy, diarrhea, or intolerance of several different foods)

    (3) *one sexual symptom:* a history of at least one sexual or reproductive symptom other than pain (e.g., sexual indifference, erectile or ejaculatory dysfunction, irregular menses, excessive menstrual bleeding, vomiting throughout pregnancy)

    (4) *one pseudoneurological symptom:* a history of at least one symptom or deficit suggesting a neurological condition not limited to pain (conversion symptoms such as impaired coordination or balance, paralysis or localized weakness, difficulty swallowing or lump in throat, aphonia, urinary retention, hallucinations, loss of touch or pain sensation, double vision, blindness, deafness, seizures; dissociative symptoms such as amnesia; or loss of consciousness other than fainting)

C. Either (1) or (2):

   (1) after appropriate investigation, none of the symptoms in Criterion B can be fully explained by a known general medical condition or the direct effects of a substance (e.g., a drug of abuse, a medication)

   (2) when there is a related general medical condition, the physical complaints or resulting social or occupational impairment are in excess of what would be expected from the history, physical examination, or laboratory findings

D. The symptoms are not intentionally feigned or produced (as in Factitious Disorder or Malingering).

❏ ❏ ❏ ❏

300.81 Undifferentiated Somatoform Disorder   (ICD-10 code F45.1)

ESSENTIAL FEATURES. This is a residual disorder that is diagnosed when an individual does not meet the full criteria for another Somatoform Disorder. *For at least a 6-month period* there is either a single symptom or, more commonly, multiple symptoms that are not explainable by a general medical disorder or the direct effects of a substance. Symptoms are apparently linked to psychological factors. Anxiety and depressed mood are commonly associated with the disorder.

DIFFERENTIAL DIAGNOSIS. Persons who present with physical complaints that are exaggerated or have no known medical origin often have a Somatoform Disorder. It is important to rule out Somatization Disorder. These individuals have a long-standing history of exaggerated physical symptoms, usually beginning during adolescence, which have no known medical origin. The medical history given by individuals who have Somatization Disorder is often selective; therefore, when this disorder is suspected, the clinician must gather all past medical records to make the diagnosis. If somatic complaints last 6 months or more and the full criteria for Somatization Disorder are not met, a diagnosis of Undifferentiated Somatoform Disorder is made. If the complaints are of shorter duration, a diagnosis of Somatoform Disorder Not Otherwise Specified is given.

Anxiety Disorders often are associated with physical symptoms and complaints. The clinician should determine whether or not the physical symptoms occur only during a Panic Attack. Individuals with General Anxiety Disorder worry and are anxious about many things (i.e., their worries are not exclusively focused on body function). Individuals with Mood Disorders, especially Depressive Disorders, often have body and pain complaints in association with a depressed mood. The person with Somatization Disorder or Undifferentiated Somatization Disorder has physical complaints regardless of, and separate from, mood states. The physical symptoms associated with Factitious Disorder and

Malingering are intentionally produced, although the motivations for symptoms are different. Individuals with Factitious Disorder desire to become patients, whereas the person with Malingering wants to escape punishment (e.g., avoid jail) or acquire some benefit (e.g., financial compensation).

DIAGNOSTIC CRITERIA FOR UNDIFFERENTIATED SOMATOFORM DISORDER (300.81)
(ICD-10 code F45.1)

A. One or more physical complaints (e.g., fatigue, loss of appetite, gastrointestinal or urinary complaints).

B. Either (1) or (2):

(1) after appropriate investigation, the symptoms cannot be fully explained by a known general medical condition or the direct effects of a substance (e.g., a drug of abuse, a medication)

(2) when there is a related general medical condition, the physical complaints or resulting social or occupational impairment is in excess of what would be expected from the history, physical examination, or laboratory findings

C. The symptoms cause clinically significant distress or impairment in social, occupational, or other important areas of functioning.

D. The duration of the disturbance is at least 6 months.

E. The disturbance is not better accounted for by another mental disorder (e.g., another Somatoform Disorder, Sexual Dysfunction, Mood Disorder, Anxiety Disorder, Sleep Disorder, or Psychotic Disorder).

F. The symptom is not intentionally produced or feigned (as in Factitious Disorder or Malingering).

▫ ▫ ▫ ▫

300.11 Conversion Disorder
(ICD-10 code F44.x)
(significantly modified from DSM-III-R)

ESSENTIAL FEATURES. The symptom is a voluntary motor or sensory loss (pseudoneurological) or a change of function that implies a physical disorder. The symptom cannot be explained by any known pathophysiological mechanism or general medical condition, and is not intentionally produced (as it is in Malingering or Factitious Disorder). The symptom is an expression of a psychological conflict or need. The complaint is not limited to pain or sexual dysfunction, nor is it merely one of the symptoms of Somatization Disorder or another mental disorder.

ASSOCIATED FEATURES. The symptom usually appears suddenly, with onset during times of extreme psychosocial stress. Associated mental disorders include Personality Disorders (especially Histrionic, Antisocial, and Dependent), Major Depressive Disorder, and Dissociative Disorders. Some individuals with Conversion Disorder show a marked lack of concern for their disability, called *la belle indifference,* and others are quite dramatic in exhibiting their disability.

DIFFERENTIAL DIAGNOSIS. Exercise clinical caution before making this diagnosis, because in a significant percentage of cases—33% in many studies—the individual diagnosed with Conversion Disorder will eventually display a neurologic or medical disorder that explains the original symptoms. The person with Somatization Disorder has conversion symptoms but will also have numerous somatic symptoms that involve other systems. Individuals with Dissociative Disorders will usually have selective physical complaints, such as amnesia and disturbances in identity. By definition, an individual with Pain Disorder has complaints that are limited to pain, and the pain complaints are either wholly psychologically based or are an exaggeration of complaints from a medical illness.

A person who experiences a Panic Attack typically has somatic and neurologic complaints. Remember that a Panic Attack occurs abruptly and is of short duration, whereas a Conversion Disorder is a relatively stable complaint that is usually not episodic, except for pseudoseizures. An individual with Schizophrenia or another Psychotic Disorder occasionally will have somatic symptoms, which are bizarre in nature, and the patient's explanation for the problem is often diagnostic (e.g., "The rays from Mars made my arm limp"). A person with Hypochondriasis has a particular complaint, such as constipation, and is not reassured by normal laboratory results or physical examinations. Individuals with Factitious Disorder desire to become patients, whereas the person with Malingering wants to escape punishment (e.g., avoid jail) or acquire some benefit (e.g., financial compensation).

> NOTE: A significant percentage of individuals diagnosed with Conversion Disorder will later be diagnosed with a general medical disorder that could explain the symptom (25 to 50% in older studies, less in more recent studies). Therefore, it is often prudent to specify that the diagnosis is "(Provisional)". An associated diagnosis of Somatization Disorder makes the diagnosis of Conversion Disorder much more likely to be correct.

DIAGNOSTIC CRITERIA FOR (ICD-10 code F44.x)
CONVERSION DISORDER (300.11)

A. One or more symptoms or deficits affecting voluntary motor or sensory function that suggest a neurological or other general medical condition.

B. Psychological factors are judged to be associated with the symptom or deficit because the initiation or exacerbation of the symptom or deficit is preceded by conflicts or other stressors.

C. The symptom or deficit is not intentionally produced or feigned (as in Factitious Disorder or Malingering).

D. The symptom or deficit cannot, after appropriate investigation, be fully explained by a general medical condition, or by the direct effects of a substance, or as a culturally sanctioned behavior or experience.

E. The symptom or deficit causes clinically significant distress or impairment in social, occupational, or other important areas of functioning or warrants medical evaluation.

F. The symptom or deficit is not limited to pain or sexual dysfunction, does not occur exclusively during the course of Somatization Disorder, and is not better accounted for by another mental disorder.

Specify type of symptom or deficit:
With Motor Symptom or Deficit

With Sensory Symptom or Deficit

With Seizures or Convulsions

With Mixed Presentation

❑ ❑ ❑ ❑

307.xx Pain Disorder   *(ICD-10 code F45.4)*
(significantly modified from DSM-III-R)

ESSENTIAL FEATURES. There is a preoccupation with pain and the pain causes significant distress or impairment. In addition, psychological factors are felt to play a significant role in the pain.

ASSOCIATED FEATURES. The individual frequently visits physicians, uses excessive pain medications, and assumes an invalid's role. Surgery may already have been performed or may be desired by the patient. A search for a "cure" is not unusual. The person usually denies that psychological factors have any role in the pain. Depressed mood is common and an associated diagnosis of Major Depression is warranted in many cases. Pain Disorders are frequently associated with insomnia. Persistent pain often develops following physical trauma. Some persons with Pain Disorder began working at an early age, had physically demanding jobs, were "workaholics," and rarely took vacations.

DIFFERENTIAL DIAGNOSIS. An exaggerated or dramatic presentation of pain can occur with an acutely worsening medical condition because the patient is anxious and afraid. Pain is a symptom that, by definition, occurs as part of Somatization Disorder. The individual's medical history and records will show many other physical symptoms without a medical explanation, as well as other exaggerated symptoms. Pain is a common complaint of persons who have a Depressive Disorder. The clinician must correlate the person's depressed mood with pain complaints to see if a relationship exists.

Pain can also occur with Anxiety or Psychotic Disorders. In the latter case, the pain complaints are often bizarre, or the individual's rationale for the pain uncovers the psychosis. The pain complaints associated with Factitious Disorder and Malingering are intentionally produced, although the motivations for symptoms are different. Individuals with Factitious Disorder desire to become patients; whereas, the person with Malingering wants to escape punishment (e.g., avoid jail) or acquire some benefit (e.g., financial compensation).

DIAGNOSTIC CRITERIA FOR PAIN DISORDER (307.xx) (SEE SUBTYPES BELOW)

(ICD-10 code F45.4)

A. Pain in one or more anatomical sites is the predominant focus of the clinical presentation and is of sufficient severity to warrant clinical attention.

B. The pain causes clinically significant distress or impairment in social, occupational, or other important areas of functioning.

C. Psychological factors are judged to have an important role in the onset, severity, exacerbation, or maintenance of the pain.

D. The symptom or deficit is not intentionally produced or feigned (as in Factitious Disorder or Malingering).

E. The pain is not better accounted for by a Mood, Anxiety, or Psychotic Disorder and does not meet criteria for Dyspareunia.

Specify subtype:
307.80 Pain Disorder Associated With Psychological Factors: psychological factors are judged to have the major role in the onset, severity, exacerbation, or maintenance of the pain. (If a general medical condition is present, it does not have a major role in the onset, severity, exacerbation, or maintenance of the pain.) This type of Pain Disorder is not diagnosed if criteria are also met for Somatization Disorder. (ICD-10 Code F45.4)

Specify subtype:
Acute: duration less than 6 months
Chronic: duration more than 6 months

307.89 Pain Disorder Associated With Both Psychological Factors and a General Medical Condition: both psychological factors and a general medical condition are judged to have important roles in the onset, severity, exacerbation, or maintenance of the pain. The associated general medical condition or anatomical site of the pain is coded on Axis III (see following). (ICD-10 code F45.4)

Specify subtype:
Acute: duration less than 6 months
Chronic: duration more than 6 months

CODING NOTE: Pain Disorder Associated With a General Medical Condition, in which a general medical condition has a major role in the onset, severity, exacerbation, or maintenance of the pain (and psychological factors, if present, are not judged to have a major role in the onset, severity, exacerbation, or maintenance of the pain), is coded on Axis III only. It is not considered a mental disorder.

CODING NOTE: The Axis III diagnostic code for the pain is based on the associated general medical condition if one has been established (see DSM-IV Appendix G) or on the anatomical location of the pain if the underlying general medical condition is not yet clearly established (e.g., low back [724.2], sciatic [724.3], pelvic [625.9], headache [784.0], facial [784.0], chest [786.50], joint [719.4], bone [733.90], abdominal [789.0], breast [611.71], renal [788.0], ear [388.70], eye [379.91], throat [784.1], tooth [525.9], and urinary [788.0]).

❑ ❑ ❑ ❑

300.7 Hypochondriasis   (ICD-10 code F45.2)

ESSENTIAL FEATURES. The person has an enduring (of at least 6 months' duration), nondelusional belief or fear that he or she has a serious illness. The person is not reassured by appropriate clinical investigation that fails to confirm the illness. The symptoms must be differentiated from those of a Panic Attack.

ASSOCIATED FEATURES. The hypochondriacal individual usually presents his or her medical history in great detail. The person is often frustrated and angry with physicians. Doctor shopping and poor physician-patient relationships are common. Anxiety and Depressive Disorders are frequently observed. Past exposure to true disease and psychosocial stressors apparently predispose to this disorder. The course is usually chronic, with waxing and waning symptoms.

DIFFERENTIAL DIAGNOSIS. An individual preoccupation with a physical symptom or complaint may represent a response to a legitimate, undiagnosed medical condition. For this reason, a thorough medical evaluation is important. In addition, the clinician must rule out many other psychiatric disorders prior to a diagnosis of Hypochondriasis. If an individual has psychotic or delusional body concerns, a diagnosis of a Psychotic Disorder (i.e., Delusional Disorder, Somatic Type, or Schizophrenia) or Major Depressive Disorder With Psychotic Features is considered. Anxiety Disorders, especially Panic Disorder and General Anxiety Disorder, are associated with somatic and other worries.

The individual with Obsessive-Compulsive Disorder can ruminate about physical complaints; however, other obsessions and compulsions are present. A person with Separation Anxiety Disorder can develop physical complaints (e.g., abdominal pain). An individual can have a disease phobia, but the fear is of exposure to or acquiring the disease, whereas the person with Hypochondriasis believes he or she already has the disease. The other Somatoform Disorders (i.e., Somatization Disorder, Body Dysmorphic Disorder, etc.) are also considered in the differential diagnosis.

DIAGNOSTIC CRITERIA FOR HYPOCHONDRIASIS (300.7)

(ICD-10 code F45.2)

A. Preoccupation with fears of having, or the idea that one has, a serious disease based on the person's misinterpretation of bodily symptoms.

B. The preoccupation persists despite appropriate medical evaluation and reassurance.

C. The belief in Criterion A is not of delusional intensity (as in Delusional Disorder, Somatic Type) and is not restricted to a circumscribed concern about appearance (as in Body Dysmorphic Disorder).

D. The preoccupation causes clinically significant distress or impairment in social, occupational, or other important areas of functioning.

E. The duration of the disturbance is at least 6 months.

F. The preoccupation is not better accounted for by Generalized Anxiety Disorder, Obsessive-Compulsive Disorder, Panic Disorder, a Major Depressive Episode, Separation Anxiety, or another Somatoform Disorder.

> **Specify if:**
> **With Poor Insight:** if, for most of the time during the current episode, the person does not recognize that the concern about having a serious illness is excessive or unreasonable

□ □ □ □

300.7 Body Dysmorphic Disorder (Dysmorphophobia)
(ICD-10 code F45.2)

(significantly modified from DSM-III-R)

ESSENTIAL FEATURES. There is marked preoccupation either with some imagined defect in appearance or, if a physical abnormality is present, the individual's concern is grossly exaggerated. In some individuals, the clinician must ensure that the somatic preoccupation is not part of another psychiatric disorder, such as Anorexia Nervosa or Gender Identity Disorder.

(94)

ASSOCIATED FEATURES. Patients may check their appearance frequently or may avoid mirrors to decrease anxiety. Repeated visits to surgeons or dermatologists in an attempt to correct the defect are common. Ideas of reference related to the "ugliness" are also common. Social or occupational situations where others might see the imagined defect may be avoided; extreme social isolation may result. Individuals are often reluctant to discuss their symptoms, especially with mental health professionals.

DIFFERENTIAL DIAGNOSIS. Excessive concerns about appearance, especially among adolescents, can be considered normal. When this concern causes significant impairment, a psychiatric disorder is often present. Individuals who have a Major Depressive Disorder occasionally develop exaggerated or even bizarre somatic concerns. The associated depressed mood and other neurovegetative symptoms help to establish the diagnosis.

Individuals who are extremely self-conscious, such as those with Avoidant Personality Disorder or a Social Phobia, also manifest exaggerated concerns about their appearance. Obsessive body concerns can occur with Obsessive-Compulsive Disorder (OCD), Anorexia Nervosa, and Gender Identity Disorder. The individual with OCD has numerous obsessions and compulsions that are not limited to the body. The person with Anorexia Nervosa is focused on fatness, and the person with Gender Identity Disorder is focused on sexual characteristics.

> NOTE: If the individual's preoccupation is of delusional intensity, an additional diagnosis of Delusional Disorder (Somatic Type) can be made.

DIAGNOSTIC CRITERIA FOR (ICD-10 code F45.2)
BODY DYSMORPHIC DISORDER (300.7)

A. Preoccupation with an imagined defect in appearance. If a slight physical anomaly is present, the person's concern is markedly excessive.

B. The preoccupation causes clinically significant distress or impairment in social, occupational, or other important areas of functioning.

C. The preoccupation is not better accounted for by another mental disorder (e.g., dissatisfaction with body shape and size in Anorexia Nervosa).

❑ ❑ ❑ ❑

300.81 Somatoform Disorder Not Otherwise Specified (NOS) (ICD-10 code F45.9)

ESSENTIAL FEATURES. Somatoform symptoms exist that do not meet the criteria for any specific Somatoform Disorder. Examples include nonpsychotic somatoform symptoms of less than 6 months' duration, such as fatigue or pseudocyesis.

❑ ❑ ❑ ❑

DIFFERENCES BETWEEN DSM-III-R AND DSM-IV SOMATOFORM DISORDERS

❑ The DSM-IV symptom list for **Somatization Disorder** was reduced significantly and is now organized into eight symptoms in four groups. These are pain (4), gastrointestinal (2), sexual (1), and pseudoneurological (1) symptoms.

❑ The diagnostic criteria for **Conversion Disorder** were narrowed to include only voluntary motor or sensory symptoms. Four subtypes were added.

❑ DSM-III-R's Somatoform Pain Disorder was replaced by **Pain Disorder**. Two types of Pain Disorder are defined: **With Psychological Factors** and **Associated With Both Psychological Factors and a General Medical Condition**. **Acute** (duration less than 6 months) and **Chronic** (6 months or longer) specifiers were added.

❑ **Hypochondriasis** now has the specifier **With Poor Insight** if the individual has little or no recognition of the unreasonable nature of his or her disease concerns.

❑ The phrase "not of delusional intensity" was eliminated from the DSM-III-R diagnostic criteria for **Body Dysmorphic Disorder**. In DSM-IV, the clinician can make this diagnosis *and* diagnose Delusional Disorder, Somatic Type in the same individual.

CASE VIGNETTE: SOMATOFORM DISORDERS

Case Vignette

P.S. is a 32-year-old woman who is currently hospitalized on a general medical ward for evaluation of right-side paralysis. The attending physician requested a psychiatric consultation when no medical reason for the paralysis was found.

On examination, P.S. is initially quite upset that anyone doubted the medical nature of her complaints. She reports the sudden onset of right-side problems while she and her boyfriend were talking with a lawyer. According to her, this complaint occurred once before: "They thought I had a stroke." She is quite dramatic in her presentation and describes a long, complex medical history. She denies prior psychiatric hospitalizations or contact with other mental health professionals, and denies drug or alcohol abuse or Panic Attacks. Her family history includes a father who was an alcoholic (she is unfamiliar with his recent whereabouts) and a brother who is currently in prison.

Review of P.S.'s many medical records reveals numerous hospitalizations and medical evaluations for a wide variety of complaints. Complaints that resulted in past hospitalizations or medical evaluations include vomiting, chronic diarrhea, chronic abdominal pain, "crippling" migraines, dysuria, shortness of breath, amnesia, double vision, loss of consciousness, seizures, paralysis (on three different occasions), dyspareunia, dysmenorrhea, dysphagia, menometror-rhagia (irregular and excessive periods), and blindness. Despite numerous extensive medical evaluations, no organic reasons were found for any of her complaints.

DIAGNOSIS AND DISCUSSION

Axis I—300.81 Somatization Disorder (ICD-10 code F45.0)
Axis II—799.9 Diagnosis Deferred (ICD-10 code R46.8)
Axis III—No Known General Medical Condition

P.S. presents in a dramatic fashion, and has a long-standing, medically complex history. She has multiorgan complaints and no evidence of any medical conditions. P.S. has all the clinical features necessary for the diagnosis of Somatization Disorder. She also meets the criteria for Conversion Disorder; however, this diagnosis is not made during the course of a more pervasive disorder, such as Somatization Disorder. The Axis II diagnosis is deferred pending additional information and observation.

CHAPTER 18

FACTITIOUS DISORDERS

300.16, 300.19 Factitious Disorder (*ICD-10 code F68.1*)
(significantly modified from DSM-III-R)

> CODING NOTE: When physical symptoms predominate, code 300.19, not 301.51 as in DSM-III-R.

ESSENTIAL FEATURES. Factitious Disorders are characterized by the intentional production of physical or psychological symptoms, not motivated by obvious external gain. The patient may lie about subjective symptoms, injure himself or herself, ingest medication, or exaggerate or exacerbate a preexisting condition. The behavior is voluntary in the sense that the act is intentional but involuntary in the sense that the impulse usually cannot be controlled. The unconscious goal is apparently to assume a "sick" role. Factitious Disorders are not Malingering, in which the goal is an externally recognizable objective (for example, money, drugs, avoiding imprisonment or military duty). The presence of factitious symptoms does not preclude true physical or psychological symptoms. The diagnosis of Factitious Disorder always implies psychopathology, frequently a severe personality disturbance.

ASSOCIATED FEATURES. Use of drugs to create symptoms, a history of multiple unnecessary hospitalizations (Munchausen syndrome), and scars or other iatrogenic sequelae of unnecessary treatment are commonly seen. The disorder is often associated with medical employment (e.g., as a nurse) and/or generally unstable social adaptation (e.g., frequent moves to avoid detection). Substance Abuse (see Differential Diagnosis) and lying to avoid detection may be seen. Lying is sometimes dramatic and pathological (*pseudologia fantastica*). Extensive treatment for childhood illness or important (positive or negative) past relationships with the medical profession may predispose one to Factitious Disorder.

DIFFERENTIAL DIAGNOSIS. True physical or mental disorders, Somatoform Disorders, Schizophrenia or Delusional Disorder, and Malingering are considered. Substance Abuse related to creating symptoms or treatment for a factitious syndrome should be differentiated from that which is associated with Malingering.

DIAGNOSTIC CRITERIA FOR
FACTITIOUS DISORDER (300.16, 300.19)

(ICD-10 code F68.1)

A. Intentional production or feigning of physical or psychological signs or symptoms.

B. The motivation for the behavior is to assume the sick role.

C. External incentives for the behavior (such as economic gain, avoiding legal responsibility, or improving physical well-being, as in Malingering) are absent.

> **Code based on type (ICD-10 code does not change):**
> **300.16 With Predominantly Psychological Signs and Symptoms:** psychological signs and symptoms predominate
>
> **300.19 With Predominantly Physical Signs and Symptoms:** physical signs and symptoms predominate
>
> **300.19 With Combined Psychological and Physical Signs and Symptoms:** both psychological and physical signs and symptoms are present; neither predominates

❑ ❑ ❑ ❑

300.19 Factitious Disorder Not Otherwise Specified (NOS)

(ICD-10 code F68.1)

This category is for factitious symptoms that do not meet criteria for a specific Factitious Disorder (e.g., Factitious Disorder by proxy, in which signs or symptoms are produced in another person who is under the individual's care). (See suggested research criteria in Appendix B of DSM-IV.)

❑ ❑ ❑ ❑

DIFFERENCES BETWEEN DSM-III-R
AND DSM-IV FACTITIOUS DISORDERS

Factitious Disorder With Predominantly Physical Symptoms is now coded 300.19 rather than 301.51. The three forms of Factitious Disorder are considered subtypes rather than separate disorders. Mixing of symptoms and signs is allowed by the modifier "Predominantly."

CASE VIGNETTE: FACTITIOUS DISORDERS

Case Vignette

J.M., a 28-year-old nurse who never married is referred for psychiatric consultation during hospitalization for a bleeding disorder. According to the internist, she has been evaluated many times and there seems to be no reasonable explanation for her disorder except ingestion of an anticoagulant. A bottle of Coumadin was found hidden in her hospital bathroom.

During the interview, J.M. is oriented and nonpsychotic but displays constant and dramatic anger. She adamantly denies taking, or owning, the Coumadin. She denies past psychiatric treatment, Substance Abuse, or family history of psychiatric problems. She does describe childhood abuse by both parents, chaotic relationships with others, chronic boredom and unhappiness with her career, and threats of suicide on several occasions. She says that she once dated and "almost married" a prominent cardiac surgeon.

DIAGNOSIS AND DISCUSSION

Axis I—300.19 Factitious Disorder With Predominantly Physical Signs and Symptoms (ICD-10 code F68.1)

Axis II—799.9 The patient may meet criteria for Borderline Personality Disorder. Code a provisional diagnosis or "Diagnosis Deferred" (ICD-10 code R46.8).

Axis III—Bleeding Disorder Secondary to Warfarin Ingestion

CHAPTER 19

DISSOCIATIVE DISORDERS

The Dissociative Disorders are all characterized by a disturbance or alteration in the normally integrative functions of identity, memory, or consciousness. Various forms of dissociation may be seen in a number of other Axis I disorders (e.g., Posttraumatic Stress Disorder, Somatization Disorder, Conversion Disorder). Although Sleepwalking Disorder has some similar features, it is classified as a Sleep Disorder.

> NOTE: If dissociative symptoms occur solely during the course of Posttraumatic Stress Disorder, Acute Stress Disorder, Somatization Disorder, Conversion Disorder, or a Sleep Disorder, those diagnoses preempt any diagnosis of Dissociative Disorder.

Nonpathological manifestations of dissociation in some religions and cultures should not be confused with Dissociative Disorders. On the other hand, if they become clinically significant, a diagnosis is warranted. DSM-IV lists criteria for a proposed Dissociative Trance Disorder in its Appendix B (see p. 221 of this book), and discusses several culture-bound syndromes in Appendix I. Dissociative traits and disorders are often associated with high scores on tests of hypnotizability.

Severe psychosocial stress (especially severe physical threat or internal conflict), wartime, and natural disaster predispose susceptible persons to dissociative syndromes and disorders.

300.12 Dissociative Amnesia   *(ICD-10 code F44.0)*
(Psychogenic Amnesia in DSM-III-R)

ESSENTIAL FEATURES. There is sudden, extensive loss of memory. The diagnosis is not made if the person travels to a new locale and/or assumes a new identity, or if the amnesia is related to Dissociative Identity Disorder. The memory loss must be extensive; simple forgetfulness is not included here. Traumatic memories are most often affected. The loss is, by definition, reversible. The most common presentation involves realization of gaps in past memory related to some trauma or stress. Acute memory loss, generally related to violent trauma or disaster, is less common.

ASSOCIATED FEATURES. During the amnestic period there may be indifference toward memory disturbance (cf., *la belle indifférence*). DSM-IV mentions several types of memory loss that may occur, including **localized** (failure to recall things that happened during a particular time period), **selective** (ability to recall only part of the events during the [usually traumatic] period), **generalized** (rare loss of memory of one's entire life), **continuous** (loss of recall from some past time to, and including, the present), and **systematized** (inability to remember particular types or categories of information).

DIFFERENTIAL DIAGNOSIS. Substance-Related Disorders, such as those found in alcohol blackouts (usually differentiated by incomplete return of memory), Substance-Induced Persisting Amnestic Disorder, and Amnestic Disorders Due to a General Medical Condition (such as a **cerebral insult, anesthesia, neurosurgery** or **ictal/postictal syndrome**, including the transient amnesia often seen after electroconvulsive therapy) preempt Dissociative Amnesia. The presence of generalized, continuous, or systematized amnesia (see above) may suggest a more severe Dissociative Disorder, such as Dissociative Identity Disorder. Catatonic stupor sometimes mimics Dissociative Amnesia. Malingering and Factitious Disorders must be differentiated as well.

DIAGNOSTIC CRITERIA FOR (ICD-10 code F44.0)
DISSOCIATIVE AMNESIA (300.12)

A. The predominant disturbance is one or more episodes of inability to recall important personal information, usually of a traumatic or stressful nature, that is too extensive to be explained by ordinary forgetfulness.

B. The disturbance does not occur exclusively during the course of Dissociative Identity Disorders, Dissociative Fugue, Posttraumatic Stress Disorder, Acute Stress Disorder, or Somatization Disorder and is not due to the direct effects of a substance (e.g., a drug of abuse, a medication) or a neurological or other general medical condition (e.g., Amnestic Disorder Due to Head Trauma).

C. The symptoms cause clinically significant distress or impairment in social, occupational, or other important areas of functioning.

❑ ❑ ❑ ❑

300.13 Dissociative Fugue (ICD-10 code F44.1)
(significantly modified from DSM-III-R);
(Psychogenic Fugue in DSM-III-R)

ESSENTIAL FEATURES. Dissociative Fugue is characterized by sudden, unexpected travel and a loss of memory for a significant portion of the past. Except for amnesia, the person usually does not appear unusual during the fugue. There may be no recollection following recovery of events that took place during the fugue. In some cases, the episode includes assumption of a new identity (without

97

memory of the old one); in others, there is little more than brief, apparently purposeful travel.

PREDISPOSING FACTORS. Heavy alcohol use and severe psychosocial stress are among the predisposing factors. The disorder is more common in wartime or in the wake of a major disaster.

DIFFERENTIAL DIAGNOSIS. Alcohol blackouts, Dissociative Identity Disorder, Dissociative Amnesia, Malingering, and Factitious Disorder With Psychological Features are considered. Similar syndromes caused by a general medical condition, trauma or substance toxicity, especially in the elderly, must also be differentiated.

DIAGNOSTIC CRITERIA FOR DISSOCIATIVE FUGUE (300.13)

(ICD-10 code F44.1)

A. The predominant disturbance is sudden, unexpected travel away from home or one's customary place of work, with inability to recall one's past.

B. Confusion about personal identity or assumption of new identity (partial or complete).

C. The disturbance does not occur exclusively during the course of Dissociative Identity Disorder and is not due to the direct physiological effects of a substance (e.g., a drug of abuse, a medication) or a general medical condition (e.g., temporal lobe epilepsy).

D. The symptoms cause clinically significant distress or impairment in social, occupational, or other important areas of functioning.

□ □ □ □

300.14 Dissociative Identity Disorder
(significantly modified from DSM-III-R)
(Multiple Personality Disorder in DSM-III-R)

(ICD-10 code F44.81)

ESSENTIAL FEATURES. There are two or more distinct identities (called "personalities" in DSM-III-R) or personality states within one person, which govern one's behavior at different times. Although it is tempting to define *identity* as similar to personality, DSM-IV does not do so. The hallmark of this disorder is a failure to integrate identity, memory, and consciousness.

The patient experiences a feeling of separate "personality states" within the self, each of which has some characteristics of an entire identity (e.g., memories, traits, attitudes), and one or more of which may be felt as an entire additional "person." The individual identities may be quite different or may differ only in their approaches to a problem area (e.g., sexuality). At least some of the alternative identities, at some time and recurrently, appear to take control of the patient's behavior. The transition is usually sudden.

In classic cases, probably very rare, there are at least two fully developed personalities. In others, more common and not universally accepted as so-called multiple personality, there is one distinct identity and one or more personality states. Each identity may be aware of some or all of the others, to varying degrees, and may experience them as friends or adversaries. Most are aware of lost periods of time or distortion in the experience of time.

Sometimes, symptoms and background information suggestive of multiple personality states are discovered only after outside suggestion, hypnosis, or other memory-retrieval techniques. In such cases, since the "memories" and other products of such techniques are often unreliable, a diagnosis of Dissociative Identity Disorder should be made only with great caution.

ASSOCIATED AND PREDISPOSING FEATURES. One or more of the identities may appear to be dysfunctional or to have a specific mental disorder while another appears relatively healthy. The patient has usually given each of the personalities a different name, which may have some symbolic meaning. Symptoms suggesting delayed posttraumatic reactions are often seen. Personality Disorders (e.g., Borderline Personality) are common, but one probably should not assume that Dissociative Identity Disorder is always associated with them. Many other Axis I disorders are often reported in these patients. Patients are usually quite suggestible, and score high on tests of hypnotizability. The disorder is very often—perhaps almost always—preceded by severe child abuse (often sexual abuse) or other serious emotional trauma in childhood. Women greatly outnumber men with the disorder.

DIFFERENTIAL DIAGNOSIS. Dissociative Identity Disorder preempts other Dissociative Disorders, such as Dissociative Fugue, Dissociative Amnesia, and Depersonalization Disorder. Syndromes, often culturally based, that include the belief that one is "possessed" by external persons or forces should not suggest this disorder. Several Personality Disorders, including Borderline Personality Disorder, may either mimic or coexist with Dissociative Identity Disorder. The distinction between this and some other disorders, especially Psychotic Disorders, is a matter of clinical dispute. A clear description of the dissociative and anmestic aspects of the history and presentation is important in differentiating it from, for example, a Psychotic Disorder. Malingering and Factitious Disorder With Psychological Features can be hard to differentiate from Dissociative Identity Disorder.

> NOTE: Although some clinicians caution against underdiagnosis of this disorder, many authorities feel that Dissociative Identity Disorder is extremely rare, and that most presentations are either subcategories of Psychotic or Borderline Disorders or inappropriately precipitated and diagnosed on the basis of (often faulty) information about past memories or events.

DIAGNOSTIC CRITERIA FOR   (ICD-10 code F44.81)
DISSOCIATIVE IDENTITY DISORDER (300.14)

A. The presence of two or more distinct identities or personality states (each with its own relatively enduring pattern of perceiving, relating to, and thinking about the environment and self).

B. At least two of these identities or personality states recurrently take control of the person's behavior.

C. Inability to recall important personal information that is too extensive to be explained by ordinary forgetfulness.

D. The disturbance is not due to the direct effects of a substance (e.g., blackouts or chaotic behavior during Alcohol Intoxication) or a general medical condition (e.g., complex partial seizures).

> **NOTE: In children, the symptoms must not be attributable to imaginary playmates or other fantasy play.**

❑ ❑ ❑ ❑

300.6 Depersonalization Disorder   (ICD-10 code F48.1)

ESSENTIAL FEATURES. There is persistent or recurrent depersonalization (a feeling of detachment or estrangement from oneself), with intact reality testing but severe enough to cause marked distress. It is not uncommon to hear patients describe feeling as if they were robots, in a dream, or somehow detached from (even outside of) their bodies.

ASSOCIATED FEATURES. Derealization, depression, rumination, somatic concerns, anxiety, and disturbance of a sense of time are often seen, as is the fear that one is "going crazy."

PREDISPOSING FACTORS. Predisposing factors often include severe stress.

DIFFERENTIAL DIAGNOSIS. Simple, even recurrent symptoms of Depersonalization that do not cause social or occupational impairment, such as those seen frequently in young adults, must be distinguished from this disorder. Depression may include periods of apathy and ennui. If the depersonalization is merely a symptom of another disorder, such as a Psychotic Disorder (in which reality testing is usually impaired), Sleep Disorder, or Anxiety Disorder (e.g., part of a Panic Attack), or is the direct physiologic result of a substance or general medical condition, Depersonalization Disorder should not be diagnosed. As in the other Dissociative Disorders, the subjective nature of the symptoms makes it important to consider Malingering and Factitious Disorder.

DIAGNOSTIC CRITERIA FOR DEPERSONALIZATION DISORDER (300.6)

(ICD-10 code F48.1)

A. Persistent or recurrent experiences of feeling detached from, and as if one is an outside observer·of, one's mental processes or body (e.g., feeling as if one is in a dream).

B. Reality testing remains intact during the depersonalization experience.

C. The depersonalization causes clinically significant distress or impairment in social, occupational, or other important areas of functioning.

D. The depersonalization experience does not appear exclusively during the course of another mental disorder, such as Schizophrenia, Panic Disorder, Acute Stress Disorder, or another Dissociative Disorder, and is not due to the direct effects of a substance (e.g., a drug of abuse, a medication) or a general medical condition (e.g., temporal lobe epilepsy).

❑ ❑ ❑ ❑

300.15 Dissociative Disorder Not Otherwise Specified (NOS)

(ICD-10 code F44.9)

These are disorders in which the predominant feature is a disturbance or alteration in the normally integrative functions of identity, memory, or consciousness, but which do not meet criteria for a specific Dissociative Disorder.

Examples include Ganser's syndrome, trance states (such as those that occur following abuse or trauma in children), states related to brainwashing or indoctrination, loss of consciousness without medical explanation, and other clinically significant dissociative states in which the symptoms are insufficient to meet all of the criteria for the diagnoses outlined above. DSM-IV particularly emphasizes Dissociative Trance Disorder, in which regionally or culturally related "possession" or trance, often with accompanying movements or ritual, appears to come from outside oneself. The condition is not accepted as a "normal" part of the culture (see Suggested Research Criteria, p. 728).

DIFFERENCES BETWEEN DSM-III-R AND DSM-IV DISSOCIATIVE DISORDERS

❑ DSM-III-R's Psychogenic Amnesia is now **Dissociative Amnesia**.

❑ In **Dissociative Fugue** (formerly Psychogenic Fugue), the criteria no longer require a change in name or identity.

❑ DSM-III-R's Multiple Personality Disorder is now **Dissociative Identity Disorder**, and criteria now require that the patient be unable to recall important personal information (as stipulated in DSM-III but deleted from DSM-III-R).

❑ A requirement that symptoms cause clinically significant distress or impairment, or interfere with social, occupational, or other important areas of functioning was added to several of the disorders.

....

CASE VIGNETTE: DISSOCIATIVE DISORDERS

Case Vignette

While checking into a motel on a fishing trip, T.R., a 36-year-old man, was distressed to find that he apparently had someone else's wallet and credit cards, and had inexplicably lost his own. While talking with the manager to arrange payment, it became apparent that he had no identifying cards or papers, he resembled the person whose picture was on the "other person's" driver's license, and—from documents in the glove box—he was driving the "other person's" car. Subsequently it was determined that T.R. was actually the "other person," and had unexpectedly left his place of work that morning.

A detailed history revealed no prior serious psychiatric symptoms. He had had no episodes of unconsciousness or altered consciousness, to his knowledge, in the past. He had been a sales manager with the same firm for 6 years, was married, and had two adolescent children. There had been some recent marital problems, and his 17-year-old son was arrested for breaking and entering on the day before the "fishing trip." The patient had a past history of significant alcohol intake, but there was no evidence of recent drinking and he was not intoxicated at the motel. Indeed, he declined a drink the manager offered him in an effort to help him "calm down while we figure this thing out." The physical workup was essentially normal.

DIAGNOSIS AND DISCUSSION
Axis I—300.13 Dissociative Fugue (ICD-10 F44.1)
Axis II—V71.09 No Diagnosis or Condition Apparent on Axis II (ICD-10 Z03.2)

This appears to be an obvious Dissociative Disorder, apparently precipitated by severe psychosocial stress, with no sign of underlying Psychotic Disorder or neurological disease. The dissociative episode was not part of an alcoholic blackout. Although another "person" was created, it does not meet criteria for Multiple Personality Disorder. The purposeful behavior and apparent creation of a new identity are inconsistent with Dissociative Amnesia. There is no indication of Malingering. Although probably a reaction to psychosocial stressors, other criteria for Adjustment Disorder are not met. Available evidence does not suggest a Personality Disorder, although the code for Deferred Axis II Diagnosis or Condition (799.9) would also be correct.

CHAPTER 20

SEXUAL AND GENDER IDENTITY DISORDERS

The Sexual Disorders are divided into three groups. The Sexual Dysfunctions are characterized by inhibitions in sexual desire or dysfunction of the psychophysiological changes that characterize the sexual response cycle. The Paraphilias are characterized by arousal in response to sexual objects or situations not part of normal arousal-activity patterns, and which may interfere with a capacity for reciprocal, affectionate sexual activity. The Gender Identity Disorders are characterized by distinct and continuous identification with the opposite sex and persistent discomfort with one's own.

SEXUAL DYSFUNCTIONS

The Sexual Dysfunctions listed below are all characterized by disturbances of the desire or psychophysiological components of the sexual response cycle. These diagnoses are ordinarily applied only when the disturbance is a major part of the clinical presentation (although it may not be the chief complaint). Whether or not the complaint/symptom is a diagnosable disorder depends largely on the extent to which it troubles the patient, on the clinician's judgment, and, in many disorders, on the adequacy of sexual stimulation. For some patients, multiple Sexual Dysfunction diagnoses are appropriate.

The Sexual Dysfunctions are divided into disorders related to **sexual desire, sexual arousal, orgasm,** and **sexual pain.** The first three of these correspond to the first three phases of the **sexual response cycle:**

1. Desire (including fantasies) for sexual activity
2. Excitement (arousal, physiological changes such as erection or lubrication, sexual pleasure)
3. Orgasm (peaking of sexual pleasure, release of sexual tension, rhythmic muscle and genital contractions, ejaculation)
4. Resolution (general and muscular relaxation, feeling of well-being, physiological refractoriness to further sexual activity in males)

223

Three categories of *subtypes* are commonly specified in this group of disorders:

1. **Lifelong** *versus* **Acquired:** this refers to whether the dysfunction has been present since the beginning of sexual functioning *or* was preceded by a period of normal sexual functioning.
2. **Generalized** *versus* **Situational:** this refers to whether the dysfunction is limited to certain kinds of stimulation, situations, or partners. It is sometimes appropriate to include dysfunction occurring during masturbation.
3. **Due to Psychological Factors** *versus* **Due to Combined Factors:** this refers to whether psychological factors have the major role in symptom production (and general medical conditions and substances [e.g., medications, drugs of abuse, alcohol] have no role), *or* both psychological and general medical/substance factors are involved. Note that if the dysfunction is due entirely to the effects of a general medical condition or substance, it is diagnosed as such (see following).

ASSOCIATED FEATURES. Sexual Dysfunction complaints often focus on, or are associated with, problems in interpersonal relationships, depression, anxiety, or somatic symptoms.

AGE AND CULTURAL FACTORS. Advancing age is often associated with decreased sexual functioning; however, broad individual differences are the rule.

PREDISPOSING FACTORS. Anxiety and excessively high subjective standards for sexual performance predispose one to the development of acquired Sexual Dysfunction. Negative attitudes toward sexuality, often due to particular past experiences, internal conflicts, inadequate education, or rigid cultural values, are predisposing, as are several mental disorders. Family values and stereotypes play a role in many disorders.

DIFFERENTIAL DIAGNOSIS. The patient's culture and social group should be considered when diagnosing Sexual Dysfunction to differentiate it from personal or social expectations. On the other hand, lack of education, opportunity, or social approval can be a source of bona fide dysfunction. Experienced clinical judgment is important. General medical conditions and Substance-Related Disorders should be sought before assuming a disorder is purely "functional." If another Axis I mental disorder is the primary cause of the sexual problems, a Sexual Dysfunction should *not* be diagnosed. V-code conditions (e.g., Relational Problems) and Personality Disorders may be comorbid with Sexual Dysfunction Disorders.

▢ ▢ ▢ ▢

Sexual Desire Disorders

302.71 Hypoactive Sexual Desire Disorder *(ICD-10 code F52.0)*

ASSOCIATED FEATURES. Problems with sexual arousal or orgasm are seen.

DIAGNOSTIC CRITERIA FOR
HYPOACTIVE SEXUAL DESIRE DISORDER
(302.71)

(ICD-10 code F52.0)

A. Persistently or recurrently deficient (or absent) sexual fantasies and desire for sexual activity. The judgment of deficiency or absence is made by the clinician, taking into account factors that affect sexual functioning, such as age and the context of the person's life.

B. The disturbance causes marked distress or interpersonal difficulty.

C. The dysfunction is not better accounted for by another Axis I disorder (except another Sexual Dysfunction) and is not due exclusively to the direct physiological effects of a substance (e.g., drug of abuse, medication) or general medical condition.

> **Specify type:**
> Lifelong or Acquired
>
> **Specify type:**
> Generalized or Situational
>
> **Specify:**
> Due to Psychological Factors or Due to Combined Factors

❏ ❏ ❏ ❏

302.79 Sexual Aversion Disorder

(ICD-10 code F52.10)

ASSOCIATED FEATURES AND DISORDERS. Panic Attacks, severely impaired relationships, and extensive strategies to avoid sexual situations are seen.

DIAGNOSTIC CRITERIA FOR
SEXUAL AVERSION DISORDER (302.79)

(ICD-10 code F52.10)

A. Persistent or recurrent extreme aversion to, and avoidance of, all (or almost all) genital sexual contact with a sexual partner.

B. The disturbance causes marked distress or interpersonal difficulty.

C. The dysfunction is not better accounted for by another Axis I disorder (except another Sexual Dysfunction).

> **Specify type:**
> Lifelong or Acquired
>
> **Specify type:**
> Generalized or Situational
>
> **Specify:**
> Due to Psychological Factors or Due to Combined Factors

❏ ❏ ❏ ❏

Sexual Arousal Disorders

302.72 Female Sexual Arousal Disorder   (ICD-10 code F52.2)
(significantly modified from DSM-III-R)

ASSOCIATED FEATURES. Painful coitus and damage to interpersonal relationships are seen.

DIAGNOSTIC CRITERIA FOR   (ICD-10 code F52.2)
FEMALE SEXUAL AROUSAL DISORDER (302.72)

A. Persistent or recurrent inability to attain, or to maintain until completion of the sexual activity, an adequate lubrication-swelling response of sexual excitement.

B. The disturbance causes marked distress or interpersonal difficulty.
   C.

The dysfunction is not better accounted for by another Axis I disorder (except another Sexual Dysfunction) and is not due exclusively to the direct physiological effects of a substance (e.g., drug of abuse, medication) or general medical condition.

Specify type:
Lifelong or Acquired

Specify type:
Generalized or Situational

Specify:
Due to Psychological Factors or Due to Combined Factors

▫ ▫ ▫ ▫

302.72 Male Erectile Disorder   (ICD-10 code F52.2)
(significantly modified from DSM-III-R)

ASSOCIATED FEATURES. Sexual anxiety, fear of failure, and disturbance of relationships are seen. Erection is often possible with some partners but not others; masturbation is rarely affected.

DIAGNOSTIC CRITERIA FOR   (ICD-10 code F52.2)
MALE ERECTILE DISORDER (302.72)

A. Persistent or recurrent inability to attain or maintain an adequate erection until completion of the sexual activity.

B. The disturbance causes marked distress or interpersonal difficulty.

C. The dysfunction is not better accounted for by another Axis I disorder (except another Sexual Dysfunction) and is not due exclusively to the direct physiological effects of a substance (e.g., a drug of abuse, a medication) or general medical condition.

> **Specify type:**
> Lifelong or Acquired
>
> **Specify type:**
> Generalized or Situational
>
> **Specify:**
> Due to Psychological Factors or Due to Combined Factors

❑ ❑ ❑ ❑

Orgasmic Disorders

302.73 Female Orgasmic Disorder   (ICD-10 code F52.3)
(Inhibited Female Orgasm in DSM-III-R)

ASSOCIATED FEATURES. Performance anxiety and damage to self-esteem are seen. Orgasm is often possible with other partners or through noncoital stimulation by self or partner.

DIAGNOSTIC CRITERIA FOR   (ICD-10 code F52.3)
FEMALE ORGASMIC DISORDER (302.73)

A. Persistent or recurrent delay in, or absence of, orgasm following a normal sexual excitement phase. Women exhibit wide variability in the type or intensity of stimulation that triggers orgasm. The diagnosis of Female Orgasmic Disorder should be based on the clinician's judgment that the woman's orgasmic capacity is less than would be reasonable for her age, sexual experience, and the adequacy of sexual stimulation she receives.

B. The disturbance causes marked distress or interpersonal difficulty.

C. The orgasmic dysfunction is not better accounted for by another Axis I disorder (except another Sexual Dysfunction) and is not due exclusively to the direct physiological effects of a substance (e.g., a drug of abuse, a medication) or general medical condition.

> **Specify type:**
> Lifelong or Acquired
>
> **Specify type:**
> Generalized or Situational
>
> **Specify:**
> Due to Psychological Factors or Due to Combined Factors

❑ ❑ ❑ ❑

302.74 Male Orgasmic Disorder (ICD-10 code F52.3)
(Inhibited Male Orgasm in DSM-III-R)

ASSOCIATED FEATURES. Covert Paraphilias and damage to relationships are seen. Ejaculation by noncoital means is often unaffected.

DIAGNOSTIC CRITERIA FOR (ICD-10 code F52.3)
MALE ORGASMIC DISORDER (302.74)

A. Persistent or recurrent delay in, or absence of, orgasm following a normal sexual excitement phase during sexual activity that the clinician, taking into account the person's age, judges to be adequate in focus, intensity, and duration.

B. The disturbance causes marked distress or interpersonal difficulty.

C. The sexual dysfunction is not better accounted for by another Axis I disorder (except another Sexual Dysfunction) and is not due exclusively to the direct physiological effects of a substance (e.g., a drug of abuse, a medication) or general medical condition.

> **Specify type:**
> **Lifelong** or **Acquired**
>
> **Specify type:**
> **Generalized** or Situational
>
> **Specify:**
> **Due to Psychological Factors** or **Due to Combined Factors**

❑ ❑ ❑ ❑

302.75 Premature Ejaculation (ICD-10 code F52.4)

ASSOCIATED FEATURES. Damage to self-esteem and relationship difficulties are seen. Premature Ejaculation is often associated with youth, new partners, and novel sexual situations.

DIAGNOSTIC CRITERIA FOR (ICD-10 code F52.4)
PREMATURE EJACULATION (302.75)

A. Persistent or recurrent ejaculation with minimal sexual stimulation before, on, or shortly after penetration and before the person wishes it. The clinician must take into account factors that affect duration of the excitement phase, such as age, novelty of the sexual partner or situation, and recent frequency of sexual activity.

B. The disturbance causes marked distress or interpersonal difficulty.

C. The premature ejaculation is not due exclusively to the direct physiological effects of a substance (e.g., withdrawal from opioids).

> **Specify type:**
> Lifelong or Acquired
>
> **Specify type:**
> Generalized or Situational
>
> **Specify:**
> Due to Psychological Factors or Due to Combined Factors

□ □ □ □

Sexual Pain Disorders

302.76 Dyspareunia   (ICD-10 code F52.6)
(Not Due to a General Medical Condition)

ASSOCIATED FEATURES. Marital disturbance and avoidance of sexual situations are seen.

DIAGNOSTIC CRITERIA FOR   (ICD-10 code F52.6)
DYSPAREUNIA (302.76)

A. Recurrent or persistent genital pain associated with sexual intercourse, in either a male or a female.

B. The disturbance causes marked distress or interpersonal difficulty.

C. The disturbance is not caused exclusively by Vaginismus or lack of lubrication, is not better accounted for by another Axis I disorder (except another Sexual Dysfunction), and is not due to the direct physiological effects of a substance or a general medical condition.

> **Specify type:**
> Lifelong or Acquired
>
> **Specify type:**
> Generalized or Situational
>
> **Specify:**
> Due to Psychological Factors or Due to Combined Factors

□ □ □ □

306.51 Vaginismus   (ICD-10 code F52.5)
(Not Due to a General Medical Condition)

ASSOCIATED FEATURES. Associated features may include intact sexual functioning except for activities involving intromission, past sexual trauma or abuse, or young age. The disorder includes spasm during penetration by a penis, finger, tampon, or speculum.

DIAGNOSTIC CRITERIA FOR VAGINISMUS (306.51)   (ICD-10 code F52.5)

A. Recurrent or persistent involuntary spasm of the musculature of the outer third of the vagina that interferes with sexual intercourse.

B. The disturbance causes marked distress or interpersonal difficulty.

C. The dysfunction is not better accounted for by another Axis I disorder (e.g., Somatization Disorder) and is not due exclusively to the direct physiological effects of a substance (e.g., drug of abuse, medication) or general medical condition.

> **Specify type:**
> Lifelong or Acquired
>
> **Specify type:**
> Generalized or Situational
>
> **Specify:**
> Due to Psychological Factors or Due to Combined Factors

❑ ❑ ❑ ❑

6xx.xx Sexual Dysfunction Due to a General Medical Condition   (ICD-10 codes follow)
(new in DSM-IV)

ESSENTIAL FEATURES. There is a clinically significant Sexual Dysfunction directly caused by the physiological effects of a general medical condition. The symptoms may be those of any of the disorders discussed in this section, but full criteria for a particular disorder need not be met.

ASSOCIATED FEATURES AND PHYSICAL AND LABORATORY FINDINGS. Associated features and findings are those of the Sexual Dysfunction and the underlying general medical condition.

DIFFERENTIAL DIAGNOSIS. The symptoms are not merely psychological reactions to the general medical condition but are caused by its physiological effects. Dysfunction related solely to normal aging is not considered "Due to a General Medical Condition." Causative mental illness (e.g., depression) and Substance-Related Disorders must be ruled out, including those caused by medications used to treat a mental illness or general medical condition. If there is convincing evidence that the dysfunction is caused by both substance use and a general medical condition, both may be diagnosed. If psychological factors play a role in the symptoms, consider a diagnosis of the relevant primary Sexual Dysfunction Due to Combined Factors. If uncertain of the source of the symptoms, Sexual Dysfunction NOS should be considered.

DIAGNOSTIC CRITERIA FOR SEXUAL DYSFUNCTION DUE TO . . . (SPECIFY GENERAL MEDICAL CONDITION) (6xx.xx)

(see ICD-10 codes below)

A. Clinically significant sexual dysfunction that results in marked distress or interpersonal difficulty dominates the clinical presentation.

B. There is evidence from the history, physical examination, or laboratory findings that the sexual dysfunction is fully explained by the direct physiological effects of a general medical condition.

C. The disturbance is not better accounted for by another mental disorder.

> **Code based on predominant Sexual Dysfunction as described earlier in this section** (e.g., 607.84 Male Erectile Disorder Due to Diabetes Mellitus):
>
> **625.8 Female Hypoactive Sexual Desire Disorder Due to . . . (specify the general medical condition)** (ICD-10 N94.8)
>
> **608.89 Male Hypoactive Sexual Desire Disorder Due to . . .** (ICD-10 N50.8)
>
> **607.84 Male Erectile Disorder Due to . . .** (ICD-10 N48.4)
>
> **625.0 Female Dyspareunia Due to . . .** (ICD-10 N94.1)
>
> **608.89 Male Dyspareunia Due to . . .** (ICD-10 N50.8)
>
> **625.8 Other Female Sexual Dysfunction Due to . . .:** used if some other (or no) sexual feature predominates (ICD-10 N94.8)
>
> **608.89 Other Male Sexual Dysfunction Due to . . .:** used if some other (or no) sexual feature predominates (ICD-10 N50.8)
>
> **CODING NOTE:** Include the name of the general medical condition on Axis I, and code the general medical condition on Axis III.

□ □ □ □

291.8 or 292.89 Substance-Induced Sexual Dysfunction (new in DSM-IV)

(ICD-10 uses substance code)

> NOTE: See special coding procedures following Diagnostic Criteria.

ESSENTIAL FEATURES. There is a clinically significant Sexual Dysfunction directly caused by the physiological effects of a substance, including prescription use, poisoning, or intoxication. The symptoms may be those of any of the Sexual Disorders discussed above, but full criteria for a particular disorder need not be met. The symptoms must be clearly in excess of those expected for the type or amount of substance, duration of use, or prior primary Sexual Dysfunctions.

ASSOCIATED FEATURES AND PHYSICAL AND LABORATORY FINDINGS. Associated features and findings are those of the underlying substance, intoxication, or withdrawal syndrome.

DIFFERENTIAL DIAGNOSIS. The Sexual Dysfunction is not merely a psychological reaction but is caused by physiological effects of the substance. If the sexual symptoms do not clearly exceed those usually associated with intoxication, Substance Intoxication is diagnosed instead. If the patient is taking medication for a general medical condition, the clinician should be certain that condition is not the source of the Sexual Dysfunction. If there is evidence that the dysfunction is caused by both substance use and a general medical condition, both may be diagnosed. Primary Sexual Dysfunctions are ruled out when symptoms are found to be fully explained by the effects of substance use. If uncertain about the source of the symptoms, consider Sexual Dysfunction NOS.

DIAGNOSTIC CRITERIA FOR　　　　　　　　　　　　(ICD-10 code uses
SUBSTANCE-INDUCED SEXUAL DYSFUNCTION　　　　substance code)
(291.8 or 292.89)

A. Clinically significant sexual dysfunction that results in marked distress or interpersonal difficulty dominates the clinical presentation.

B. There is evidence from the history, physical examination, or laboratory findings that the sexual dysfunction is fully explained by substance, as manifested by either (1) or (2):
   (1) the symptoms in Criterion A developed during, or within a month of, Substance Intoxication
   (2) medication use is etiologically related to the disturbance

C. The disturbance is not better accounted for by a Sexual Dysfunction that is not substance induced. Evidence that the symptoms are better accounted for by a Sexual Dysfunction that is not substance induced might include the following: the symptoms precede the onset of the substance use or dependence (or medication use); the symptoms persist for a substantial period of time (e.g., about a month) after the cessation of intoxication, or are substantially in excess of what would be expected given the type or amount of the substance used, or the duration of use; or there is other evidence that suggests the existence of an independent non-substance-induced Sexual Dysfunction (e.g., a history of recurrent non-substance-related episodes).

Specify if: (based on symptoms dominating the clinical presentation)

With Impaired Desire

With Impaired Arousal

With Impaired Orgasm

With Sexual Pain

Specify if:
With Onset During Intoxication: DSM-IV criteria met for Intoxication and the symptoms develop during intoxication

(See table in DSM-IV, p.177 or p. 99 in this *Guide*, for applicability by substance.)

CODING NOTE: Code the (Specific Substance)-Induced Sexual Dysfunction as follows: 291.8 Alcohol (ICD-10 F10.8); 292.89 for all others: Amphetamine or Related Substance (ICD-10 F15.8); Cocaine (ICD-10 F14.8); Opioid (ICD-10 F11.8); Sedative/Hypnotic/Anxiolytic (ICD-10 F13.8); Other or Unknown Substance (ICD-10 F19.8).

CODING NOTE: Also code Substance-Specific Intoxication if criteria are met.

□ □ □ □

302.70 Sexual Dysfunction Not Otherwise Specified (NOS)   *(ICD-10 code F52.9)*

This category includes clinically significant Sexual Dysfunctions that result in marked distress or interpersonal difficulty but do not meet criteria for any specific Sexual Dysfunction. Sexual Dysfunction NOS includes, but is not limited to, situations in which the clinician is unable to determine whether the symptoms are primary, due to a general medical condition, or substance induced.

□ □ □ □

....

PARAPHILIAS
(significantly modified From DSM-III-R)

All the Paraphilias are characterized by recurrent, intense sexual urges and sexually arousing fantasies generally involving nonhuman objects, suffering or humiliation, or children or other nonconsenting persons. The diagnosis is made only if the urges have been acted on or if there is marked distress or impairment, *and* the symptoms have been present for at least 6 months. The paraphiliac impulses and behaviors, in order to be diagnosed, must be preferred avenues of sexual excitement and expression (whether or not there is opportunity to act on them), and not simply sexual experimentation.

102

ASSOCIATED FEATURES. People with Paraphilias may have extreme guilt, shame, or depression, or may overtly see their activities as normal. Sexual Dysfunctions and/or problems with interpersonal relationships may be present. The patient may have a job or hobby that allows pursuit, in fantasy or reality, of the Paraphilia. Personality disturbances, often severe enough to warrant an Axis II diagnosis, are common. The existence of more than one Paraphilia in the same patient is common. The disorders are usually chronic, although severity may decrease with age. Stressors may be associated with exacerbation but generally should not be used to justify inappropriate behavior.

ASSOCIATED PHYSICAL AND LABORATORY FINDINGS. Associated findings can include sexually transmitted diseases, injury to self or others, and (although not always reliable) abnormalities on penile plethysmography.

SPECIFIC CULTURE AND GENDER DIFFERENCES. Cultural differences with regard to what constitutes acceptable, or deviant, sexual behavior should be considered. DSM-IV states that females with Paraphilia are unusual to extremely rare. Other sources suggest that sex differences are not so great, and that case reporting does not necessarily reflect prevalence.

DIFFERENTIAL DIAGNOSIS. Normal variants of sexual activity and nonpathological sexual experimentation should be ruled out before diagnosing any Paraphilia. Paraphilia-like behaviors that are carried out for nonarousing purposes (e.g., collecting fetishistic items) should not be confused with Paraphilia, even if the purpose is to arouse someone else (as in prostitution). Rape or other sexual assault may or may not involve a Paraphilia. Although the Paraphilias can be diagnosed in addition to other mental disorders, paraphiliac behavior arising impulsively and/or temporarily from such disorders, Intoxication, Dementia, or other general medical conditions should be considered a symptom of the underlying disorder rather than a separate diagnosis. If more than one Paraphilia is present, all should be diagnosed.

□ □ □ □

302.4 Exhibitionism   (ICD-10 code F65.2)

ESSENTIAL FEATURES. There is exposure of the genitals to a stranger in a context of sexual fantasy and arousal. Although DSM-IV implies that Exhibitionism occurs only in males, many authors report that it does occur in females. Forensic and clinical populations are almost entirely male.

DIFFERENTIAL DIAGNOSIS. Accidental exposure and exposure not related to sexual activity should be ruled out. Either may also be offered as a rationalization for Exhibitionism. See general differential diagnosis, above.

DIAGNOSTIC CRITERIA FOR   (ICD-10 code F65.2)
EXHIBITIONISM (302.4)

A. Over a period of at least 6 months, recurrent, intense sexually arousing fantasies, sexual urges, or behaviors involving the exposure of one's genitals to an unsuspecting stranger.

B. The fantasies, sexual urges, or behaviors cause clinically significant distress or impairment in social, occupational, or other important areas of functioning.

□ □ □ □

302.81 Fetishism

(ICD-10 code F65.0)

ESSENTIAL FEATURES. There are recurrent, intense sexual urges and sexually arousing fantasies involving the use of nonliving objects (fetishes). Women's apparel are common fetish objects. Some authors include nonsexual body parts ("partialism").

DIFFERENTIAL DIAGNOSIS. Transvestic Fetishism is included in the differential diagnosis. See general differential diagnosis of Paraphilias, preceding.

DIAGNOSTIC CRITERIA FOR FETISHISM (302.81)

(ICD-10 code F65.0)

A. Over a period of at least 6 months, recurrent, intense, sexually arousing fantasies, sexual urges, or behaviors involving the use of nonliving objects (e.g., female undergarments).

B. The fantasies, sexual urges, or behaviors cause clinically significant distress or impairment in social, occupational, or other important areas of functioning.

C. The fetish objects are not limited to articles of female clothing used in cross-dressing (as in Transvestic Fetishism) or devices designed for the purpose of tactile genital stimulation (e.g., a vibrator).

□ □ □ □

302.89 Frotteurism

(ICD-10 code F65.8)

ESSENTIAL FEATURES. There are recurrent, intense sexual urges and sexually arousing fantasies involving touching and rubbing against a nonconsenting person.

DIFFERENTIAL DIAGNOSIS. Touching or fondling associated with poor judgment or impulse control (as in certain mental disorders or some children who have been sexually abused) are considered. See general differential diagnosis of Paraphilias, preceding.

DIAGNOSTIC CRITERIA FOR FROTTEURISM (302.89)

(ICD-10 code F65.8)

A. Over a period of at least 6 months, recurrent, intense sexually arousing fantasies, sexual urges, or behaviors involving touching and rubbing against a nonconsenting person.

B. The fantasies, sexual urges, or behaviors cause clinically significant distress or impairment in social, occupational, or other important areas of functioning.

□ □ □ □

302.2 Pedophilia

(ICD-10 code F65.4)

ESSENTIAL FEATURES. There are recurrent, intense, sexual urges and sexually arousing fantasies involving sexual activity with a prepubescent child. The age of the perpetrator is arbitrarily set at 16 years or older, and at least 5 years older than the child. For perpetrators in late adolescence, clinical judgment must take into account both the sexual maturity of the child and the age difference. Pedophiles may be attracted to children of the same sex, the opposite sex, or both. Actions related to pedophilic urges may be limited to relatively nonintrusive activities (e.g., exposing oneself, masturbating) or to touching and fondling, but in some perpetrators may involve genital contact or penetration, with varying degrees of force. The behavior may be rationalized as "educational" or responding to "seduction" by the child (who is unable to consent meaningfully or legally to the activity).

DIFFERENTIAL DIAGNOSIS. See general differential diagnosis of Paraphilias.

DIAGNOSTIC CRITERIA FOR PEDOPHILIA (302.2)

(ICD-10 code F65.4)

A. Over a period of at least 6 months, recurrent, intense sexually arousing fantasies, sexual urges, or behaviors involving sexual activity with a prepubescent child or children (generally age 13 years or younger).

B. The fantasies, sexual urges, or behaviors cause clinically significant distress or impairment in social, occupational, or other important areas of functioning.

C. The person is at least age 16 years and at least 5 years older than the child or children in Criterion A.

NOTE: Do not include an individual in late adolescence involved in an ongoing relationship with a 12- or 13-year-old.

Specify if:
Sexually Attracted to Males

Sexually Attracted to Females

Sexually Attracted to Both

Specify if:
Limited to Incest

Specify if:
Exclusive Type: attracted to children only

Nonexclusive Type

▢ ▢ ▢ ▢

302.83 Sexual Masochism

(ICD-10 code F65.5)

ESSENTIAL FEATURES. There are recurrent, intense, sexual urges and sexually arousing fantasies involving the act of being humiliated, beaten, bound, or otherwise made to suffer. The masochistic fantasies may be invoked during intercourse or masturbation but are not otherwise acted on. The fantasies are of real masochistic situations, not simulations.

ASSOCIATED FEATURES. When consenting partners engage in sadomasochistic sexual activity, their roles are often overtly or covertly "scripted" to prevent serious injury. In other cases, the disorder can be quite dangerous (e.g., in autoerotic asphyxia, in which accidental death during masochistic self-stimulation may occur and may be mistaken for suicide or homicide).

DIFFERENTIAL DIAGNOSIS. Masochistic fantasies without marked distress or recurrent masochistic behavior are considered. Transvestic Fetishism may be associated with Sexual Masochism, if the cross-dressing is humiliating and the humiliation is the sexually arousing feature. Masochistic or "self-defeating" personality traits are distinguished from this disorder by their lack of association with sexual excitement. See general differential diagnosis of Paraphilias.

DIAGNOSTIC CRITERIA FOR
SEXUAL MASOCHISM (302.83)

(ICD-10 code F65.5)

A. Over a period of at least 6 months, recurrent, intense sexually arousing fantasies, sexual urges, or behaviors involving the act (real, not simulated) of being humiliated, beaten, bound, or otherwise made to suffer.

B. The fantasies, sexual urges, or behaviors cause clinically significant distress or impairment in social, occupational, or other important areas of functioning.

▢ ▢ ▢ ▢

302.84 Sexual Sadism

(ICD-10 code F65.5)

ESSENTIAL FEATURES. There are recurrent, intense, sexual urges and sexually arousing fantasies involving acts in which the psychological or physical suffering (including humiliation) of the victim is sexually exciting. The fantasies are of real sadistic situations, not simulations. Some people with this disorder are bothered by their sadistic fantasies or actions; others are not. The fantasies usually involve having control over the victim, who is terrified. Some persons act with a consenting partner, who may have Sexual Masochism.

ASSOCIATED FEATURES. Cruel or sadistic fantasies or actions, with or without a sexual complement, have commonly been present since childhood. Other Paraphilias may be present but are not as common as in some other paraphiliac disorders. When consenting partners engage in sadomasochistic sexual activity, their roles are often overtly or covertly scripted to prevent serious injury. Sexual Sadism is particularly dangerous when combined with antisocial personality traits or Antisocial Personality Disorder. Some persons use animals (e.g., dogs or cats from an animal shelter) as substitutes for unavailable human victims.

DIFFERENTIAL DIAGNOSIS. Rape or other nonparaphiliac sexual assault may or may not involve Sexual Sadism. Sadistic acts not repeatedly associated with sexual arousal should be differentiated from Sexual Sadism. See the general differential diagnosis for Paraphilias.

DIAGNOSTIC CRITERIA FOR SEXUAL SADISM (302.84)

(ICD-10 code F65.5)

A. Over a period of at least 6 months, recurrent, intense sexually arousing fantasies, sexual urges, or behaviors involving acts (real, not simulated) in which the psychological or physical suffering (including humiliation) of a victim is sexually exciting to the person.

B. The fantasies, sexual urges, or behaviors cause clinically significant distress or impairment in social, occupational, or other important areas of functioning.

□ □ □ □

302.3 Transvestic Fetishism

(ICD-10 code F65.1)

ESSENTIAL FEATURES. There are recurrent, intense, sexual urges and sexually arousing fantasies involving cross-dressing. The person, virtually always male, usually keeps a collection of women's clothes used to cross-dress when alone (during which he generally masturbates and may imagine himself to be both the male subject and the female object of his fantasy). Some men wear only a single item of women's clothing; others dress up completely. The basic sexual preference is heterosexual, although the patient may have engaged in occasional homosexual acts.

ASSOCIATED FEATURES. Sexual Masochism may be present.

DIFFERENTIAL DIAGNOSIS. This disorder should not be diagnosed in the presence of Gender Identity Disorders. Masquerading as a female in a theatrical fashion should not be confused with this disorder, even if the cross-dresser is homosexual. Female impersonators, unless showing other signs of Transvestic Fetishism, should not receive this diagnosis. Persons with Sexual Masochism whose humiliation is associated with cross-dressing should not be given this diagnosis unless the garments themselves cause sexual arousal. See preceding for the general differential diagnosis of Paraphilia.

DIAGNOSTIC CRITERIA FOR TRANSVESTIC FETISHISM (302.3)

(ICD-10 code F65.1)

A. Over a period of at least 6 months, in a heterosexual male, recurrent, intense sexually arousing fantasies, sexual urges, or behaviors involving cross-dressing.

B. The fantasies, sexual urges, or behaviors cause clinically significant distress or impairment in social, occupational, or other important areas of functioning.

Specify if:
With Gender Dysphoria: if the person has persistent discomfort with gender role or identity

❑ ❑ ❑ ❑

302.82 Voyeurism

(ICD-10 code F65.3)

ESSENTIAL FEATURES. There are recurrent, intense, sexual urges and sexually arousing fantasies involving the observing of unsuspecting people, usually strangers, who are naked, in the process of undressing and/or engaging in sexual activity. The act of looking itself, with no other sexual activity sought, is the focus of the sexual excitement (although the patient may have fantasies of sexual experience with the observed person).

ASSOCIATED FEATURES. Other Paraphilias, rarely ones that cause physical injury to others, are sometimes seen.

DIFFERENTIAL DIAGNOSIS. Normal sexual peeking or looking, but not with an unsuspecting, unconsenting partner, and/or not as the primary mode of excitement is considered. The use of pornography, including observing live sexual entertainment, is not, by itself, sufficient for this diagnosis. See preceding for general differential diagnosis of the Paraphilias.

DIAGNOSTIC CRITERIA FOR VOYEURISM (302.82)

(ICD-10 code F65.3)

A. Over a period of at least 6 months, recurrent, intense, sexually arousing fantasies, sexual urges, or behaviors involving the act of observing an unsuspecting person who is naked, in the process of disrobing, or engaged in sexual activity.

B. The fantasies, sexual urges, or behaviors cause clinically significant distress or impairment in social, occupational, or other important areas of functioning.

❑ ❑ ❑ ❑

302.9 Paraphilia Not Otherwise Specified (NOS) (ICD-10 code F65.9)

This diagnostic code is reserved for syndromes that meet the general criteria for Paraphilia but do not meet the criteria for any of the specific categories just discussed. Examples include telephone scatologia (obscene phone calls), necrophilia (corpses), partialism (exclusive focus on body part), zoophilia (bestiality), klismaphilia (enemas), coprophilia (feces), and urophilia (urine).

....

GENDER IDENTITY DISORDERS

302.6, 302.85 Gender Identity Disorder (significantly modified from DSM-III-R) (ICD-10 codes F64.2, F64.0)

NOTE: See special coding procedures under Diagnostic Criteria.

ESSENTIAL FEATURES. There is sufficiently strong and persistent cross-gender identification that one desires to be, or believes one should be, a member of the opposite sex. A feeling of discomfort or inappropriateness with the current sex or sex role is also required. In children, the disorder is accompanied by strong preference for behaviors and activities related to the opposite sex while avoiding those of one's own sex. Adults with the disorder function in the opposite-sex role whenever possible, and often alter their bodies in some way (e.g., with hormonal treatment or surgery, including genital-change procedures).

ASSOCIATED FEATURES. Social problems or ostracism, often beginning in childhood, are seen. Male patients sometimes have childhood memories of a parent encouraging "cute" dressing in women's clothing and mimicking female mannerisms.

PHYSICAL AND LABORATORY FINDINGS. Findings are usually normal, unless altered by hormone treatments or surgery.

COURSE. Most children with the disorder will not continue to meet all criteria for Gender Identity Disorder in adulthood, although some evidence indicates that up to 75% of young boys with the diagnosis will describe homosexual or bisexual gender preference in late adolescence or adulthood.

DIFFERENTIAL DIAGNOSIS. The differential diagnosis includes wanting to change sex solely for perceived social or cultural advantage and simple nonconformity with common sex roles and behavior. Physical "intersex" conditions such as chromosomal or congenital abnormality should not be diagnosed here; if gender discomfort or identity is a clinically significant issue, consider Gender Identity Disorder NOS. Psychotic symptoms, such as delusions of being the opposite sex, should not be used to support this diagnosis. Some men meet criteria for both Gender Identity Disorder and Transvestic Fetishism, and they may be comorbid; however, most do not meet criteria for the latter. See preceding for a general discussion of differential diagnosis of Paraphilia.

DIAGNOSTIC CRITERIA FOR GENDER IDENTITY DISORDER (302.6, 302.85)

(ICD-10 codes F64.2, F64.0)

A. A strong and persistent cross-gender identification (not merely a desire for any perceived cultural advantages of being the other sex).

In children, the disturbance is manifested by four (or more) of the following:
   (1) repeatedly stated desire to be, or insistence that he or she is, the other sex
   (2) in boys, preference for cross-dressing or simulating female attire; in girls, insistence on wearing only stereotypical masculine clothing
   (3) strong and persistent preferences for cross-sex roles in make-believe play or persistent fantasies of being the other sex
   (4) intense desire to participate in the stereotypical games and pastimes of the other sex
   (5) strong preference for playmates of the other sex

In adolescents and adults, the disturbance is manifested by symptoms such as a stated desire to be the other sex, frequent passing as the other sex, desire to live or be treated as the other sex, or the conviction that one has the typical feelings and reactions of the other sex.

B. Persistent discomfort with one's sex or a sense of inappropriateness in the gender role of that sex.

In children, the disturbance is manifested by any of the following: *In a boy,* assertion that his penis or testes are disgusting or will disappear or assertion that it would be better not to have a penis, *or* aversion toward rough-and-tumble play and rejection of male stereotypical toys, games, and activities. *In a girl,* rejection of urinating in a sitting position, assertion that she has or will grow a penis, or assertion that she does not want to grow breasts or menstruate, *or* marked aversion toward normative feminine clothing.

In adolescents and adults, the disturbance is manifested by symptoms such as preoccupation with getting rid of one's primary and secondary sex characteristics (e.g., request for hormones, surgery, or other procedures to physically alter sexual characteristics to simulate the other sex) *or* belief that he or she was born the wrong sex.

C. The disturbance is not concurrent with a physical intersex condition.

D. The disturbance causes clinically significant distress or impairment in social, occupational, or other important areas of functioning.

> **CODING NOTE: Code based on current age.**
> **302.6 Gender Identity Disorder in Children (ICD-10 F64.2)**
> **302.85 Gender Identity Disorder in Adolescents or Adults (ICD-10 F64.0)**

Specify, if for sexually mature individuals
Sexually Attracted to Males

Sexually Attracted to Females

Sexually Attracted to Both

Sexually Attracted to Neither

❏ ❏ ❏ ❏

302.6 Gender Identity Disorder Not Otherwise Specified (NOS)

(ICD-10 code F64.9)

This residual category should be used for persons with clinically significant Gender Identity Disorders not classifiable in the categories outlined and not subsumed under other major psychiatric or physical disorders. Examples include children with persistent cross-dressing without other Gender Identity Disorder criteria; adults with transient, stress-related cross-dressing; and adults with clinical features of transsexualism that have lasted less than 2 years.

❏ ❏ ❏ ❏

302.9 Sexual Disorder Not Otherwise Specified (NOS)

(ICD-10 code F52.9)

This category is for sexual disturbances that do not meet the criteria for any specific Sexual Disorder and are neither Sexual Dysfunctions nor Paraphilias. Examples include clinically significant distress about one's sexual orientation (e.g., homosexuality).

❏ ❏ ❏ ❏

DIFFERENCES BETWEEN DSM-III-R AND DSM-IV SEXUAL AND GENDER IDENTITY DISORDERS

Sexual Dysfunctions

❏ All Sexual Dysfunctions now require clinically significant distress or interpersonal problems to be considered mental disorders.

❏ In **Female Sexual Arousal Disorder** and **Male Erectile Disorder,** subjective complaints alone are insufficient for the diagnosis; physiological signs are required.

❑   Criteria for **Female Orgasmic Disorder** are simplified.

❑   **Sexual Dysfunctions Due To Medical Conditions** and **Substance-Induced Sexual Dysfunctions** are new in DSM-IV.

Paraphilias

❑   Severity criteria are no longer specified. In the text and criteria for specific Paraphilias, DSM-IV suggests that if there is no distress or impairment in functioning, Paraphilia should not be diagnosed even if the urges have been acted upon. DSM-IV implies, however, that "clinically significant distress or impairment" is meant to include participation of nonconsenting persons or illegal behavior (p. 525).

❑   Criteria for **Transvestic Fetishism** are similar; the **With Gender Dysphoria** specifier added.

Gender Identity Disorders

❑   DSM-IV places the three former DSM-III-R Gender Identity Disorders (Gender Identity Disorder of Childhood; Gender Identity Disorder of Adolescence and Adulthood, Nontranssexual Type [GIDAANT], and Transsexualism) in this single diagnosis, which accommodates all ages and both sexes. No DSM-IV Gender Identity Disorders are listed in Disorders Usually First Diagnosed in Infancy, Childhood, or Adolescence.

CASE VIGNETTES: SEXUAL AND GENDER IDENTITY DISORDERS

Case Vignette 1

G.W., a 36-year-old shoe salesman, was referred for evaluation soon after a female customer complained that he was behaving inappropriately. She stated that G.W. appeared to be fondling her feet as he fit her with new shoes. Upon questioning, he initially said he was merely fitting a delicate shoe and admiring the leather; however, he eventually agreed that his hands might have lingered on her shoes, and that he was acting unprofessionally. He made no attempt to fondle other parts of her body or otherwise assault her.

A college graduate, G.W. appeared ashamed and contrite. He had been disciplined for similar reasons in previous jobs at other shoe stores, and was concerned that he might lose his job. He showed signs of clinical depression which, he said, had not been present before this complaint. He described trouble sleeping, recent weight loss, and guilt that he might never be able to conquer his impulses and lead a normal life.

Later in therapy, G.W. spoke of having a large collection of women's shoes and magazines related to them, which he often used in masturbation.

Masturbation is his primary sexual outlet, although he occasionally dates and enjoys heterosexual relationships. His sexual fantasies are almost exclusively about women's shoes, on or off their feet. He was married once, for about a year, but the relationship was "unsatisfying." He does not dress in women's clothing.

DIAGNOSIS AND DISCUSSION

Axis I—302.81 Fetishism (ICD-10 F65.0) 309.0 Adjustment Disorder With Depressed Mood (ICD-10 F43.20)
Axis II—799.9 Diagnosis Deferred on Axis II (ICD-10 R46.8)

G.W. meets all criteria for Fetishism. His fantasies and impulses exceed those of ordinary sexual experimentation and are the primary focus of his sexual life. There is no indication of Transvestic Fetishism or other Paraphilias. Adjustment Disorder With Depressed Mood may be an appropriate additional diagnosis. Personality Disorders are commonly associated with Paraphilias, and should be considered; however, no criteria are met in this vignette.

Case Vignette 2

V.F., a 22-year-old woman, seeks psychiatric consultation because of concerns that she is "frigid." She has not been able to attain orgasm with her husband of 3 months, although she feels attracted to him, has arousing fantasies about him, and describes normal physiological signs of arousal. Intercourse is not painful for her. Her husband has no difficulty with erections or orgasm, and in fact often ejaculates in only a few minutes. This signals the end of their lovemaking for the evening. She has not discussed this with him, but she confided in her mother who recommended she seek medical help. Her gynecologist found no physical abnormality, either in her genitalia or her general health. He said, in effect, "Some women are more sexually responsive than others. Perhaps a psychiatrist can help."

A careful history reveals that V.F. was brought up in a protected, but not overly restrictive environment. She has masturbated to orgasm many times, but had no other sexual experience prior to marriage. Her husband is from the same sociocultural group and had little or no sexual experience before marriage (except for masturbation). Sex education, for both, was limited to clinically oriented books and church-sponsored premarital counseling. There is no history of drug or alcohol use.

DIAGNOSIS AND DISCUSSION

Axis I—799.9 Diagnosis or Condition Deferred on Axis I (ICD-10 R69)

V.F. does not describe an inability to attain orgasm in general, but only during intercourse with her husband. She does not meet criteria for Female Orgasmic Disorder. There is no Dyspareunia or sexual aversion, and no apparent physical problem with the excitement phase of sexual response. There is an implication that arousal is possible, but perhaps is inhibited by insufficient stimulation or lack of education on the part of her husband. There may be interpersonal or communication difficulty consistent with Partner Relational Problem (V61.1). Further information is needed before making a diagnosis, which in any case is not likely to be an Axis I Sexual Dysfunction. For example, the husband may suffer from Premature Ejaculation.

CHAPTER 21

EATING DISORDERS

This is a new section in DSM-IV. In DSM-III-R, Anorexia Nervosa, Bulimia Nervosa, and Eating Disorder Not Otherwise Specified were in the section "Disorders Usually First Evident in Infancy, Childhood and Adolescence."

These disorders are severe disturbances in eating behavior, typically beginning in adolescence or early adult life. Simple obesity is not considered a mental disorder. If circumstances warrant, it should be coded as a physical disorder (Axis III). If emotional symptoms related to simple obesity merit clinical attention, see Psychological Factors Affecting Medical Condition (316).

307.1 Anorexia Nervosa (ICD-10 code F50.0)
(significantly modified from DSM-III-R)

ESSENTIAL FEATURES. Anorexia Nervosa is characterized by refusal to maintain body weight over a minimal normal weight for age and height, intense fear of gaining weight or becoming fat even though underweight, distorted body image, and amenorrhea in postmenarcheal females. The disturbance of body image is manifested by the way in which the patient's weight, size, and shape are experienced. Patients often state that they "feel fat" despite signs of starvation.

ASSOCIATED FEATURES. Self-induced vomiting or use of purgatives is common, but the primary mode of weight loss is reduction in food intake. Significant weight loss is frequently associated with metabolic signs such as hypothermia, bradycardia, hypotension, edema, lanugo (neonatal-like body hair), and amenorrhea. Depressive symptoms are common. Binge-eating episodes are usually followed by vomiting. Food is a frequent topic of thought, conversation, or fantasy, and unusual hoarding or concealing of food is also seen. Patients almost always deny or minimize the severity of their illness and are resistant to therapy. Delayed psychosexual development is common in adolescence, as is decreased libido in adults. Compulsive behaviors may be present and may justify an additional diagnosis of Obsessive-Compulsive Disorder.

LABORATORY FINDINGS. Findings can include leukopenia, mild anemia, dehydration (elevated blood urea nitrogen), metabolic alkalosis (with induced vomiting), and metabolic acidosis (with laxative abuse). Physical findings are consistent with starvation. Occasionally, onset is associated with stressful life situations. Perfectionistic behavior and mild obesity are common before onset. More than 90% of patients are female. Onset typically occurs in adolescent and early adulthood. Course is variable and long-term mortality is over 10%.

DIFFERENTIAL DIAGNOSIS. Weight loss occurs commonly with certain psychiatric disorders, especially Mood Disorders such as Major Depressive Disorder, and general medical conditions. Individuals with Schizophrenia can develop bizarre eating patterns. (NOTE: Although quite rare, if the full Anorexia Nervosa syndrome is also present, both diagnoses are given.) The clinician must also rule out Bulimia Nervosa. If an individual with Anorexia Nervosa exhibits binge eating and purging, this is *not* considered Bulimia Nervosa, but is a subtype of the diagnosis (i.e., Anorexia Nervosa, Binge-Eating/Purging Type).

A person who has a Social Phobia may exhibit self-consciousness about eating habits, but should not have profound weight loss. The obsessions and compulsions that occur in Obsessive-Compulsive Disorder sometimes involve food, body appearance, or excessive exercise. In addition, an individual with Body Dysmorphic Disorder has a distorted body image that involves a specific body part but does not have the marked weight loss and body distortion associated with Anorexia Nervosa.

DIAGNOSTIC CRITERIA FOR ANOREXIA NERVOSA (307.1)   (ICD-10 code F50.0)

A. Refusal to maintain body weight at or above a minimally normal weight for age and height (e.g., weight loss leading to maintenance of body weight less than 85% of that expected; or failure to make expected weight gain during period of growth, leading to body weight less than 85% of that expected).

B. Intense fear of gaining weight or becoming fat, even though underweight.

C. Disturbance in the way in which one's body weight or shape is experienced, undue influence of body weight or shape on self-evaluation, or denial of the seriousness of the current low body weight.

D. In postmenarcheal females, amenorrhea, i.e., the absence of at least three consecutive menstrual cycles. (A woman is considered to have amenorrhea if her periods occur only following hormone, e.g., estrogen, administration.)

> **Specify type:**
> **Restricting Type:** during the current episode of Anorexia Nervosa, the person has not regularly engaged in binge-eating or purging behavior (i.e., self-induced vomiting or the misuse of laxatives, diuretics, or enemas)
>
> **Binge-Eating/Purging Type:** during the current episode of Anorexia Nervosa, the person has regularly engaged in binge-eating or purging behavior (i.e., self-induced vomiting or the misuse of laxatives, diuretics, or enemas)

□ □ □ □

307.51 Bulimia Nervosa   *(ICD-10 code F50.2)*

ESSENTIAL FEATURES. There are recurrent episodes of binge eating (rapid eating of large amounts of food over a 2-hour period of time), with a feeling of lack of control over eating behavior during these binges. The food consumed is often sweet and of high caloric content, and is usually eaten inconspicuously or secretly. The binge is followed by inappropriate compensatory behaviors (e.g., enemas, laxative, diuretics, and especially self-induced vomiting). Vomiting allows either continued eating or termination of the binge, and also reduces unpleasant feelings.

ASSOCIATED FEATURES. Although the individual is usually of normal weight, a history of being overweight during adolescence is not uncommon. Depression, anxiety, Substance Abuse or Dependence, and Personality Disorder(s) (especially Borderline Personality Disorder) are often present. About 90% of patients are female.

LABORATORY FINDINGS. Findings may include fluid and electrolyte abnormalities, metabolic alkalosis (self-induced vomiting), or metabolic acidosis (laxative abuse). Physical findings may include signs of chronic self-induced vomiting, such as loss of teeth enamel and calluses or scars on the dorsal surface of the hand.

DIFFERENTIAL DIAGNOSIS. The clinician must determine whether the binge eating and compensatory behaviors, such as self-induced vomiting and laxatives, are part of another eating disorder, specifically Anorexia Nervosa, Binge-Eating/Purging Type. If criteria for Anorexia Nervosa are met, a diagnosis of Bulimia Nervosa is not made. Other diagnoses to consider are Major Depression With Atypical Features (e.g., excessive eating but no compensatory behaviors); Schizophrenia, which can involve bizarre eating behaviors; and certain medical disorders, such as Kleine-Levin syndrome. Binge eating is sometimes a feature of Borderline Personality Disorder; both diagnoses are given if criteria are met.

DIAGNOSTIC CRITERIA FOR   *(ICD-10 code F50.2)*
BULIMIA NERVOSA (307.51)

A. Recurrent episodes of binge eating. An episode of binge eating is characterized by both of the following:
   (1) eating, in a discrete period of time (e.g., within any 2-hour period), an amount of food that is definitely larger than most people would eat during a similar period of time and under similar circumstances
   (2) a sense of lack of control over eating during the episode (e.g., a feeling that one cannot stop eating or control what or how much one is eating)

B. Recurrent inappropriate compensatory behavior in order to prevent weight gain, such as self-induced vomiting; misuse of laxatives, diuretics, enemas, or other medications; fasting; or excessive exercise.

C. The binge eating and inappropriate compensatory behaviors both occur, on average, at least twice a week for 3 months.

D. Self-evaluation is unduly influenced by body shape and weight.

E. The disturbance does not occur exclusively during episodes of Anorexia Nervosa.

Specify type:
Purging Type: during the current episode of Bulimia Nervosa, the person has regularly engaged in self-induced vomiting or the misuse of laxatives, diuretics, or enemas

Nonpurging Type: during the current episode of Bulimia Nervosa, the person has used other inappropriate compensatory behaviors, such as fasting or excessive exercise, but has not regularly engaged in self-induced vomiting or the misuse of laxatives, diuretics, or enemas

□ □ □ □

307.50 Eating Disorder Not Otherwise Specified (NOS) *(ICD-10 code F50.9)*

This residual category is for clinically significant disorders that do not meet criteria for a specific Eating Disorder (e.g., all features of Anorexia Nervosa in a female except regular menses; features of Bulimia Nervosa except the required frequency of binge-eating episodes).

□ □ □ □

DIFFERENCES BETWEEN DSM-III-R AND DSM-IV EATING DISORDERS

❑ This section is new in DSM-IV. The diagnoses listed here were formerly located in DSM-III-R section "Disorders Usually First Evident in Infancy, Childhood or Adolescence."

❑ Individuals who are binge eating and purging exclusively during the course of **Anorexia Nervosa** should no longer receive both diagnoses, since DSM-IV contains new subtypes for Anorexia Nervosa (**Restricting Type** and **Binge-Eating/Purging Type**) and **Bulimia Nervosa (Purging Type and Nonpurging Type)** which allow for such patients.

....

CASE VIGNETTE: EATING DISORDERS

Case Vignette

B.R. is a 19-year-old college freshman who is brought in for evaluation by her parents; she is attending college while living with them. B.R.'s parents are very concerned about her declining weight. Two weeks ago B.R.'s mother found a large supply of diuretic hidden in her daughter's closet. The parents also report that B.R. is a perfectionist; when not in class, she spends her time studying in her room. She has never dated, has no friends, and is a straight *A* student. The mother reluctantly reports that large boxes of cookies, pies, and a cake have disappeared from the kitchen.

On examination, B.R. appears extremely thin. She weighs 85 pounds and is 5 feet 7 inches tall. She denies any problems with food intake, and denies use of diuretics, laxatives, amphetamine-like substances, or enemas. She does admit that her last menstrual period was more than 4 months ago. She does not agree with her parents' concerns about her weight; she angrily states, "I don't have a problem!"

DIAGNOSIS AND DISCUSSION

Axis I—307.1 Anorexia Nervosa, Binge-Eating/Purging Type (Provisional) (ICD-10 F50.0)
Axis II—Obsessive-Compulsive Traits; Rule out Obsessive-Compulsive
Personality Disorder (ICD-10 F60.5)
Axis III—Diuretic Use

The history and presentation are consistent with Anorexia Nervosa. Because B.R. has not had a medical evaluation, the clinician chooses to add "(Provisional)" to the diagnosis. B.R. is apparently using diuretics, and is probably binge eating high-calorie foods, thus, she is considered a Binge-Eating/Purging Type. By history, she also has obsessive-compulsive traits. As more history is gathered and additional observations are made, the clinician may find that B.R. has an Obsessive-Compulsive Personality Disorder.

CHAPTER 22

SLEEP DISORDERS

DSM-IV organizes the sleep disorders differently from DSM-III-R and provides more information about their evaluation and diagnosis. The organization is by presumed etiology (primary, caused by another mental disorder, caused by a general medical condition, and substance induced).

Polysomnography is a procedure that measures important characteristics of the five sleep stages. The stages, which will not be examined in detail here, are **rapid eye movement or REM sleep, stage 1 non-REM (NREM)** (the transition from wakefulness to sleep), **stage 2 NREM**, and **stages 3 and 4 NREM** (deepest, "slow-wave" sleep). Other polysomnographic terms used include **sleep continuity** (balance of sleep and wakefulness; "better" refers to fewer interruptions of sleep), **sleep latency** (time required to fall asleep), **intermittent wakefulness** (amount of time awake after initially falling asleep), **sleep efficiency** (portion of time spent asleep *versus* awake in bed), and **sleep architecture** (distribution of, and amount of time spent in, the various sleep stages). The DSM-IV text that refers to the relationship of each disorder to the International Classification of Sleep Disorders is not summarized in this Training Guide.

PRIMARY SLEEP DISORDERS

Dyssomnias

Dyssomnias are concerned with the amount, quality, or schedule of sleep, including insomnia, unwanted awakening, and excessive sleep. They are primary disorders in that they are not caused by known mental or physical illness or substances.

307.42 Primary Insomnia   (ICD-10 code F51.0)
(new in DSM-IV)

ESSENTIAL FEATURES. The essential feature of the insomnias is a predominant complaint of difficulty initiating or maintaining sleep, or of not feeling rested after apparently adequate sleep (nonrestorative sleep). The clinician should be familiar with normal variations related to age and other factors.

Associated Features. Nonspecific complaints are common, including disturbances of concentration or mood. Stress is often a factor.

Physical and Laboratory Findings. Physical examination is usually negative. Polysomnography may indicate poor sleep continuity, increased stage 1, decreased stages 3 and 4, increased muscle tension, and/or increased *alpha* activity during sleep.

Complications. Complications are few, and are primarily related to treatment (including self-treatment) with substances taken either to induce sleep or increase alertness.

Differential Diagnosis. Normal variations in sleep needs and patterns should be considered first. Many other mental disorders can cause insomnia; in such cases, Primary Insomnia should not be additionally diagnosed unless it is the predominant complaint, is judged not to be caused by the other mental disorder, and warrants independent clinical attention. Circadian Rhythm Sleep Disorder is alleviated when the sleep-wake pattern is restored. Daytime sleepiness often associated with insomnia must be differentiated from the greater sleepiness of hypersomnia, narcolepsy, and Breathing-Related Sleep Disorders. When the sleep disturbance is caused by a physical disorder or substance (e.g., caffeine), Primary Insomnia should not be diagnosed.

Diagnostic Criteria for   (ICD-10 code F51.0)
Primary Insomnia (307.42)

A. The predominant complaint is difficulty initiating or maintaining sleep, or nonrestorative sleep, for at least 1 month.

B. The sleep disturbance (or associated daytime fatigue) causes clinically significant distress or impairment in social, occupational, or other important areas of functioning.

C. The sleep disturbance does not occur exclusively during the course of narcolepsy, Breathing-Related Sleep Disorder, a Circadian Rhythm Sleep Disorder, or a Parasomnia.

D. The disturbance does not occur exclusively during the course of another mental disorder (e.g., Major Depressive Disorder, Generalized Anxiety Disorder, a Delirium).

E. The disturbance is not due to the direct physiological effects of a substance (e.g., a drug of abuse, a medication) or a general medical condition.

□ □ □ □

307.44 Primary Hypersomnia   (ICD-10 code F51.1)
(new in DSM-IV)

ESSENTIAL FEATURES. There is clinically significant excessive sleepiness or episodic daytime attacks of sleepiness not accounted for by inadequate sleep or another Sleep Disorder. Nighttime sleep appears normal, and may not be excessive.

ASSOCIATED FEATURES. Associated features can include the severe and recurrent Hypersomnia of Kleine-Levin syndrome or sleep-wake transition symptoms (e.g., sleep drunkenness). Many patients with hypersomnia disorders become demoralized or depressed. Accidental injury is common, as are social and vocational problems. Some patients abuse, or develop tolerance to, stimulant medication. Family history may be positive for Sleep Disorders or autonomic dysfunction.

PHYSICAL AND LABORATORY FINDINGS. Polysomnography is usually normal (except for short sleep latency). General EEG slowing and paroxysmal *theta* activity are characteristic of Kleine-Levin syndrome, as are occasional neurological signs (e.g., depressed reflexes, nystagmus).

DIFFERENTIAL DIAGNOSIS. Normal sleep variations, Circadian Rhythm Sleep Disorder, and sleep deprivation should be easily ruled out. If hypersomnia symptoms appear related to Primary Insomnia, this diagnosis should not be made. In Narcolepsy, the daytime symptoms are more discrete and seizurelike; Narcolepsy often includes cataplexy and characteristic polysomnographic architecture in the sleep-wake periods. Primary Hypersomnia should not be diagnosed if it is always associated with another mental disorder. When the sleep disturbance is caused by a physical disorder or substance, Primary Hypersomnia should not be diagnosed.

DIAGNOSTIC CRITERIA FOR   (ICD-10 code F51.1)
PRIMARY HYPERSOMNIA (307.44)

A. The predominant complaint is excessive sleepiness for at least 1 month (or less if recurrent) as evidenced by either prolonged sleep episodes or daytime sleep episodes occurring almost daily.

B. The excessive sleepiness causes clinically significant distress or impairment in social, occupational, or other important areas of functioning.

C. The excessive sleepiness is not better accounted for by insomnia, does not occur exclusively during the course of another Sleep Disorder (e.g., Narcolepsy, Breathing-Related Sleep Disorder, Circadian Rhythm Sleep Disorder, or a Parasomnia) and cannot be accounted for by an inadequate amount of sleep.

D. The disturbance does not occur exclusively during the course of another mental disorder.

E. The disturbance is not due to the direct physiological effects of a substance (e.g., a drug of abuse, a medication) or a general medical condition.

Specify if:
Recurrent: if there are periods of excessive sleepiness lasting at least 3 days occurring several times a year for at least 2 years

▢ ▢ ▢ ▢

347 Narcolepsy *(ICD-10 code G47.4)*
(new in DSM-IV)

ESSENTIAL FEATURES. Features include at least 3 months of repetitive, brief (usually a few minutes), seizure-like sleep attacks, in addition to cataplexy and/or interruption of the sleep-wake transition period by REM episodes. The episodes are refreshing, and may include dreaming. Some authors diagnose Narcolepsy in the absence of the cataplexy or REM intrusion if certain characteristic findings are present during multiple sleep latency testing (MSLT).

ASSOCIATED FEATURES. Patients with Narcolepsy often have other sleep signs and symptoms, such as cataplexy, hypnagogic or hypnopompic hallucinations, or sleep paralysis. The sleep attacks cannot be controlled by the patient, and thus may be associated with serious accidents or injury.

PHYSICAL AND LABORATORY FINDINGS. Findings include obvious sleepiness, slurring of speech, or episodes of cataplexy. Short sleep latency and REM sleep during test naps are found on multiple sleep latency testing (MSLT).

PREDISPOSING FACTORS. Sleep deprivation and boring settings may be associated with increased attacks. Cataplexy is often triggered by strong emotional feelings.

DIFFERENTIAL DIAGNOSIS. Sleep deprivation should be easily ruled out. Primary Hypersomnia can appear early in the course (see preceding). Breathing-Related Sleep Disorder can produce severe daytime sleepiness, and may coexist with the disorder. Some other mental disorders may cause daytime sleepiness or behaviors that are superficially similar. Certain forms of psychomotor epilepsy mimic narcoleptic sleep attacks; when the sleep disturbance is caused by another physical disorder or a substance, Narcolepsy should not be diagnosed.

DIAGNOSTIC CRITERIA FOR (ICD-10 code G47.4)
NARCOLEPSY (347)

A. Irresistible attacks of refreshing sleep that occur daily over at least 3 months.

B. The presence of one or both of the following:
   (1) cataplexy (i.e., brief episodes of sudden bilateral loss of muscle tone, most often in association with intense emotion)

(2) recurrent intrusions of elements of rapid eye movement (REM) sleep into the transition between sleep and wakefulness, as manifested by either hypnopompic or hypnagogic hallucinations or sleep paralysis at the beginning or end of sleep episodes

C. The disturbance is not due to the direct physiological effects of a substance (e.g., a drug of abuse, a medication) or another general medical condition.

❑ ❑ ❑ ❑

780.59 Breathing-Related Sleep Disorder (ICD-10 code G47.3)
(new in DSM-IV)

ESSENTIAL FEATURES. There is abnormal breathing that interferes with sleep. The ventilation disorder may be due to obstructive sleep apnea, central sleep apnea, or central alveolar hypoventilation syndrome.

ASSOCIATED FEATURES. Sleep is typically not refreshing; daytime sleepiness is common. Obstructive sleep apnea is characterized by snoring or gasping. Both obstructive sleep apnea and central alveolar hypoventilation syndrome are often associated with obesity. Central sleep apnea is more often associated with neurological or cardiac dysfunction.

PHYSICAL AND LABORATORY FINDINGS. In sleep apneas, findings include apneic episodes of more than 10 seconds and often reduced arterial blood oxygen during sleep. Airway obstruction may be observed via imaging or endoscopy. Nocturnal cardiac arrhythmias are common.

DIFFERENTIAL DIAGNOSIS. Nonpathological snoring and other Sleep Disorders should be ruled out. Nocturnal anxiety or Panic Attacks may appear similar but do not include apneic episodes or lowered blood oxygen saturation.

DIAGNOSTIC CRITERIA FOR (ICD-10 code G47.3)
BREATHING-RELATED SLEEP
DISORDER (780.59)

A. Sleep disruption, leading to excessive sleepiness or insomnia, that is judged to be due to a sleep-related breathing condition (e.g., obstructive or central sleep apnea syndrome or central alveolar hypoventilation syndrome).

B. The disturbance is not better accounted for by another mental disorder and not due to the direct physiological effects of a substance (e.g., a drug of abuse, a medication) or another general medical condition (other than a breathing-related disorder).

> **CODING NOTE: Also code the Breathing-Related Sleep Disorder on Axis III.**

❑ ❑ ❑ ❑

307.45 Circadian Rhythm Sleep Disorder   (ICD-10 code F51.2)
(Sleep-Wake Schedule Disorder in DSM-III-R)

ESSENTIAL FEATURES. There is a mismatch between the sleep-wake schedule demanded by the person's environment and his or her endogenous circadian rhythm. The usual result is either insomnia or hypersomnia, which generally disappears if the patient is allowed to follow his or her own sleep-wake schedule.

ASSOCIATED FEATURES. Nonspecific dysphoria is common.

PREDISPOSING FACTORS. Lifestyles that include frequently changing or irregular patterns of sleep and wakefulness, whether related to erratic schedules or frequent travel across several time zones, are predisposing.

DIFFERENTIAL DIAGNOSIS. Normal or transient sleep adjustments after changes in sleep schedules and voluntary delaying of sleep are considered. Primary Insomnia and Primary Hypersomnia are easily ruled out. If the sleep disturbance is limited to the course of another mental disorder, the diagnosis should not be made.

DIAGNOSTIC CRITERIA FOR   (ICD-10 code F51.2)
CIRCADIAN RHYTHM SLEEP
DISORDER (307.45)

A. A persistent or recurrent pattern of sleep disruption leading to excessive sleepiness or insomnia that is due to a mismatch between the sleep-wake schedule required by a person's environment and his or her circadian sleep-wake pattern.

B. The sleep disturbance causes clinically significant distress or impairment in social, occupational, or other important areas of functioning.

C. The disturbance does not occur exclusively during the course of another Sleep Disorder or other mental disorder.

D. The disturbance is not due to the direct physiological effects of a substance (e.g., a drug of abuse, a medication) or a general medical condition.

Specify type:
Delayed Sleep Phase Type: a persistent pattern of late sleep onset and late awakening times, with an inability to fall asleep and awaken at a desired earlier time

Jet Lag Type: sleepiness and alertness that occur at an inappropriate time of day relative to local time, occurring after repeated travel across more than one time zone

Shift Work Type: insomnia during the major sleep period or excessive sleepiness during the major wake period, associated with night-shift work or frequently changing shift work

Unspecified Type

❑ ❑ ❑ ❑

307.47 Dyssomnia Not Otherwise Specified (NOS)

(ICD-10 code F51.9)

This category is for insomnias, hypersomnias, or circadian rhythm disturbances that do not meet criteria for any specific Dyssomnia. Examples include nocturnal myoclonus, symptoms of chronic sleep deprivation, and situations in which the clinician has concluded that a Dyssomnia is present but is unable to determine whether it is primary, due to a general medical condition, or substance induced.

PARASOMNIAS

The parasomnias are characterized by abnormal events—especially autonomic arousal, motor activity, or cognitive processes—that occur either during sleep or at the interface of wakefulness and sleep. The predominant complaint focuses on this disturbance and not on its effects on sleep or wakefulness. Some disorders that meet these criteria are classified elsewhere (e.g., Enuresis Not Due to a General Medical Condition).

307.47 Nightmare Disorder
(Dream Anxiety Disorder in DSM-III-R)

(ICD-10 code F51.5)

ESSENTIAL FEATURES. There are vivid, very frightening dreams that repeatedly awaken the patient and for which he or she has detailed recall. The episodes occur during REM sleep and thus involve little motor movement.

ASSOCIATED FEATURES. Severe psychopathology is, by definition, absent; however, the disorder may be associated with stressors, anxiety, and depression that do not meet DSM-IV criteria for another mental disorder. Sleeplessness after awakening from the nightmare is common.

DIFFERENTIAL DIAGNOSIS. Occasional nightmares which do not impair function or cause significant distress are considered. Sleep Terror Disorder is differentiated by a number of factors (see following). Breathing-Related Sleep Disorder and nocturnal anxiety or Panic Attacks are not associated with frightening dreams. If nightmare symptoms are restricted to the course of another mental disorder, the diagnosis should not be made. If the disturbance was initiated and maintained by a known general medical condition or substance (e.g., a medication), Nightmare Disorder should not be diagnosed.

DIAGNOSTIC CRITERIA FOR   (ICD-10 code F51.5)
NIGHTMARE DISORDER (307.47)

A. Repeated awakenings from the major sleep period or naps with detailed recall of extended and extremely frightening dreams, usually involving threats to survival, security, or self-esteem. The awakenings generally occur during the second half of the sleep period.

B. On awakening from the frightening dreams, the person rapidly becomes oriented and alert (in contrast to the confusion and disorientation seen in Sleep Terror Disorder and some forms of epilepsy).

C. The dream experience, or the sleep disturbance resulting from the awakening, causes clinically significant distress or impairment in social, occupational, or other important areas of functioning.

D. The nightmares do not occur exclusively during the course of another mental disorder (e.g., a delirium, Posttraumatic Stress Disorder) and are not due to the direct physiological effects of a substance (e.g., a drug of abuse, a medication) or a general medical condition.

□ □ □ □

307.46 Sleep Terror Disorder   (ICD-10 code F51.4)

ESSENTIAL FEATURES. There are repeated episodes of abrupt awakening from sleep with vague but intense anxiety. The patient typically sits up abruptly with a frightened expression, emits a cry or scream, and shows both emotional and physiological signs of anxiety and confusion. If a dream is recalled, it is obscure and fragmented. The episodes are also called *pavor nocturnus*.

ASSOCIATED FEATURES. In children, there is no consistently associated psychopathology. In adults, Axis I disorders are often present and predisposing, including situational stress, sleep deprivation, alcohol or other drug use, fatigue, and Anxiety Disorders (e.g., Posttraumatic Stress Disorder, Generalized Anxiety Disorder). Sleep Terror Disorder may be diagnosed in addition to other mental disorders. The disorder is more common in children than adults, and usually remits before adulthood.

PHYSICAL AND LABORATORY FINDINGS. The disorder is usually associated with stages 3 and 4 non-REM sleep, consistent with their occurring more often during the first third of the sleep period. Episodes are routinely preceded by high-voltage *delta* activity on EEG, often with tachycardia. In persons with this diagnosis, such premonitory signs may occur without an actual night terror.

PREDISPOSING FACTORS. Many patients with this disorder have had a serious fe-brile illness in the past. Family history of the disorder is also common.

DIFFERENTIAL DIAGNOSIS. Nightmare Disorder is distinguished by its appearance during REM sleep and concomitant differences in presentation. REM phenom-ena such as so-called REM Sleep Behavior Disorder, in which dreams are re-ported and awakening is more complete, may be coded under Parasomnia NOS. Hypnagogic hallucinations differ in that they occur at sleep onset and consist of vivid images at the transition period. Sleepwalking Disorder may be comorbid but is generally free of fear or significant autonomic arousal. Epileptic seizures during sleep may appear similar to sleep terrors.

DIAGNOSTIC CRITERIA FOR   (ICD-10 code F51.4)
SLEEP TERROR DISORDER (307.46)

A. Recurrent episodes of abrupt awakening from sleep, usually occurring during the first third of the major sleep episode and beginning with a panicky scream.

B. Intense fear and signs of autonomic arousal, such as tachycardia, rapid breathing, and sweating, during each episode.

C. Relative unresponsiveness to efforts of others to comfort the person during the episode.

D. No detailed dream is recalled and there is amnesia for the episode.

E. The episodes cause clinically significant distress or impairment in social, occu-pational, or other important areas of functioning.

F. The disturbance is not due to the direct physiological effects of a substance (e.g., a drug of abuse, a medication) or a general medical condition.

❑ ❑ ❑ ❑

307.46 Sleepwalking Disorder   (ICD-10 code F51.3)

ESSENTIAL FEATURES. There are repeated episodes of complex dissociative motor behaviors, including leaving the bed and walking about, associated with non-REM sleep stages 3 and 4 (occasionally stage 2 in older adults) and usually lasting less than 30 minutes. Perseverative movements are common, which may proceed to semipurposeful motor acts. The patient may engage in complex be-haviors, rarely including leaving the home, driving, and so forth. Although out-wardly seeming awake, the person is in an altered state of consciousness and cannot exercise the judgment or coordination expected during wakefulness. Fragments of dreams or memories of behaviors during sleepwalking may occur but are commonly absent; the patient almost never recalls the entire episode.

ASSOCIATED FEATURES. The disorder is much more common in children than adults. Adult sleepwalkers almost always have a childhood history of sleepwalking (often with an interval of several years without symptoms). People with Sleepwalking Disorder have a higher than normal incidence of other non-REM Sleep Disorders. Children have not been observed to have any consistently associated psychopathology; however, adults frequently have situational stress, Adjustment Disorders, or Anxiety Disorders. DSM-IV states that personality disorders are common; however, other authors feel that sleepwalking in adults is not consistently associated with serious psychopathology.

PHYSICAL AND LABORATORY FINDINGS. Findings sometimes include high-voltage *delta* waves on EEG prior to episodes.

PREDISPOSING FACTORS. Febrile illness in childhood and family history of sleepwalking or other non-REM Sleep Disorders are common. In persons already predisposed, fatigue, external stress, and unconscious conflict increase the likelihood of sleepwalking.

DIFFERENTIAL DIAGNOSIS. First rule out clinically insignificant isolated sleepwalking episodes. Escape behaviors associated with sleep terrors should be distinguished by their fear and extreme autonomic arousal. Substance-related sleepwalking or that due to general medical conditions should not be diagnosed here. Psychomotor epilepsy may manifest itself at night; it should be ruled out in patients whose symptoms are especially troublesome and in those with neurological signs or symptoms. Dissociative Fugue is distinguishable in a number of ways, notably by its lack of disturbed consciousness. Sleep drunkenness may resemble sleepwalking but occurs after awakening and is often associated with aggressive behavior. REM Sleep Behavior Disorder occurs during REM sleep, usually later in the night, and is associated with reportable dreams.

DIAGNOSTIC CRITERIA FOR SLEEPWALKING DISORDER (307.46)   (ICD-10 code F51.3)

A. Repeated episodes of rising from bed during sleep and walking about, usually occurring during the first third of the major sleep episode.

B. While sleepwalking, the person has a blank, staring face, is relatively unresponsive to the efforts of others to communicate with him or her, and can be awakened only with great difficulty.

C. On awakening (either from the sleepwalking episode or the next morning), the person has amnesia for the episode.

D. Within several minutes after awakening from the sleepwalking episode, there is no impairment of mental activity or behavior (although there may initially be a short period of confusion or disorientation).

E. The sleepwalking causes clinically significant distress or impairment in social, occupational, or other important areas of functioning.

F. The disturbance is not due to the direct physiological effects of a substance (e.g., a drug of abuse, a medication) or a general medical condition.

❑ ❑ ❑ ❑

307.47 Parasomnia Not Otherwise Specified (NOS)

(ICD-10 code F51.8)

This category is for abnormal sleep physiology or behavior that does not meet criteria for a specific Parasomnia. Examples include hypnagogic or hypnopompic "sleep paralysis"; REM Sleep Behavior Disorder; and situations in which a Parasomnia is present but it is unclear whether it is primary, due to a general medical condition, or substance induced.

❑ ❑ ❑ ❑

SLEEP DISORDERS RELATED TO ANOTHER MENTAL DISORDER

307.42 Insomnia Related to Another Mental Disorder

(ICD-10 code F51.0)

ESSENTIAL FEATURES. There is clinically significant insomnia caused by an Axis I or II mental disorder and lasting for at least 1 month. The diagnosis is not used if the disturbance is related to a substance or general medical condition.

DIAGNOSTIC CRITERIA FOR INSOMNIA RELATED TO . . . (SPECIFY AXIS I OR II MENTAL DISORDER) (307.42)

(ICD-10 code F51.0)

NOTE: Code the causative mental disorder as well.

A. The predominant complaint is difficulty initiating or maintaining sleep, or nonrestorative sleep, for at least 1 month, that is associated with daytime fatigue or impaired daytime functioning.

B. The sleep disturbance (or daytime sequelae) causes clinically significant distress or impairment in social, occupational, or other important areas of functioning.

C. The insomnia is judged to be related to another Axis I or Axis II disorder (e.g., Major Depressive Disorder, Generalized Anxiety Disorder, Adjustment Disorder With Anxiety), but is sufficiently severe to warrant independent clinical attention.

D. The disturbance is not better accounted for by another Sleep Disorder (e.g., Narcolepsy, Breathing-Related Sleep Disorder, a Parasomnia).

E. The disturbance is not due to the direct physiological effects of a substance (e.g., a drug of abuse, a medication) or a general medical condition.

❑ ❑ ❑ ❑

307.44 Hypersomnia Related to Another Mental Disorder
(ICD-10 code F51.1)

ESSENTIAL FEATURES. There is clinically significant hypersomnia caused by an Axis I or II mental disorder and lasting for at least 1 month. The diagnosis is not used if the disturbance is related to a substance or general medical condition.

DIAGNOSTIC CRITERIA FOR HYPERSOMNIA RELATED TO . . . (SPECIFY AXIS I OR II MENTAL DISORDER) (307.44)
(ICD-10 code F51.1)

A. The predominant complaint is excessive sleepiness for at least 1 month as evidenced by either prolonged sleep episodes or daytime sleep episodes occurring almost daily.

B. The excessive sleepiness causes clinically significant distress or impairment in social, occupational, or other important areas of functioning.

C. The hypersomnia is judged to be related to another Axis I or Axis II disorder (e.g., Major Depressive Disorder, Dysthymic Disorder) but is sufficiently severe to warrant independent clinical attention.

D. The disturbance is not better accounted for by another Sleep Disorder (e.g., Narcolepsy, Breathing-Related Sleep Disorder, a Parasomnia) or by inadequate sleep.

E. The disturbance is not due to the direct physiological effects of a substance (e.g., a drug of abuse, a medication) or a general medical condition.

CODING NOTE: Code the causative mental disorder as well.

❑ ❑ ❑ ❑

OTHER SLEEP DISORDERS

780.xx Sleep Disorder Due to a General Medical Condition
(ICD-10 code G47.x)

(includes DSM-III-R non-substance-related Insomnia or Hypersomnia Related to a Known Organic Factor [780.50])
(new in DSM-IV)

ESSENTIAL FEATURES. Sleep disturbance caused by general medical condition and sufficiently severe to warrant independent clinical attention is seen.

DIAGNOSTIC CRITERIA FOR   (ICD-10 code G47.x)
SLEEP DISORDER DUE TO . . . (SPECIFY
GENERAL MEDICAL CONDITION) (780.xx)

A. A prominent disturbance in sleep that is sufficiently severe to warrant independent clinical attention.

B. There is evidence from the history, physical examination, or laboratory findings that the sleep disturbance is the direct physiological consequence of a general medical condition.

C. The disturbance is not better accounted for by another mental disorder (e.g., an Adjustment Disorder in which the stressor is a serious medical illness).

D. The disturbance does not occur exclusively during the course of a delirium.

E. The disturbance does not meet criteria for Breathing-Related Sleep Disorder or Narcolepsy.

F. The sleep disturbance causes clinically significant distress or impairment in social, occupational, or other important areas of functioning.

Specify type:
.52 Insomnia Type: if the predominant sleep disturbance is insomnia (ICD-10 G47.0)

.54 Hypersomnia Type: if the predominant sleep disturbance is hypersomnia (ICD-10 G47.1)

.59 Parasomnia Type: if the predominant sleep disturbance is a Parasomnia (ICD-10 G47.8)

.59 Mixed Type: if more than one sleep disturbance is present and none predominates (ICD-10 G47.8)

CODING NOTE: Include the name of the general medical condition in the Axis I diagnosis (e.g., "780.54, Sleep Disorder Due to Acquired Hypothyroidism, Hypersomnia Type), and also code the general medical condition on Axis III. (See DSM-IV Appendix G for ICD-9-CM disease and E codes.)

❑ ❑ ❑ ❑

291.8, 292.89 Substance-Induced   *(ICD-10 code uses*
Sleep Disorder   *substance code)*
(includes DSM-III-R's Substance-related Insomnia or
Hypersomnia Related to a Known Organic Factor
[formerly 780.50])
(new in DSM-IV)

ESSENTIAL FEATURES. There is sleep disturbance caused by the direct physiological effects of a substance (e.g., medication, toxin, drug of abuse), and it is sufficiently severe to warrant independent clinical attention.

DIAGNOSTIC CRITERIA FOR SUBSTANCE-INDUCED SLEEP DISORDER (291.8, 292.89)

(ICD-10 code uses substance code)

A. A prominent disturbance in sleep that is sufficiently severe to warrant independent clinical attention.

B. There is evidence from the history, physical examination, or laboratory findings of either (1) or (2), below:
   (1) The symptoms in Criterion A developed during, or within a month of, Substance Intoxication or Withdrawal.
   (2) Medication use is etiologically related to the sleep disturbance.

C. The disturbance is not better accounted for by a Sleep Disorder that is not substance induced. Evidence that the symptoms are better accounted for by a Sleep Disorder that is not substance induced might include the following: the symptoms precede the onset of the substance use (or medication use); the symptoms persist for a substantial period of time (e.g., about a month) after the cessation of acute withdrawal or severe intoxication, or are substantially in excess of what would be expected given the type or amount of the substance used or the duration of use; or there is other evidence that suggests the existence of an independent non-substance-induced Sleep Disorder (e.g., a history of recurrent non-substance-related episodes).

D. The disturbance does not occur exclusively during the course of a delirium.

E. The sleep disturbance causes clinically significant distress or impairment in social, occupational, or other important areas of functioning.

Specify type:
Insomnia Type: if the predominant sleep disturbance is insomnia

Hypersomnia Type: if the predominant sleep disturbance is hypersomnia

Parasomnia Type: if the predominant sleep disturbance is a Parasomnia

Mixed Type: if more than one sleep disturbance is present and none predominates

Specify if:
With Onset During Intoxication: if the criteria are met for Intoxication with the substance and the symptoms develop during Intoxication syndrome.

With Onset During Withdrawal: if criteria are met for withdrawal from the substance and symptoms develop during, or shortly after, a withdrawal syndrome.

(See table in DSM-IV, p. 177, for applicability by substance.)

CODING NOTE: Code the (Specific Substance)-Induced Sleep Disorder as follows: 291.8 Alcohol (ICD-10 F10.8); **292.89 for all of the following: Amphetamine or Related Substance** (ICD-10 F15.8); **Caffeine** (ICD-10 F15.8); **Cocaine** (ICD-10 F14.8); **Opioid** (ICD-10 F11.8); **Sedative/Hypnotic/Anxiolytic** (ICD-10 F13.8); **Other or Unknown Substance** (ICD-10 F19.8).

CODING NOTE: Also code Substance-Specific Intoxication or Withdrawal if criteria are met.

❑ ❑ ❑ ❑

··

DIFFERENCES BETWEEN DSM-III-R AND DSM-IV SLEEP DISORDERS

The Sleep Disorders in DSM-IV are organized differently from those in DSM-III-R, and are now compatible with the 1990 International Classification of Sleep Disorders. Considerably more information is included.

❑ **Primary Insomnia, Primary Hypersomnia, Sleep Terror Disorder,** and **Sleepwalking Disorder** require the symptoms to be clinically significant before making a diagnosis of mental disorder.

❑ **Narcolepsy, Breathing-Related Sleep Disorder, Sleep Disorder Due To a General Medical Condition,** and **Substance-Induced Sleep Disorder** are new in DSM-IV.

❑ **Primary Insomnia** no longer must occur three times a week. A clinical significance criterion has been added.

❑ **Primary Hypersomnia** can be preempted by Primary Insomnia with daytime hypersomnia. Sleep drunkenness is no longer sufficient to imply hypersomnia. The **Recurrent** subtype has been added.

❑ The subtypes of **Circadian Rhythm Sleep Disorder** have been revised (now **Delayed Sleep Phase, Jet Lag, Shift Work, Unspecified**).

❑ **Nightmare Disorder** (DSM-III-R's Dream Anxiety Disorder) is not diagnosed if the symptoms are better accounted for by another mental or physical disorder.

❑ **Sleep Terror Disorder** no longer has a criterion for duration of awakening.

❑ **Insomnia** or **Hypersomnia Related To an Axis I or II Mental Disorder**, **Sleep Disorders Due To a General Medical Condition**, and **Substance-Induced Sleep Disorder** must be of sufficient severity to warrant clinical attention separate from the causative mental disorder, general medical condition, or substance abuse.

❑ **Sleep Disorders Due To a General Medical Condition** includes the former DSM-III-R non-substance-related Organic Insomnia and Organic Hypersomnia, but adds the specifiers **Insomnia Type, Hypersomnia Type, Parasomnia Type**, and **Mixed Type**.

❑ **Substance-Induced Sleep Disorders** includes the former DSM-III-R substance-related Organic Insomnia and Organic Hypersomnia, but adds the specifiers **Insomnia Type, Hypersomnia Type, Parasomnia Type**, and **Mixed Type**, as well as **Onset Related to Intoxication** and **Onset Related to Withdrawal**.

....

CASE VIGNETTES: SLEEP DISORDERS

Case Vignette 1

P.C., a very obese, 42-year-old man, presented with complaints of irritability, poor concentration, and fatigue. His wife believed he was depressed. He described insomnia, restless sleep, and daytime listlessness, but most other signs of mood disorder were lacking. He has twice fallen asleep during boring meetings at work. On weekends he spends much of his time napping.

Careful history indicated that P.C. gained much of his weight during the past year, and that his sleep disturbance increased with his weight. His wife reported that when sleeping he often becomes very still for 10–20 seconds, then emits a gasping snore. "It sounds like he's choking," but he rarely awakens completely. The episodes seem worse when he has been drinking, but they are not limited to intoxication. Except for his obesity, superficial physical examination was normal.

Referral for polysomnography revealed apneic episodes of 20–30 seconds, punctuated at the end by snorts and gasps, many times a night. Respirations are otherwise normal. The episodes aroused P.C. from sleep, but he did not recall them the next morning. An otolaryngology consultant found excessive soft tissue surrounding the upper airway.

DIAGNOSIS AND DISCUSSION

Axis I—780.59 Breathing-Related Sleep Disorder, Obstructive Sleep Apnea Syndrome (ICD-10 G47.3)
Axis II—V71.09 No Diagnosis or condition on Axis II (ICD-10 Z03.2)
Axis III—Obstructive Sleep Apnea Syndrome

This is a classic presentation of obstructive sleep apnea. Criteria for a Depressive Disorder are not met; most or all mood symptoms seem related to the Sleep Disorder. He does not have signs of central sleep apnea. Central alveolar hypoventilation syndrome is unlikely, but arterial blood gases have not been measured. There is no indication of anxiety symptoms which might suggest nocturnal Panic Attacks. There is no mention of Axis II symptoms.

Case Vignette 2

F.W., a 19-year-old military recruit, was referred to the psychiatrist after he walked in his sleep in his barracks on at least three occasions. Other trainees in his company said that he had a "blank" look on his face when sleepwalking, that he didn't seem aware of the occurrences, and that he returned to bed after a few minutes. F.W. said he was not aware of this behavior and did not recall any dream associated with it the next morning.

F.W. walked in his sleep as a young child, as did one of his sisters, but he had not done so since about age 7. There was no personal history of significant dysphoria, adjustment problems, or other psychiatric symptoms. He had been doing well in his basic training and did not want a medical discharge: "Both my brothers were Marines, and I'm going to be a Marine, too." Physical examination, including neurological exam and EEG, was negative.

DIAGNOSIS AND DISCUSSION
Axis I—307.46 Sleepwalking Disorder (ICD-10 F51.3)
Axis II—V71.09 No Diagnosis or Condition on Axis II (ICD-10 Z03.2)

Some clinicians might consider diagnosing an Adjustment Disorder related to becoming a military trainee; however, the patient does not perceive basic training as a significant psychosocial stressor. Malingering seems unlikely. The symptoms are better explained by a Sleepwalking Disorder, probably preexisting and perhaps precipitated by the new environment.

CHAPTER 23

IMPULSE CONTROL DISORDERS NOT ELSEWHERE CLASSIFIED

This is a residual diagnostic category for disorders of impulse control not elsewhere classified. The essential feature of these disorders is the individual's failure to resist performing a potentially harmful act. The individual usually has a sense of tension or arousal before committing the act, and a sense of relief or pleasure at the time the act is committed. Other features may or may not be present. These include conscious resistance to the impulse, preplanning, and guilt, regret, or self-reproach after committing the act.

312.34 Intermittent Explosive Disorder   (ICD-10 code F63.8)
(significantly modified from DSM-III-R)

ESSENTIAL FEATURES. The individual experiences several discrete episodes in which loss of control of aggressive impulse results in serious assaultive acts or destruction of property. The aggressiveness is grossly out of proportion to the precipitating events. Aggressiveness appears usually within minutes to hours and, regardless of duration, disappears quickly. The clinician must be sure that these episodes do not occur during the course of other mental disorders.

ASSOCIATED FEATURES. Genuine regret often follows aggressive episodes. Between aggressive episodes, there may be signs of impulsiveness or aggressiveness. Nonspecific EEG changes and abnormalities on neuropsychological testing are sometimes present.

DIFFERENTIAL DIAGNOSIS. A number of psychiatric disorders are potentially associated with angry outbursts. For example, individuals with a Delirium or Dementia become confused, are often paranoid, and are therefore prone to misinterpret situations and react aggressively. Similarly, a person who is in the midst of a Manic Episode, especially when his or her mood is irritable, or anyone who has a Psychotic Disorder, is more prone to have an angry outburst.

Some individuals with Personality Change Due to a General Medical Disorder are disinhibited and react with anger, as are individuals with certain

Personality Disorders, such as Antisocial Personality Disorder and Borderline Personality Disorder. Additional psychiatric disorders commonly associated with excessive or uncontrolled anger are Conduct Disorder, Oppositional Defiant Disorder, and Substance-Induced Intoxication or Withdrawal. Occasionally, a person will try to cover up a violent act by feigning Intermittent Explosive Disorder or another psychiatric disorder (i.e., the person is Malingering); unfortunately, angry behavior not associated with a psychiatric disorder is common in our society.

DIAGNOSTIC CRITERIA FOR INTERMITTENT EXPLOSIVE DISORDER (312.34)

(ICD-10 code F63.8)

A. Several discrete episodes of failure to resist aggressive impulses that result in serious assaultive acts or destruction of property.

B. The degree of aggressiveness expressed during the episodes is grossly out of proportion to any precipitating psychosocial stressors.

C. The aggressive episodes are not better accounted for by another mental disorder (e.g., Antisocial Personality Disorder, Borderline Personality Disorder, a Psychotic Disorder, a Manic Episode, Conduct Disorder, or Attention-Deficit/Hyperactivity Disorder) and are not due to the direct physiological effects of a substance (e.g., a drug of abuse, a medication) or a general medical condition (e.g., head trauma, Alzheimer's disease).

❑ ❑ ❑ ❑

312.32 Kleptomania

(ICD-10 code F63.2)

ESSENTIAL FEATURES. The person cannot resist the impulse to steal objects. The object is not stolen for its monetary value, its utility, or to express anger or gain revenge. There is a sense of tension immediately before the theft and a sense of relief or pleasure afterward. The stealing is not due to a Conduct Disorder, Antisocial Personality Disorder, or a Manic Episode.

ASSOCIATED FEATURES. The person often has signs of depression, anxiety, guilt, and personality disturbance.

DIFFERENTIAL DIAGNOSIS. The most common form of stealing is ordinary theft or shoplifting; in contrast, Kleptomania is quite rare. Certain psychiatric disorders are commonly associated with individuals who steal, particularly Conduct Disorder and Antisocial Personality Disorder. Less commonly, individuals with impaired reality testing, such as during a Manic Episode or Schizophrenia, may steal. Rarely, a person with brain dysfunction, like Dementia, will steal. An individual can also lie and report an irresistible urge to steal in order to escape punishment (i.e., Malinger).

DIAGNOSTIC CRITERIA FOR (ICD-10 code F63.2)
KLEPTOMANIA (312.32)

A. Recurrent failure to resist impulses to steal objects that are not needed for personal use or for their monetary value.

B. Increasing sense of tension immediately before committing the theft.

C. Pleasure, gratification, or relief at the time of committing the theft.

D. The stealing is not committed to express anger or vengeance and is not in response to a delusion or a hallucination.

E. The stealing is not better accounted for by Conduct Disorder, a Manic Episode, or Antisocial Personality Disorder.

□ □ □ □

312.31 Pathological Gambling (ICD-10 code F63.0)
(significantly modified from DSM-III-R)

ESSENTIAL FEATURES. There is a chronic, progressive failure to resist impulses to gamble. Gambling eventually disrupts and damages personal, family, or vocational pursuits. Characteristic problems include severe indebtedness, default on debts, family disruption, inattention to work, and illegal activities to finance gambling.

ASSOCIATED FEATURES. As indebtedness from gambling activities increases, the individual is forced to lie, embezzle, steal, or perform other illegal acts. Pathological gamblers have been described as overconfident, very energetic, easily bored, and "big spenders." At times of increased stress, anxiety and depression may be seen; suicide attempts are not uncommon.

DIFFERENTIAL DIAGNOSIS. Most individuals who gamble do so simply for pleasure (social gamblers); occasionally, people earn their living by gambling (professional gamblers). The clinician must determine whether the individual who meets the criteria for Pathological Gambling is having a Manic Episode. This is a difficult distinction because gambling itself can cause cocaine-like highs and depressive lows for the Pathological Gambler. A past history of Manic Episodes not associated with gambling helps the clinician separate these two diagnoses. Antisocial Personality Disorder is also considered in the differential diagnosis.

DIAGNOSTIC CRITERIA FOR (ICD-10 code F63.0)
PATHOLOGICAL GAMBLING (312.31)

A. Persistent and recurrent maladaptive gambling behavior as indicated by five (or more) of the following:

(1) is preoccupied with gambling (e.g., preoccupied with reliving past gambling experiences, handicapping or planning the next venture, or thinking of ways to get money with which to gamble)

(2) needs to gamble with increasing amounts of money in order to achieve the desired excitement

(3) has repeated unsuccessful efforts to control, cut back, or stop gambling

(4) is restless or irritable when attempting to cut down or stop gambling

(5) gambles as a way of escaping from problems or of relieving a dysphoric mood (e.g., feelings of helplessness, guilt, anxiety, depression)

(6) after losing money gambling, often returns another day to get even ("chasing" one's losses)

(7) lies to family members, therapist, or others to conceal the extent of involvement with gambling

(8) has committed illegal acts such as forgery, fraud, theft, or embezzlement to finance gambling

(9) has jeopardized or lost a significant relationship, job, or educational or career opportunity because of gambling

(10) relies on others to provide money to relieve a desperate financial situation caused by gambling

B. The gambling behavior is not better accounted for by a Manic Episode.

❑ ❑ ❑ ❑

312.33 Pyromania   (ICD-10 code F63.1)

ESSENTIAL FEATURES. There has been deliberate fire setting on more than one occasion, accompanied by increased tension prior to fire setting and intense pleasure or relief during fire setting or as a result of witnessing or participating in its aftermath. The fire setting is not motivated by monetary gain, sociopolitical ideology, anger or revenge, psychotic thinking (delusions or hallucinations), or to conceal criminal activity.

ASSOCIATED FEATURES. There may be considerable advance preparation, and the person may leave clues. Persons with this disorder may be regular fire watchers, set off false alarms, show interest in firefighting paraphernalia, seek employment as a firefighter, or work as a volunteer firefighter.

DIFFERENTIAL DIAGNOSIS. Youngsters commonly experiment with fire; individuals who meet the diagnostic criteria for Pyromania are exceedingly rare. Individuals with certain psychiatric disorders, such as Conduct Disorder and Antisocial Personality Disorder, are prone to set fires for personal gain (arson) or to conceal evidence after a crime. Less frequently, individuals with Psychotic Disorders or a Manic Episode might set a fire while actively psychotic. Individuals with impaired cognitive function, such as Dementia and Mental Retardation, can set fires also. Occasionally, a person who has Substance Intoxication will start a fire.

DIAGNOSTIC CRITERIA FOR PYROMANIA (312.33)

(ICD-10 code F63.1)

A. Deliberate and purposeful fire setting on more than one occasion.

B. Tension or affective arousal before the act.

C. Fascination with, interest in, curiosity about, or attraction to fire and its situational contexts (e.g., paraphernalia, uses, consequences).

D. Pleasure, gratification, or relief when setting fires, or when witnessing or participating in their aftermath.

E. The fire setting is not done for monetary gain, as an expression of sociopolitical ideology, to conceal criminal activity, to express anger or vengeance, to improve one's living circumstances, in response to a delusion or hallucination, or as a result of impaired judgment (e.g., in dementia, Mental Retardation, Substance Intoxication).

F. The fire setting is not better accounted for by Conduct Disorder, a Manic Episode, or Antisocial Personality Disorder.

□ □ □ □

312.39 Trichotillomania

(ICD-10 code F63.3)

ESSENTIAL FEATURES. This is recurrent failure to resist the impulse to pull out one's own hair. The individual experiences increased tension before the act or when trying to resist hair pulling. There is gratification or relief during or immediately after the act. The scalp is the most common area involved, although hair pulling can involve any body region (e.g., pubic or axillary hair). The affected scalp areas have an irregular "patchy" pattern of hair loss and hair of varying lengths exist within the patch. There is no evidence of scarring or pigmentary change. Other areas commonly involved are eyebrows, eyelashes, and beard. Other medical reasons for hair loss must be ruled out.

ASSOCIATED FEATURES. Rituals may develop, such as mouthing the hair (trichophagy) or swallowing the hair. Denial of the behavior is common. When onset of the disorder occurs in adulthood, a Psychotic Disorder should be ruled out.

DIFFERENTIAL DIAGNOSIS. The clinician must first rule out medical disorders that cause hair loss (alopecia). Then, the clinician can inquire whether the person has repetitive, "driven" behavior or thoughts (e.g., Obsessive Compulsive Disorder). Very rarely, an individual with Factitious Disorder With Predominantly Physical Signs and Symptoms will simulate Trichotillomania. Occasionally, a person who has a Psychotic Disorder will repetitively pull out hair during a psychotic episode. The clinician can also look for other repetitive behavior which might be part of Stereotypic Movement Disorder.

DIAGNOSTIC CRITERIA FOR   (ICD-10 code F63.3)
TRICHOTILLOMANIA (312.39)

A. Recurrent pulling out of one's hair resulting in noticeable hair loss.

B. An increasing sense of tension immediately before pulling out the hair or when attempting to resist the behavior.

C. Pleasure, gratification, or relief when pulling out the hair.

D. The disturbance is not better accounted for by another mental disorder and is not due to a general medical condition (e.g., a dermatological condition).

E. The disturbance causes clinically significant distress or impairment in social, occupational, or other important areas of functioning,

❑ ❑ ❑ ❑

312.30 Impulse Control Disorder Not   (ICD-10 code F63.9)
Otherwise Specified

This is a residual category for disorders of impulse control that do not meet the diagnostic criteria for other specific Impulse Control Disorders.

❑ ❑ ❑ ❑

DIFFERENCES BETWEEN DSM-III-R AND DSM-IV IMPULSE CONTROL DISORDERS NOT ELSEWHERE CLASSIFIED

❑   **Intermittent Explosive Disorder** was retained in DSM-IV despite reservations about its validity. The DSM-III-R criterion that required no signs of impulsiveness or aggressiveness between episodes was deleted.

❑   The diagnostic criteria for **Pathological Gambling** were revised by adding a tenth criterion, and the threshold for diagnosis was raised from four to five symptoms.

❑   The exclusion criterion for each diagnosis in the section was revised to include at least Conduct Disorder, a Manic Episode, and Antisocial Personality Disorder.

CASE VIGNETTE: DISORDERS OF IMPULSE CONTROL NOT ELSEWHERE SPECIFIED

Case Vignette

C.M. is a 27-year-old house painter who is brought by his wife for evaluation. She states that C.M. is unable to control his gambling, despite efforts by both to stop his behavior. He reports that his gambling began about 3 years ago during a vacation in Las Vegas. During that trip he spent increasing amounts of time gambling and was a big winner. Upon his return, he began placing bets, first on major league sports events and later on horse races. The amounts of his betting gradually grew from five or ten dollars to several hundred dollars per bet. He spent more and more time either gambling or trying to obtain money to sustain his wagering. C.M. states, "At this point I would bet on anything if the odds are right."

About 12 months ago, he began having severe financial problems. He borrowed money from his relatives and friends to cover his debts: "The further behind I got, the more I would bet to try to cover my losses." He is now deeply in debt to his bookie, who is threatening harm if C.M. doesn't at least pay the interest on the money.

C.M. denies prior psychiatric history, drug or alcohol abuse, and is in excellent health, except for mild hypertension. He is currently taking hydrochlorothiazide. He is unaware of his family's psychiatric history, because his mother abandoned him when he was 3. He reports going from foster home to foster home until he joined the army at age 17. He has been employed as a house painter since his discharge from the army.

DIAGNOSIS AND DISCUSSION
Axis I—312.31 Pathological Gambling (ICD-10 F63.0)
Axis II—V71.09 No Diagnosis or 799.9 Diagnosis Deferred (ICD-10 Z03.2, R46.8)
Axis III—Mild Hypertension

C.M. exhibits many of the symptoms of Pathological Gambling. These symptoms include preoccupation with gambling; increasing size and frequency of wagers, failure to stop gambling; borrowing money from others to relieve his severe financial problems; and continued, even increased, gambling despite mounting debts. There is no indication of an Axis II diagnosis from the history.

CHAPTER 24

ADJUSTMENT DISORDERS

NOTE: Adjustment Disorders are significantly modified from DSM-III-R.

ESSENTIAL FEATURES. An Adjustment Disorder is a maladaptive reaction to a psychosocial stressor(s). The reaction manifests itself as impairment in occupational functioning, social activities, or interpersonal relationships. The symptoms are in excess of a normal or expected reaction to the stressor(s), and are not part of a pattern of overreaction to stress (e.g., a Personality Disorder) or an exacerbation of a mental disorder.

(114)

The disturbance must begin within 3 months after the onset of the psychosocial stress and last no longer than 6 months after the stressor or its consequences have ceased. The severity of the reaction is not altogether predictable from the intensity of the stressor. Certain individuals may have a severe disturbance with a seemingly mild stressor; others may have a mild reaction to a severe stressor. Stressors may be single, recurrent, or continuous.

Six different Adjustment Disorders are listed in DSM-IV, classified according to the predominant symptoms. Note that Adjustment Disorders are partial syndromes of more specific disorders. For example, Adjustment Disorder With Depressed Mood is a depressive syndrome that develops after a psychosocial stressor and does not meet the full criteria for a Major Depression.

DIFFERENTIAL DIAGNOSIS. Adjustment Disorders are subthreshold diagnoses in that the individual does not meet criteria for a major psychiatric disorder (e.g., a person with an Adjustment Disorder With Depressed Mood does not have sufficient symptoms to meet the criteria for a Major Depressive Episode). Because individuals with Personality Disorders frequently react to stress in an abnormal way, an Adjustment Disorder diagnosis is not made unless the reaction is atypical. Other disorders that are precipitated by stress to rule out include Posttraumatic Stress Disorder, Acute Stress Disorder, and Bereavement. The clinician should also consider in the differential diagnosis Psychological Factors Affecting a Medical Condition in patients who have medical illness. When no impairment is present, the proper diagnosis is normal or a non-pathologic response to stress.

DIAGNOSTIC CRITERIA FOR ADJUSTMENT DISORDERS (309.xx) (CODE BASED ON SUBTYPE, BELOW)

(ICD-10 code F43.xx)

A. The development of emotional or behavioral symptoms in response to an identifiable stressor(s) occurring within 3 months of the onset of the stressor(s).

B. These symptoms or behaviors are clinically significant as evidenced by either of the following:
   (1) marked distress that is in excess of what would be expected from exposure to the stressor
   (2) significant impairment in social or occupational (academic) functioning

C. The stress-related disturbance does not meet the criteria for another specific Axis I disorder and is not merely an exacerbation of a preexisting Axis I or Axis II disorder.

D. The symptoms do not represent Bereavement.

E. Once the stressor (or its consequences) has terminated, the symptoms do not persist for more than an additional 6 months.

Specify if:
Acute: if the disturbance lasts less than 6 months

Chronic: if the disturbance lasts for 6 months or longer

CODING NOTE: Adjustment Disorders are coded based on the subtype, which is selected according to the predominant symptoms. Specific stressor(s) are recorded on Axis IV.

Subtypes:

309.0 Adjustment Disorder with Depressed Mood

(ICD-10 code F43.20)

ESSENTIAL FEATURES. The predominant manifestations are symptoms such as depressed mood, feelings of worthlessness, and decreased self-esteem.

309.24 Adjustment Disorder With Anxiety

(ICD-10 code F43.28)

ESSENTIAL FEATURES. The predominant manifestations are symptoms such as nervousness, worry, and trouble falling asleep. In children, the clinician might see fears of separation.

309.28 Adjustment Disorder With Mixed Anxiety and Depressed Mood   (ICD-10 code F43.22)

ESSENTIAL FEATURES. The predominant manifestations are a combination of anxiety and depressive symptoms, such as those found in Adjustment Disorders With Anxiety and With Depressed Mood.

309.3 Adjustment Disorder With Disturbance of Conduct   (ICD-10 code F43.24)

ESSENTIAL FEATURES. There is violation of the rights of others or violation of age-appropriate norms and rules. The predominant manifestations are such symptoms as truancy, fighting, or reckless driving.

309.4 Adjustment Disorder With Mixed Disturbance of Emotions and Conduct   (ICD-10 code F43.25)

ESSENTIAL FEATURES. The predominant manifestations are a combination of emotional symptoms, such as those found in Adjustment Disorder With Anxiety or Depressed Mood, concurrent with behavior found in Adjustment Disorder With Disturbance of Conduct.

309.9 Adjustment Disorder Unspecified   (ICD-10 code F43.9)

ESSENTIAL FEATURES. There is a maladaptive reaction to stress with a symptom or symptoms not classified by the other Adjustment Disorder subtypes (e.g., physical complaints, social withdrawal, and work inhibition).

□ □ □ □

DIFFERENCES BETWEEN DSM-III-R AND DSM-IV ADJUSTMENT DISORDERS

- The maximum duration of an **Adjustment Disorder** is no longer limited to 6 months. The Adjustment Disorder can continue for as long as 6 months after the stress, or its consequences, ceases.

- Four diagnoses—Adjustment Disorder with Physical Complaints, Adjustment Disorder With Withdrawal, Adjustment Disorder With Work (Or Academic) Inhibition, and Adjustment Disorder NOS—were eliminated. These symptoms are all now classified as **Adjustment Disorders Unspecified**, which is a new diagnosis.

- Acute (less than 6 months) and Chronic (6 months or longer) specifiers were added to the diagnosis.

....

CASE VIGNETTE: ADJUSTMENT DISORDERS

Case Vignette

R.B., a 44-year-old business executive with chest pains, was admitted to a coronary care unit (CCU) to rule out a myocardial infarction (MI). In the CCU,
he was anxious, jittery, and had marked nervousness. In spite of strict instructions to remain in bed, he paced at the bedside.

Clinical evaluation revealed a nervous man who was concerned about
his own anxiety. His mental status, except for the aforementioned anxiety, was
normal. Prior to hospitalization, R.B. was on no medications and had no past
psychiatric history.

DIAGNOSIS AND DISCUSSION

Axis I—309.24 Adjustment Disorder With Anxiety, Acute (ICD-10 code
F43.28)

Axis II—V71.09 No Diagnosis or Condition or 799.9 Diagnosis Deferred (ICD-
10 codes Z03.2. R46.8)

Axis III—Rule out myocardial infarction

Axis IV—Psychosocial Stressors: Acute, potentially serious medical illness, admission to a coronary care unit

R.B. has a clear stressor: admission to the CCU to rule out an MI. His behavior
is maladaptive and potentially dangerous. His increased anxiety and pacing place
him at higher risk of medical complications. Since there is no evidence of any
other mental disorder, the diagnosis of an Adjustment Disorder is appropriate.
The predominant symptom is acute onset of anxiety; therefore, the diagnosis
would be Adjustment Disorder With Anxiety.

> NOTE: When a diagnosis of an Adjustment Disorder is made, it
> is appropriate to list the stressor(s) on Axis IV.

CHAPTER *25*

PERSONALITY DISORDERS

CODING NOTE: All Personality Disorders are coded on Axis II.

NOTE: Passive-Aggressive Personality Disorder (formerly 301.84) has been deleted from the main body of DSM-IV. A revised form is listed in DSM-IV Appendix B "for further study."

Personality *traits* are enduring patterns of perceiving, relating to, and thinking about the environment and oneself. They are global in their presentation, rather than being limited to specific situations or times of life. Personality *Disorders* may be diagnosed when such traits reflect persistent patterns of self- or other-perception and behavior, are inflexible and maladaptive, cause significant functional impairment or subjective distress, and are markedly abnormal for the person's culture.

Personality Disorders are recognizable by adolescence or early adulthood, although some should not be diagnosed until the patient is an adult. The disorders continue through most or all of adult life. The traits that define the disorder are often ego-syntonic, and thus may not be apparent to the person as "symptoms." They sometimes become troublesome to him or her only after a significant life change (e.g., loss of a spouse, due to aging).

PERSONALITY DISORDER CLUSTERS. DSM-IV continues the DSM-III-R clustering of the Personality Disorders but notes that the clusters are poorly validated. Cluster A includes Paranoid, Schizoid, and Schizotypal Personality Disorders, characterized by odd or eccentric behaviors. Cluster B includes Antisocial, Borderline, Histrionic, and Narcissistic Personality Disorders, which have in common frequent dramatic, emotional, or erratic behaviors. Cluster C includes Avoidant, Dependent, and Obsessive-Compulsive Personality Disorders, all frequently characterized by anxiety and fearfulness.

DIAGNOSIS OF PERSONALITY DISORDERS IN CHILDREN AND ADOLESCENTS. Provided relevant specific criteria are met, and the symptoms and signs are not thought to be related to a developmental stage or Axis I disorder, most Personality Disorders may be diagnosed in children and adolescents as well as adults. The diagnosis should be made only with caution, and then only after the maladaptive

(115)

traits have been present and stable for at least 1 year. The clinician should note that traits and behaviors may change significantly between childhood and adolescence, and between adolescence and adulthood. Antisocial Personality Disorder should not be diagnosed if the person is under 18 (see following).

ASSOCIATED FEATURES AND DIFFERENTIAL DIAGNOSIS. *Axis I disorders* may coexist with Personality Disorders. However, a Personality Disorder should be diagnosed only when the characteristic features are typical of long-term functioning, and not limited to discrete periods of illness. Features suggestive of a Personality Disorder may be seen during episodes of Axis I disorders (e.g., dependency in major depression). When a history of Personality Disorder appears to blend into a severe Axis I disorder (e.g., Schizoid Personality into Schizophrenia), the Personality Disorder may be diagnosed and specified as "premorbid." If the Personality Disorder has not existed in the absence of the Axis I disorder, it should not be diagnosed or coded. Personality Disorders are not caused by episodes of extreme stress, although they may be uncovered by them. Symptoms that arise after such experiences must be differentiated from Posttraumatic Stress Disyorders. Maladaptive traits that manifest themselves suddenly or late in life demand thorough evaluation to rule out Personality Change Due to a General Medical Condition.

GENERAL DIAGNOSTIC CRITERIA FOR
PERSONALITY DISORDERS (CODE ON AXIS II)

A. An enduring pattern of inner experience and behavior that deviates markedly from the expectations of the individual's culture. The pattern is manifested in two or more of the following areas:
   (1) cognition (i.e., ways of perceiving and interpreting self, other people, and events)
   (2) affectivity (i.e., the range, intensity, lability, and appropriateness of emotional response)
   (3) interpersonal functioning
   (4) impulse control

(116)

B. The enduring pattern is inflexible and pervasive across a broad range of personal and social situations.

C. The enduring pattern leads to clinically significant distress or impairment in social, occupational, or other important areas of functioning.

D. The pattern is stable and of long duration and its onset can be traced back at least to adolescence or early adulthood.

E. The enduring pattern is not better accounted for as a manifestation or consequence of another mental disorder.

F. The enduring pattern is not due to the direct physiological effects of a substance (e.g., a drug of abuse, a medication) or a general medical condition (e.g., head trauma).

NOTE: If criteria for more than one Personality Disorder are met, list all in order of importance. If an Axis I disorder is also present but an Axis II personality disorder is the main focus of clinical attention, "principal diagnosis" or "reason for clinic visit" may be specified.

▯ ▯ ▯ ▯

CLUSTER A

301.0 Paranoid Personality Disorder   (ICD-10 code F60.0)

ESSENTIAL FEATURES. This disorder is characterized by a pervasive and unwarranted tendency to interpret the actions of other people as deliberately threatening or malevolent. There is a general expectation of being exploited or harmed by others in some way. When persons with paranoid personality are confronted with new situations, they search intensely for confirmation of their paranoid expectations, and conclude what they expected all along.

These people have great difficulty with interpersonal relationships, being argumentative, usually very intense, and tending to counterattack when they perceive any threat. They are critical of others and often litigious, and accept criticism only with great difficulty. They routinely lack passive, sentimental, tender, or humorous feelings.

ASSOCIATED FEATURES. During severe stress, transient psychotic symptoms may occur; however, these are brief and do not warrant an additional diagnosis. The disorder may predispose one to Axis I disorders such as Delusional Disorder and Schizophrenia, Paranoid Type. Substance Abuse is common, as are depression and other Axis I disorders.

DIFFERENTIAL DIAGNOSIS. Delusional Disorder, Schizophrenia, Paranoid Type, and Mood Disorder With Psychotic Symptoms are differentiated by their persistent psychotic symptoms and other features. Antisocial Personality Disorder shares some symptoms with Paranoid Personality Disorder; however, the latter is not generally associated with lifelong history of antisocial behavior. Schizoid Personality Disorder suggests eccentricity and does not have prominent paranoid ideation. Schizotypal Personality Disorder suggests thinking, behavior, speech, or perceptions that are more odd or magical than paranoid. Some sensory impairments, especially deafness, produce paranoid traits associated with the development of physical handicaps; these must be differentiated from paranoid personality. Substance Abuse Disorders often coexist with this disorder, but one should be cautious to differentiate the personality from paranoia related to intoxication, chronic drug abuse, or worries about the abuse being discovered. Other Axis I and Axis II comorbidity is discussed in the general Personality Disorder section.

DIAGNOSTIC CRITERIA FOR   (ICD-10 code F60.0)
PARANOID PERSONALITY DISORDER (301.0)

A. A pervasive distrust and suspiciousness of others such that their motives are interpreted as malevolent, beginning by early adulthood and present in a variety of contexts, as indicated by four (or more) of the following:

   (1) suspects, without sufficient basis, that others are exploiting, harming, or deceiving him or her

   (2) is preoccupied with unjustified doubts about the loyalty or trustworthiness of friends or associates

   (3) is reluctant to confide in others because of unwarranted fear that the information will be used maliciously against him or her

   (4) reads hidden demeaning or threatening meanings into benign remarks or events

   (5) persistently bears grudges (i.e., is unforgiving of insults, injuries, or slights)

   (6) perceives attacks on his or her character or reputation that are not apparent to others and is quick to react angrily or to counterattack

   (7) has recurrent suspicions, without justification, regarding fidelity of spouse or sexual partner

B. Does not occur exclusively during the course of Schizophrenia, a Mood Disorder With Psychotic Features, or another Psychotic Disorder, and is not due to the direct effects of a general medical condition.

> **NOTE: If criteria are met prior to the onset of Schizophrenia, specify "Paranoid Personality Disorder (premorbid)."**

□ □ □ □

301.20 Schizoid Personality Disorder   (ICD-10 code F60.1)

ESSENTIAL FEATURES. There is pervasive indifference to social relationships and a restricted range of emotional experience and expression in social and interpersonal settings. These patients prefer to be loners, and apparently neither desire nor enjoy sexual or personal (even family) relationships. Their outward appearance may be aloof, without strong emotions. They are somewhat socially inadequate and appear self-absorbed. Although males are rarely assertive enough to date and marry, females may passively accept a marital relationship. The social impairment may not preclude intellectual or occupational achievement, provided the individual can maintain a comfortable isolation.

DIFFERENTIAL DIAGNOSIS. Schizotypal Personality Disorder involves more eccentricity, with Schizophreniform features. People with Avoidant Personality Disorder avoid, but desire, social relationships. Psychotic Disorders and Syndromes have psychotic symptoms not characteristic of this disorder. Some mild Pervasive Developmental Disorders appear similar but can be distinguished by history. Chronic Substance Abuse or a medical disorder causing personality change (especially in mid- or late life) should be ruled out. Other Axis I and Axis II comorbidity is discussed in the general Personality Disorder section.

DIAGNOSTIC CRITERIA FOR SCHIZOID PERSONALITY DISORDER (301.20)

(ICD-10 code F60.1)

A. A pervasive pattern of detachment from social relationships and a restricted range of expression of emotions in interpersonal settings, beginning by early adulthood and present in a variety of contexts, as indicated by four (or more) of the following:

    (1) neither desires nor enjoys close relationships, including being part of a family

    (2) almost always chooses solitary activities

    (3) little, if any, interest in having sexual experiences with another person

    (4) takes pleasure in few, if any, activities

    (5) lacks close friends or confidants other than first-degree relatives

    (6) appears indifferent to the praise or criticism of others

    (7) shows emotional coldness, detachment, or flattened affectivity

B. Does not occur exclusively during the course of Schizophrenia, a Mood Disorder With Psychotic Features, another Psychotic Disorder, or a Pervasive Developmental Disorder, and is not due to the direct effects of a general medical condition.

    NOTE: If criteria are met prior to the onset of Schizophrenia, specify "Schizoid Personality Disorder (premorbid)."

❏ ❏ ❏ ❏

301.22 Schizotypal Personality Disorder

(ICD-10 code F21)

ESSENTIAL FEATURES. There is a pervasive pattern of peculiar ideation and behavior, with deficits in social and interpersonal relatedness, none of which is severe enough to meet criteria for Schizophrenia. Paranoia, ideas of reference, odd beliefs, rituals and/or magical thinking are common, but they do not reach chronic delusional proportions. Close relationships are difficult and uncomfortable.

ASSOCIATED FEATURES. Interpersonal relatedness is impaired, with inappropriate or constricted affect and rare reciprocation of the expressions or gestures of others (such as passing smiles or nods). Like persons with schizoid personality, they have very few close friends other than first-degree relatives, and may be quite anxious in unfamiliar social situations. Features of Borderline Personality Disorder are often present, and may justify both diagnoses. Transient psychotic symptoms are not unusual but rarely meet criteria for Axis I Psychotic Disorders. Schizotypal personality may coexist with such disorders, but should not be separately diagnosed unless its symptoms predate them ("premorbid"). A history of Major Depressive Episode is common.

DIFFERENTIAL DIAGNOSIS. Schizophrenia, Delusional Disorder, and Mood Disorder With Psychotic Features all imply nontransient psychotic symptoms. In Schizoid and Avoidant Personality Disorders the eccentricities and oddities of Schizotypal Personality Disorder are absent. In Paranoid Personality, suspiciousness and paranoid ideation may be present, but the remaining schizotypal criteria are not. Some mild Pervasive Developmental Disorders appear similar but can be distinguished by history and severity. Chronic Substance Abuse or a medical disorder causing personality change (especially in mid- or late life) should be ruled out. Adolescents may exhibit schizotypal traits without the Personality Disorder. Other Axis I and/or Axis II comorbidity is discussed in the general Personality Disorder section.

DIAGNOSTIC CRITERIA FOR (ICD-10 code F21)
SCHIZOTYPAL PERSONALITY DISORDER
(301.22)

A. A pervasive pattern of social and interpersonal deficits marked by acute discomfort with, and reduced capacity for, close relationships, as well as by cognitive or perceptual distortions and eccentricities of behavior, beginning by early adulthood and present in a variety of contexts, as indicated by five (or more) of the following:
   (1) ideas of reference (excluding delusions of reference)
   (2) odd beliefs or magical thinking that influences behavior and is inconsistent with subcultural norms (e.g., superstitiousness, belief in clairvoyance, telepathy, or "sixth sense"; in children and adolescents, bizarre fantasies or preoccupations)
   (3) unusual perceptual experiences, including bodily illusions
   (4) odd thinking and speech (e.g., vague, circumstantial, metaphorical, over-elaborate, or stereotyped)
   (5) suspiciousness or paranoid ideation
   (6) inappropriate or constricted affect
   (7) behavior or appearance that is odd, eccentric, or peculiar
   (8) lack of close friends or confidants other than first-degree relatives
   (9) excessive social anxiety that does not diminish with familiarity and tends to be associated with paranoid fears rather than negative judgments about self

B. Does not occur exclusively during the course of Schizophrenia, a Mood Disorder With Psychotic Features, another Psychotic Disorder, or a Pervasive Developmental Disorder.

NOTE: If criteria are met prior to the onset of Schizophrenia, specify "Schizotypal Personality Disorder (premorbid)."

▫ ▫ ▫ ▫

CLUSTER B

301.7 Antisocial Personality Disorder
(significantly modified from DSM-III-R)

(ICD-10 code F60.2)

ESSENTIAL FEATURES. There is a pervasive pattern, since childhood, of irresponsibility and antisocial behavior, with disregard for the rights of others. The disorder is limited to adults.

ASSOCIATED FEATURES. Irritability and aggressiveness, including domestic aggression, are commonly associated with Antisocial Personality Disorder. Reckless behavior that does not consider the rights or safety of others is often seen. These individuals lack true empathy and usually have little or no remorse about the effects of their behavior on others, but are rarely sadistic. Antisocial behavior often diminishes in midlife, although the other characteristics generally remain. Early-life substance abuse and voluntary sexual experience are common. There may be signs of personal distress, such as intolerance for boredom or dysphoric affects. There is almost invariably an inability to sustain close, responsible, warm relationships with others (e.g., spouses, children, friends).

PREDISPOSING FACTORS. Attention-Deficit Hyperactivity Disorder (AD/HD) and Conduct Disorder during childhood are predisposing factors. Evidence of childhood Conduct Disorder is necessary for the diagnosis, but one should be cautious about predicting that all children with antisocial or ADHD symptoms will develop the pervasive adult pattern required for this diagnosis. Although DSM-III-R mentions child abuse, other authorities do not see clear correlations between physical, social, or socioeconomic environment and development of true antisocial personality. Serious antisocial behavior in the father, including criminality, may be predisposing.

DIFFERENTIAL DIAGNOSIS. Child/adolescent syndromes such as Conduct Disorder should not be confused with antisocial personality. Some authorities feel that people over 18 who still show characteristics of adolescence (e.g., some college students) should not receive the diagnosis until their adulthood is established. V-code Adult Antisocial Behavior should be considered when antisocial behavior cannot be attributed to any other mental disorder, and the individual does not meet criteria for antisocial personality.

Substance abuse and related disorders should not be equated with Antisocial Personality, although they may be associated with it. Some patients with Mental Retardation, Schizophrenia, or Delusional Disorder occasionally exhibit antisocial behavior; however, the criteria for an additional diagnosis of Antisocial Personality Disorder are rarely met. Manic Episodes often have antisocial characteristics, but the nature and course of the disorder are easy to differentiate; an additional diagnosis of Antisocial Personality Disorder is rarely indicated.

Other Axis II disorders, such as Narcissistic or Paranoid Personality Disorder, can contain arrogance, indifference to others, aggression and/or apparent superficiality. Some authorities have a separate definition for psychopathy, viewing it as a more severe disorder along the antisocial, nonempathic spectrum (cf., Cleckley or Hare criteria); DSM-IV does not separate the two concepts.

DIAGNOSTIC CRITERIA FOR ANTISOCIAL PERSONALITY DISORDER (301.7)

(ICD-10 code F60.2)

A. There is a pervasive pattern of disregard for and violation of the rights of others occurring since age 15, as indicated by three (or more) of the following:
   (1) failure to conform to social norms with respect to lawful behaviors as indicated by repeatedly performing acts that are grounds for arrest
   (2) deceitfulness, as indicated by repeated lying, use of aliases, or conning others for personal profit or pleasure
   (3) impulsivity or failure to plan ahead
   (4) irritability and aggressiveness, as indicated by repeated physical fights or assaults
   (5) reckless disregard for safety of self or others
   (6) consistent irresponsibility, as indicated by repeated failure to sustain consistent work behavior or honor financial obligations
   (7) lack of remorse, as indicated by being indifferent to or rationalizing having hurt, mistreated, or stolen from another

B. Current age is at least age 18 years.

C. There is evidence of DSM-IV **Conduct Disorder** (see p. 85) with onset before age 15.

D. The occurrence of antisocial behavior is not exclusively during the course of Schizophrenia or a Manic Episode.

□ □ □ □

301.83 Borderline Personality Disorder
(significantly modified from DSM-III-R)

(ICD-10 code F60.31)

ESSENTIAL FEATURES. There is a pervasive pattern of instability of self-image, interpersonal relationships, and mood. There is almost always a marked, persistent disturbance of identity, which is frequently manifested by uncertainty about more than one important personal issue (e.g., self-image, sexual orientation, values, career). Concerns, sometimes subtle but often blatant, about real or imagined *abandonment* may give rise to an almost constant state of emotion perceived by others as quantitatively or qualitatively inappropriate (e.g., appearing fearful, jealous, angry, suicidal).

ASSOCIATED FEATURES. Interpersonal relationships are usually unstable and intense, quickly become pseudointimate, and are characterized by extremes of idealization or devaluation. Although they may describe a wish to be alone (or left alone), patients make physical and emotional efforts to avoid loss or abandonment. Impulsivity is common, and may include Substance Abuse or other destructive habits, placing oneself in dangerous situations, self-mutilation, or suicidal behavior. Although their suicide attempts frustrate clinicians and loved ones alike, and are often dismissed as manipulative, up to 10% of persons with Borderline Personality Disorder eventually die by their own hand.

Affective instability is often associated with Borderline Personality. Marked mood shifts, usually to depression, irritability, or anxiety, are routine but often unpredictable. These are usually transient, intense, and may lead to the dangerous behaviors just described. Undermining one's own success, often described as "snatching defeat from the jaws of victory," is common. Some symptoms (e.g., instability) may improve by midlife. Childhood abuse or neglect may be predisposing.

DIFFERENTIAL DIAGNOSIS. Borderline Personality is often accompanied by features of Axis I disorders or other Personality Disorders. If their DSM-IV criteria are met, they should be added to the diagnosis. Transient psychotic symptoms occur in many patients but are rarely associated with complete criteria for Psychotic Disorders. If Borderline Personality precedes development of Schizophrenia, the Personality Disorder should be specified as "premorbid." Although, unlike DSM-III-R, DSM-IV does not specify that Borderline Personality preempts Dissociative Identity Disorder, this seems reasonable. Cyclothymic Disorder is characterized by affective instability, but Borderline Personality Disorder is rarely associated with hypomania. Both disorders may be present in some patients. Chronic substance abuse or a medical disorder causing personality change (especially in mid- or late life) should be ruled out.

DIAGNOSTIC CRITERIA FOR BORDERLINE PERSONALITY DISORDER (301.83)
(ICD-10 code F60.31)

A pervasive pattern of instability of interpersonal relationships, self-image, and affects, and marked impulsivity beginning by early adulthood and present in a variety of contexts, as indicated by five (or more) of the following:

(1) frantic efforts to avoid real or imagined abandonment. **Note:** Do not include suicidal or self-mutilating behavior covered in Criterion 5.

(2) a pattern of unstable and intense interpersonal relationships characterized by alternating between extremes of idealization and devaluation

(3) identity disturbance: markedly and persistently unstable self–image or sense of self

(4) impulsivity in at least two areas that are potentially self-damaging (e.g., spending, sex, substance abuse, reckless driving, binge eating). **Note:** Do not include suicidal or self-mutilating behavior covered in Criterion 5.

(5) recurrent suicidal behavior, gestures, or threats, or self-mutilating behavior

(6) affective instability due to a marked reactivity of mood (e.g., intense epi-sodic dysphoria, irritability, or anxiety usually lasting a few hours and only rarely more than a few days)

(7) chronic feelings of emptiness

(8) inappropriate, intense anger or difficulty controlling anger (e.g., fre-quent displays of temper, constant anger, recurrent physical fights)

(9) transient, stress-related paranoid ideation or severe dissociative symptoms

□ □ □ □

301.50 Histrionic Personality Disorder (ICD-10 code F60.4)

ESSENTIAL FEATURES. There is a pervasive pattern of excessive emotionality and attention seeking. Emotions are often inappropriately exaggerated in response to minor stimuli. Patients are sometimes physically provocative and at other times more obviously attempting to gain the attention, caring, and regard that is the underlying objective of their physical and/or pseudosexual seductive be-havior. When the phrase *attention seeking* is used in describing these individuals, this refers not so much to a wish to be looked at as to a need for others to *attend to* and have regard for him or her.

ASSOCIATED FEATURES. Attempts to control other persons while establishing a dependent relationship with them are common, as are expressions of romantic fantasy. The quality of emotional and sexual relationships is often shallow and/ or immature. Dramatic, impressionistic (i.e., nonspecific) speech is usual. Sug-gestibility, being overly trusting (especially of authority figures, even temporary ones), and inappropriate pseudointimacy are common. Somatization and oc-casional dissociation may occur.

DIFFERENTIAL DIAGNOSIS. In Somatization Disorder, the physical complaints dom-inate the clinical picture. Some patients with Somatization Disorder or other Somatoform Disorders (e.g., Conversion Disorder) also meet the criteria for Histrionic Personality Disorder. Borderline Personality Disorder may be co-morbid. In dependent personality, one sees similar excessive dependency and wishes for praise and guidance but without exaggerated emotional features. Nar-cissistic Personality implies a similar self-centeredness, but grandiosity and in-tense envy are the rule.

DIAGNOSTIC CRITERIA FOR (ICD-10 code F60.4)
HISTRIONIC PERSONALITY DISORDER (301.50)

A pervasive pattern of excessive emotionality and attention seeking, beginning by early adulthood and present in a variety of contexts, as indicated by five (or more) of the following:

(1) is uncomfortable in situations in which he or she is not the center of attention

(2) interaction with others is often characterized by inappropriate sexually seductive or provocative behavior

(3) displays rapidly shifting and shallow expression of emotions

(4) consistently uses physical appearance to draw attention to self

(5) has a style of speech that is excessively impressionistic and lacking in detail

(6) shows self-dramatization, theatricality, and exaggerated expression of emotion

(7) is suggestible i.e., easily influenced by others or circumstances

(8) Considers relationships to be more intimate than they actually are

□ □ □ □

301.81 Narcissistic Personality Disorder *(ICD-10 code F60.8)* *(significantly modified from DSM-III-R)*

ESSENTIAL FEATURES. There is a pervasive pattern of grandiosity (in fantasy or in behavior), hypersensitivity to others' evaluations and criticisms of oneself, and lack of empathy. Feeling and professing grandiosity may alternate with (or lead to) an exaggerated feeling of failure when one does not live up to the expected perfection. Although there are fantasies of great success, brilliance, or beauty (with envy of those who are truly successful), reality is often quite different. Many patients attain significant achievements, but they rarely accept them as "enough" or derive genuine pleasure from them. Self-esteem, while outwardly appearing high, is actually quite fragile, with a need for constant attention and admiration.

Although persons with Narcissistic Personality Disorder expect special regard from others, they often devalue others' abilities or achievements. Thus, a physician or therapist who is sought out as "the best" is likely to be criticized later, especially when challenging the patient's narcissism. Close relationships, including relationships with spouses or psychotherapists, invariably suffer from lack of empathy, unreasonable expectations of continuously "special" treatment, or the unreasonable expectation that the other person will supply perfectly the patient's needs.

ASSOCIATED FEATURES. Features of other Personality Disorders are often present, and sometimes more than one Axis II diagnosis is warranted. Adjustment Disorders, generally associated with depression and frustration, are common. Psychotic Disorders, such as Brief Reactive Psychosis, occasionally occur, as do significant Mood Disorders as the person becomes older and narcissistic expectations are more often frustrated. "Narcissistic injury," in which the defensive shell of arrogance is penetrated by disapproval or setback, is often deeply felt but not outwardly expressed.

DIFFERENTIAL DIAGNOSIS. Narcissistic symptoms are seen in many other Personality Disorders (e.g., Borderline, Histrionic, Antisocial). If additional diagnosis is not indicated, careful attention to the diagnostic criteria will allow differentiation (or may suggest Personality Disorder NOS). Narcissistic traits are frequently associated with social or vocational success, and should not be confused with Narcissistic Personality. Other Axis I and Axis II comorbidity is discussed in the general Personality Disorder section.

DIAGNOSTIC CRITERIA FOR NARCISSISTIC PERSONALITY DISORDER (301.81)

(ICD-10 code F60.8)

A pervasive pattern of grandiosity (in fantasy or behavior), need for admiration, and lack of empathy, beginning by early adulthood and present in a variety of contexts, as indicated by five (or more) of the following:

(1) has a grandiose sense of self-importance (e.g., exaggerates achievements and talents, expects to be recognized as superior without commensurate achievements)
(2) is preoccupied with fantasies of unlimited success, power, brilliance, beauty, or ideal love
(3) believes that he or she is "special" and unique and can only be understood by, or should associate with, other special or high-status people (or institutions)
(4) requires excessive admiration
(5) has a sense of entitlement (i.e., unreasonable expectations of especially favorable treatment or automatic compliance with his or her expectations)
(6) is interpersonally exploitative, i.e., takes advantage of others to achieve his or her own ends
(7) lacks empathy: unwilling to recognize or identify with the feelings or needs of others
(8) often envies others or believes that others are envious of him or her
(9) shows arrogant, haughty behaviors or attitudes

❑ ❑ ❑ ❑

CLUSTER C

301.82 Avoidant Personality Disorder
(significantly modified from DSM-III-R)

(ICD-10 code F60.6)

ESSENTIAL FEATURES. There is a pervasive pattern of social discomfort, fear of negative evaluation, timidity, and feelings of inadequacy. These individuals are usually unwilling to enter into relationships without strong guarantees of unrelenting acceptance. Since this is difficult to attain, they often have very few close friends or confidants. Their social avoidance may preclude rewards for which they are otherwise qualified (e.g., job promotions). Acute sensitivity to criticism is usual and routinely leads to unjustified fear or hurt from the most trivial slight.

ASSOCIATED FEATURES. The patient may appear to have general or specific phobias, and may exhibit depression, anxiety, or anger at herself or himself for a perceived lack of social success. The avoidant behavior may give rise to teasing from others, especially in adolescence, which seems to confirm the person's self-doubt.

PREDISPOSING FACTORS. Unusual physical characteristics or living within an unfamiliar racial, language, or cultural environment may predispose one to avoidant behavior; however, the clinician should be careful to evaluate the patient based on the specific diagnostic criteria.

DIFFERENTIAL DIAGNOSIS. Schizoid Personality Disorder is characterized by little desire for social involvement and an indifference to criticism. In Social Phobias or Panic Disorder With Agoraphobia, the phobic situation is usually specific, rather than involving personal relationships. Chronic Substance Abuse or a medical disorder causing personality change (especially in mid- or late life) should be considered. Other Axis I and Axis II comorbidity is discussed in the general Personality Disorder section.

DIAGNOSTIC CRITERIA FOR
AVOIDANT PERSONALITY DISORDER (301.82)

(ICD-10 code F60.6)

A pervasive pattern of social inhibition, feelings of inadequacy, and hypersensitivity to negative evaluation, beginning by early adulthood and present in a variety of contexts, as indicated by four (or more) of the following:

(1) avoids occupational activities that involve significant interpersonal contact, because of fears of criticism, disapproval, or rejection
(2) is unwilling to get involved with people unless certain of being liked
(3) shows restraint within intimate relationships because of the fear of being shamed or ridiculed
(4) is preoccupied with being criticized or rejected in social situations
(5) is inhibited in new interpersonal situations because of feelings of inadequacy
(6) views self as socially inept, personally unappealing, or inferior to others
(7) is unusually reluctant to take personal risks or to engage in any new activities because they may prove embarrassing

□ □ □ □

301.6 Dependent Personality Disorder
(significantly modified from DSM-III-R)

(ICD-10 code F60.7)

ESSENTIAL FEATURES. There is a pervasive pattern of dependence and submissive behavior. Clinging to others and fear of separation (even when there are no grounds for concern) are usual. When separation is forced, the person may panic and indiscriminately seek another attachment.

ASSOCIATED FEATURES. Because of their dread of functioning alone, persons with this disorder routinely avoid any expression or behavior that threatens their attachment to, or support from, others (e.g., arguing, independent action, or initiative). Self-deprecation is common and is generally aimed at getting others to care for them or take over their lives. Symptoms of other Personality Disorders are common, as are disorders involving adjustment, anxiety, and depression.

PREDISPOSING FACTORS. Chronic physical illness and Separation Anxiety Disorder may be predisposing factors.

DIFFERENTIAL DIAGNOSIS. Although dependent behavior is common in Agoraphobia, there is little other similarity. Other Personality Disorders have characteristics of inadequacy and passivity that may be confused with dependent personality. Additional diagnosis may be indicated. Although dependency or dependent traits associated with chronic illness, depression, Substance Abuse, Mental Retardation, victims of crime or other severe trauma, and ordinary social need (e.g., in the elderly or refugees) should not be confused with Dependent Personality Disorder, when the symptoms are chronic, pervasive, and exceed those expected for the other condition(s), it may be diagnosed.

DIAGNOSTIC CRITERIA FOR
DEPENDENT PERSONALITY DISORDER (301.6)

(ICD-10 code F60.7)

A pervasive and excessive need to be taken care of that leads to submissive and clinging behavior and fears of separation, beginning by early adulthood and present in a variety of contexts, as indicated by five (or more) of the following:

(1) has difficulty making everyday decisions without an excessive amount of advice and reassurance from others

(2) needs others to assume responsibility for most major areas of his or her life

(3) has difficulty expressing disagreement with others because of fear of loss of support or approval. **NOTE:** Do not include realistic fears of retribution.

(4) has difficulty initiating projects or doing things on his or her own (because of a lack of self-confidence in judgment or abilities, rather than a lack of motivation or energy)

(5) goes to excessive lengths to obtain nurturance and support from others, to the point of volunteering to do things that are unpleasant

(6) feels uncomfortable or helpless when alone because of exaggerated fears of being unable to care for himself or herself

(7) urgently seeks another relationship as a source of care and support when a close relationship ends

(8) is unrealistically preoccupied with fears of being left to take care of himself or herself

□ □ □ □

301.4 Obsessive-Compulsive Personality Disorder
(significantly modified from DSM-III-R)

(ICD-10 code F60.5)

ESSENTIAL FEATURES. There is pervasive preoccupation with perfectionism, inflexibility, and control. The patient's overly strict, often unattainable personal standards frequently interfere with completion of tasks or projects, although she or he strives for perfection. Preoccupation with rules, efficiency, or trivia interferes with the ability to take a broad view of situations. There is often a preoccupation with work, to the exclusion of pleasure and interpersonal relationships. Logic and intellect are frequently substituted for affective behavior (for which there may be little tolerance, particularly to affect in others). One may fantasize about relaxation, pleasure, or finishing a task but postpone such rewards in favor of focus on the form or process of the work. Decision making is difficult and fraught with ambivalence and avoidance. Harsh judgments of oneself and others are common, as is reluctance to delegate tasks. Some persons with the disorder are unable to discard even unimportant objects.

(123)

ASSOCIATED FEATURES AND DISORDERS. Associated features include difficulty expressing tender feelings (often expressed in distress or complaints about being "unable to love"). Depression is fairly common, as is frustration when the patient's strong need to be in control of both self and environment is thwarted. In addition to psychiatric complications, such as Obsessive-Compulsive Disorder, Mood Disorder, or Hypochondriasis, Type A personality traits sometimes associated with increased incidence of myocardial infarction are frequently found in individuals with Obsessive-Compulsive Personality Disorder.

DIFFERENTIAL DIAGNOSIS. Obsessive-Compulsive Disorder, by definition, involves true obsessions or compulsions, associated with marked distress, which are not present in this personality disorder. A minority of patients fill criteria for both diagnoses, in which case both should be coded.

DIAGNOSTIC CRITERIA FOR OBSESSIVE-COMPULSIVE PERSONALITY DISORDER (301.4)

(ICD-10 code F60.5)

A pervasive pattern of preoccupation with orderliness, perfectionism, and mental and interpersonal control, at the expense of flexibility, openness, and efficiency, beginning by early adulthood and present in a variety of contexts, as indicated by four (or more) of the following:

   (1) is preoccupied with details, rules, lists, order, organization, or schedules to the extent that the major point of the activity is lost
   (2) shows perfectionism that interferes with task completion (e.g., is unable to complete a project because his or her own overly strict standards are not met)

(3) is excessively devoted to work and productivity to the exclusion of leisure activities and friendships (not accounted for by obvious economic
necessity)

(4) is overconscientious, scrupulous, and inflexible about matters of moral-
ity, ethics, or values (not accounted for by cultural or religious
identification)

(5) is unable to discard worn-out or worthless objects even when they have
no sentimental value

(6) is reluctant to delegate tasks or to work with others unless they submit
to exactly his or her way of doing things

(7) adopts a miserly spending style toward both self and others; money is
viewed as something to be hoarded for future catastrophes

(8) shows rigidity and stubbornness

□ □ □ □

301.9 Personality Disorder Not Otherwise Specified (NOS)

(ICD-10 code F60.9)

This is a residual category for patients not classifiable as having any of the specific
personality disorders listed, yet who have pervasive, persistent personality traits,
beginning by early adulthood and present in a variety of contexts, which cause
significant social, academic, or occupational impairment, or subjective distress.
Such disorders may contain features of several personality disorders but not be
sufficient for any specific one.

When requirements of pervasiveness, breadth of presentation, chronicity, and impairment or distress are met, this NOS category may also be used to
describe unclassified personality syndromes (e.g., those listed in DSM-IV Appendix B), based on the clinician's judgment. The clinician may note the specific
disorder in parentheses, such as **301.9 Personality Disorder NOS (Passive-
Aggressive Personality Disorder)** (ICD-10 F60.9).

□ □ □ □

·····

DIFFERENCES BETWEEN DSM-III-R
AND DSM-IV PERSONALITY DISORDERS

General

□ The DSM-IV Personality Disorder criteria allow increased latitude in
diagnosing children or adolescents.

□ DSM-III-R's Passive-Aggressive Personality was moved to Appendix B
in DSM-IV.

□ There is decreased emphasis on Clusters A, B, and C.

Specific Disorders

- **Antisocial Personality Disorder**: Fewer criteria are required. The requirement for no "monogamous relationship" and the separate requirement for lack of remorse have been removed (the latter now being one choice of seven). Disregard for family obligations is no longer a separate choice or criterion. DSM-IV views these changes as a condensation and simplification; however, the criteria are easier to meet and criminals will make up a larger proportion of persons who meet them than was the case for DSM-III-R.

- **Borderline Personality Disorder**: Criterion 9 (paranoia or severe dissociative symptoms) is an added choice. The identity disturbance criterion is less specific.

- **Histrionic Personality Disorder**: Specific criteria of physical appearance, dramatization/exaggeration, and suggestibility have been substituted for former DSM-III-R criteria of seeking reassurance/approval, attractiveness, self-centeredness, and difficulty delaying gratification. Current criteria imply much of what was deleted, however.

- **Narcissistic Personality Disorder**: Criterion 9 (arrogant, haughty behaviors or attitudes) is new. Reaction to criticism with rage, shame, or humiliation was omitted from the nine criterion choices.

- **Avoidant Personality Disorder**: DSM-IV criteria focus on fears of what *others* might do (e.g., criticize, ridicule, reject), in contrast to DSM-III-R's inclusion of things the person fears *he or she* might do (e.g., blush, cry, say something foolish).

- **Dependent Personality Disorder**: A ninth criterion choice, "easily hurt by criticism or disapproval," has been deleted. "Unable" to make everyday decisions (Criterion 1) is now "difficulty making everyday decisions."

- **Obsessive-Compulsive Personality Disorder**: Four (not five) criteria are required. Specific criterion reference to indecisiveness and restricted expression of emotion was deleted.

....

CASE VIGNETTES: PERSONALITY DISORDERS

Case Vignette 1

For as long as the local residents can remember, H.R., a 56-year-old, single, high school graduate, has lived alone a couple of miles outside of town. Although frequently seen along the road, and occasionally in town, he doesn't frequent the local bars or cafes and has never been known to socialize. H.R. makes his living fixing things, at which he is quite adept, but chooses not to open a shop in town. He seems indifferent to praise, advice, or complaints from his customers, generally answering with a nondescript shrug and continuing his work. He never married, and did not attend either his sister's wedding or his parents' funerals, all of which occurred nearby. When passersby offer greetings or friendly conversation, H.R. remains aloof, barely acknowledging their comments. He has no complaints or psychiatric symptoms that bother him. He has never been in trouble with the law, and has had no known hallucinations, delusions, or psychiatric treatment.

DIAGNOSIS AND DISCUSSION
Axis I— V71.09 No Diagnosis or Condition on Axis I (ICD-10 code Z03.2)
Axis II—301.20 Schizoid Personality Disorder (ICD-10 code F60.1)

The chronic, pervasive Personality Disorder has some paranoid and avoidant characteristics, but the diagnosis is clear. There is no indication of an accompanying Axis I disorder.

Case Vignette 2

D.T., a middle-aged, successful businessman, comes to the clinician's office to inquire about psychotherapy because others "have trouble getting along with me." He has noticed this for many years but felt no need for change or treatment until the recent breakup of his third marriage. For the first time, D.T. wonders about his ability to be a husband and father and worries about growing old alone: "That never bothered me before. I've always thought I was my own best partner."

Since childhood, D.T. has been "obsessed" with money and power. This has come fairly easily, because, in his words, "everyone else is weak or incompetent; I just step in and take over." He has extraordinary confidence in his ability to succeed, but not to a psychotic or hypomanic extent. Nevertheless, all his life his self-image has been grandiose, and his demeanor arrogant: "Everyone else wishes they were in my shoes." Others' regard and admiration for him is important but "never enough." In spite of D.T.'s very exploitative personal and business style, he expects others to appreciate his brilliance and success: "I don't understand why my wife and kids aren't grateful to have me around. I'm not trying to brag, but my reflected glory makes the whole town treat them with respect." D.T. comments that he had trouble being a warm parent or husband, and seems not to understand his children's needs or feelings. His prior wives were both "idiots."

DIAGNOSIS AND DISCUSSION
Axis I—V Code, V62.89 Phase of Life Problem (Divorce or Marital Separation) (ICD-10 code Z60.0)
Axis II—301.81 Narcissistic Personality Disorder (ICD-10 code F60.8)

The narcissistic traits appear to be more than mere trappings of a driven and successful man. His age may have contributed to the development of discomfort in an otherwise resilient character facade.

OTHER CONDITIONS THAT MAY BE A FOCUS OF CLINICAL ATTENTION

This broadened category refers to conditions or problems not considered "psychiatric disorders" per se, but which may be a focus of clinical attention and require appropriate coding on Axis I (except for Borderline Intellectual Functioning, coded on Axis II). The condition or problem either may be related to a mental disorder but be severe enough to warrant independent clinical consideration (e.g., repeated abuse of a child by a parent with Borderline Personality Disorder), or may be unrelated to any DSM-IV diagnosis (which may or may not also be present in the patient) (e.g., Tardive Dyskinesia caused by medication prescribed for a mental disorder; marital discord between persons with no psychiatric diagnosis). Clinical significance or functional impairment is necessary for coding in almost all conditions.

(124)

PSYCHOLOGICAL FACTORS AFFECTING MEDICAL CONDITION

316 [Psychological Factor . . .] Affecting Medical Condition
(ICD-10 code F54)
(significantly modified from DSM-III-R)

(125)

ESSENTIAL FEATURES. There are psychological factors or functioning that adversely affect the onset, exacerbation, treatment, or course of a general medical condition.

DIAGNOSTIC CRITERIA FOR [PSYCHOLOGICAL FACTOR . . .] AFFECTING MEDICAL CONDITION (316)
(ICD-10 code F54)

CODING NOTE: Code the general medical condition on Axis III.

A. A general medical condition (coded on Axis III) is present.

B. Psychological factors adversely affect the general medical condition in one of the following ways:

(1) the factors have influenced the course of the general medical condition as shown by a close temporal association between the psychological factors and the development or exacerbation of, or delayed recovery from, the general medical condition

(2) the factors interfere with the treatment of the general medical condition

(3) the factors constitute additional health risks for the individual

(4) Stress-related physiological responses precipitate or exacerbate symptoms of the general medical condition

Choose name based on the nature of the psychological factors (if more than one factor is present, indicate the most prominent):
Mental Disorder Affecting Medical Condition (e.g., an Axis I disorder delaying recovery from a myocardial infarction)

Psychological Symptoms Affecting Medical Condition (e.g., symptoms delaying recovery from surgery; anxiety exacerbating asthma)

Personality Traits or Coping Style Affecting Medical Condition (e.g., pathological denial of the need for surgery in a cancer patient; pressured behavior contributing to cardiovascular disease)

Maladaptive Health Behaviors Affecting Medical Condition (e.g., noncompliance with medication or diet)

Stress-Related Physiological Response Affecting Medical Condition (e.g., tension headache, hypertension, arrythmia)

Unspecified Psychological Factors Affecting Medical Condition (e.g., interpersonal, cultural, or religious factors)

❏ ❏ ❏ ❏

MEDICATION-INDUCED MOVEMENT DISORDERS
(All New in DSM-IV)

ESSENTIAL FEATURES. Although these are coded disorders in both DSM-IV and ICD-10, their diagnostic criteria are not official in DSM-IV. Suggested research criteria are listed in DSM-IV Appendix B, "Criteria Sets and Axes Provided for Further Study" (pp. 703–761). Those tentative criteria are summarized here for clinical convenience only.

CODING NOTE: Optional ICD-9-CM E codes describing the drug or drug class for Medication-Induced Disorders (DSM-IV Appendix G) are listed on Axis I.

332.1 Neuroleptic-Induced Parkinsonism (ICD-10 code G21.0)
(new in DSM-IV)

DIFFERENTIAL DIAGNOSIS. Several neurological disorders, including cerebellar disease, Parkinson's disease, essential tremor, focal lesions, and Tardive Dyskinesia, can mimic this disorder and should be ruled out by history, examination, and/or briefly discontinuing neuroleptic medication (when feasible). Psychiatric symptoms such as catatonia and psychomotor retardation are often mistaken for Neuroleptic-Induced Parkinsonism.

SUGGESTED RESEARCH CRITERIA FOR (ICD-10 code G21.0)
NEUROLEPTIC-INDUCED
PARKINSONISM (332.1)

A. One (or more) of the following signs or symptoms has developed in association with use of neuroleptic medication:
- (1) parkinsonian tremor (i.e., a coarse, rhythmic, resting tremor with a frequency between 3 and 6 cycles/second) affecting the limbs, head, mouth, or tongue
- (2) parkinsonian muscular rigidity (i.e., cogwheel rigidity or continuous "lead-pipe" rigidity)
- (3) akinesia (i.e., a decrease in spontaneous facial expression, gestures, speech, or body movements)

B. The symptoms in Criterion A developed within a few weeks of starting or raising the dose of a neuroleptic medication, or of reducing a medication used to treat (or prevent) acute extrapyramidal symptoms (e.g., anticholinergic agents).

C. The symptoms in Criterion A are not better accounted for by a mental disorder (e.g., catatonic or negative symptoms in Schizophrenia, psychomotor retardation in a Major Depressive Episode). Evidence that the symptoms are better accounted for by a mental disorder might include the following: the symptoms precede the exposure to neuroleptic medication or are not compatible with the pattern of pharmacological intervention (e.g., no improvement after lowering the neuroleptic dose or administering anticholinergic medication).

D. The symptoms in Criterion A are not due to a nonneuroleptic substance or to a neurological or other general medical condition (e.g., Parkinson's disease, Wilson's disease). Evidence that the symptoms are due to a general medical condition might include the following: the symptoms precede exposure to neuroleptic medication, unexplained focal neurological signs are present, or the symptoms progress despite a stable medication regimen.

> NOTE: When other, nonneuroleptic medications cause Parkinson-like symptoms, consider Medication-Induced Postural Tremor or Medication-Induced Movement Disorder NOS.

❑ ❑ ❑ ❑

333.92 Neuroleptic Malignant Syndrome   (ICD-10 code G21.0)
(new in DSM-IV)

DIFFERENTIAL DIAGNOSIS. The differential diagnosis must be addressed quickly and includes other sources of hyperthermia (e.g., acute infection, malignant hyperthermia, and neurological disease or injury of temperature-regulating mechanisms). Dopamine-depleting medications other than neuroleptics can precipitate similar reactions. So-called malignant catatonia or lethal catatonia is occasionally seen in Schizophrenia or Mania in the absence of neuroleptic medication.

SUGGESTED RESEARCH CRITERIA FOR   (ICD-10 code G21.0)
NEUROLEPTIC MALIGNANT SYNDROME
(333.92)

A. The development of severe muscular rigidity and elevated temperature associated with use of neuroleptic medication.

B. Two (or more) of the following:
  - **(1)** diaphoresis
  - **(2)** dysphagia
  - **(3)** tremor
  - **(4)** incontinence
  - **(5)** changes in level of consciousness, ranging from confusion to coma
  - **(6)** mutism
  - **(7)** tachycardia
  - **(8)** elevated or labile blood pressure
  - **(9)** leukocytosis
  - **(10)** laboratory evidence of muscle injury (e.g., elevated CPK)

C. The symptoms in Criteria A and B are not due to another substance (e.g., phencyclidine) or a neurological or other general medical condition (e.g., viral encephalitis).

D. The symptoms in Criteria A and B are not better accounted for by a mental disorder (e.g., Mood Disorder With Catatonic Features).

❑ ❑ ❑ ❑

333.7 Neuroleptic-Induced Acute Dystonia   (ICD-10 code G24.0)
(new in DSM-IV)

DIFFERENTIAL DIAGNOSIS. Neurological sources of dystonia, catatonic symptoms of mental disorders, and reactions to other, nonneuroleptic medications are considered in the differential diagnosis.

SUGGESTED RESEARCH CRITERIA FOR NEUROLEPTIC-INDUCED ACUTE DYSTONIA (333.7)

(ICD-10 code G24.0)

A. One (or more) of the following signs or symptoms has developed in association with the use of neuroleptic medication:
   (1) abnormal positioning of the head and neck in relation to the body (e.g., retrocollis, torticollis)
   (2) spasms of the jaw muscles (e.g., trismus, gaping, grimacing)
   (3) impaired swallowing (dysphagia), speaking, or breathing (laryngeal-pharyngeal spasm, dysphonia)
   (4) thickened or slurred speech due to hypertonic or enlarged tongue (dysarthria, macroglossia)
   (5) tongue protrusion or dysfunction
   (6) eyes deviated up, down, or sideward (oculogyric crisis)
   (7) abnormal positioning of the distal limbs or trunk

B. The signs or symptoms in Criterion A developed within 7 days of starting or rapidly raising the dose of neuroleptic medication, or of reducing a medication used to treat (or prevent) acute extrapyramidal symptoms (e.g., anticholinergic agents).

C. The symptoms in Criterion A are not better accounted for by a mental disorder (e.g., catatonic symptoms in Schizophrenia). Evidence that the symptoms are better accounted for by a mental disorder might include the following: the symptoms precede the exposure to neuroleptic medication or are not compatible with the pattern of pharmacological intervention (e.g., no improvement after neuroleptic lowering or anticholinergic administration).

D. The symptoms in Criterion A are not due to a nonneuroleptic substance or to a neurological or other general medical condition. Evidence that the symptoms are due to a general medical condition might include the following: the symptoms precede the exposure to the neuroleptic medication, unexplained focal neurological signs are present, or the symptoms progress in the absence of change in medication.

> NOTE: When other, nonneuroleptic medications cause dystonia, consider Medication-Induced Movement Disorder NOS.

▫ ▫ ▫ ▫

333.99 Neuroleptic-Induced Acute Akathisia
(new in DSM-IV)

(ICD-10 code G21.1)

DIFFERENTIAL DIAGNOSIS. Other sources of akathisia, such as Parkinson's disease, severe iron deficiency, idiopathic myoclonus, "restless leg syndrome," and some other medical conditions are considered. Symptoms can be confused with those of Axis I mental disorders, such as Schizophrenia, agitated depression or hypomania, Substance Withdrawal, or Hyperactivity-Related Disorders.

SUGGESTED RESEARCH CRITERIA FOR NEUROLEPTIC-INDUCED ACUTE AKATHISIA (333.99)

(ICD-10 code G21.1)

A. The development of subjective complaints of restlessness after exposure to a neuroleptic medication.

B. At least one of the following is observed:
    (1) fidgety movement or swinging of the legs
    (2) rocking from foot to foot while standing
    (3) pacing to relieve restlessness
    (4) inability to sit or stand still for at least several minutes

C. The onset of the symptoms in Criteria A and B occurs within 4 weeks of initiating or increasing the dose of the neuroleptic, or of reducing medication used to treat (or prevent) extrapyramidal symptoms (e.g., anticholinergic agents).

D. The symptoms in Criterion A are not better accounted for by a mental disorder (e.g., Schizophrenia, Substance Withdrawal, agitation from a Major Depressive or Manic Episode, hyperactivity in Attention-Deficit/Hyperactivity Disorder). Evidence that symptoms may be better accounted for by a mental disorder might include the following: the onset of symptoms preceding the exposure to the neuroleptics, the absence of increasing restlessness with neuroleptic doses, and the absence of relief with pharmacological interventions (e.g., no improvement after decreasing the neuroleptic dose or treatment with medication intended to treat the akathisia).

E. The symptoms in Criterion A are not due to a nonneuroleptic substance or to a neurological or other general medical condition. Evidence that symptoms are due to a general medical condition might include the onset of the symptoms preceding the exposure to neuroleptics or the progression of symptoms in the absence of a change in medication.

> NOTE: When other, nonneuroleptic medications cause akathisia, consider Medication-Induced Movement Disorder NOS.

☐ ☐ ☐ ☐

333.82 Neuroleptic-Induced Tardive Dyskinesia
(new in DSM-IV)

(ICD-10 code G24.0)

DIFFERENTIAL DIAGNOSIS. A number of dyskinesias and other neuromuscular disorders associated with neurological disease, deficiency states, and toxins (e.g., Huntington's chorea, Wilson's disease, heavy metal toxicity) are considered.

Neuroleptic-Induced Acute Dyskinesia, dystonia, and akathisia have a similar etiology but very different implications. Some simple, benign sources of oro-buccal movements, such as poorly fitting dentures, mouth irritation, or (not always benign) mouth or jaw pathology, must also be ruled out.

SUGGESTED RESEARCH CRITERIA FOR NEUROLEPTIC-INDUCED TARDIVE DYSKINESIA (333.82)

(ICD-10 code G24.0)

A. Involuntary movements of the tongue, jaw, trunk, or extremities have developed in association with use of neuroleptic medication.

B. The involuntary movements are present over a period of at least 4 weeks and occur in any of the following patterns:
   (1) choreiform movements (i.e., rapid, jerky, nonrepetitive)
   (2) athetoid movements (i.e., slow, sinuous, continual)
   (3) rhythmic movements (i.e., stereotypies)

C. The signs or symptoms in Criteria A and B develop during exposure to a neuroleptic medication or within 4 weeks of withdrawal from an oral (8 weeks from a depot) neuroleptic medication.

D. There has been exposure to neuroleptic medication for at least 3 months (1 month if age 60 years or older).

E. The symptoms are not due to a neurological or general medical condition (e.g., Huntington's disease, Sydenham's chorea, spontaneous dyskinesia, hyperthyroidism, Wilson's disease), ill-fitting dentures, or exposure to other medications that cause acute reversible dyskinesia (e.g., L-dopa, bromocriptine). Evidence that the symptoms are due to one of these etiologies might include the following: the symptoms precede the exposure to the neuroleptic medication or unexplained focal neurological signs are present.

F. The symptoms are not better accounted for by a neuroleptic-induced acute movement disorder (e.g., Neuroleptic-Induced Acute Dystonia, Neuroleptic-Induced Acute Akathisia).

> NOTE: When other, nonneuroleptic medications cause Tardive Dyskinesia, consider Medication-Induced Movement Disorder NOS.

333.1 Medication-Induced Postural Tremor (new in DSM-IV)

(ICD-10 code G25.1)

DIFFERENTIAL DIAGNOSIS. Tremors caused by neurological or general medical conditions or nonmedication toxic substances must be considered. Existence prior to medication use mitigates against a medication-related etiology. A tremor caused by Neuroleptic-Induced Parkinsonism has different characteristics (see p. 299, Criterion A(1)).

SUGGESTED RESEARCH CRITERIA FOR MEDICATION-INDUCED POSTURAL TREMOR (333.1)

(ICD-10 code G25.1)

A. A fine postural tremor that has developed in association with use of a medication (e.g., lithium, antidepressant medication, valproic acid).

B. The tremor (i.e., a regular, rhythmic oscillation of the limbs, head, mouth, or tongue) has a frequency between 8 and 12 cycles per second.

C. The symptoms are not due to a preexisting nonpharmacologically induced tremor. Evidence that the symptoms are due to a preexisting tremor might include the following: the tremor was present prior to the introduction of the medication, the tremor does not correlate with serum levels of the medication, and the tremor persists after discontinuation of the medication.

D. The symptoms are not better accounted for by Neuroleptic-Induced Parkinsonism.

□ □ □ □

333.90 Medication-Induced Movement Disorder NOS
(new in DSM-IV)

(ICD-10 code G25.9)

This category may be used for Medication-Induced Movement Disorders not listed above, when they are a focus of clinical attention. DSM-IV suggests that presentations similar to Neuroleptic Malignant Syndrome that are associated with nonneuroleptic medications may be coded here; however, if movement symptoms are not predominant, consider 995.2 Adverse Effects of Medication NOS (ICD-10 code T88.7), below.

□ □ □ □

OTHER MEDICATION-INDUCED DISORDERS

995.2 Adverse Effects of Medication NOS
(new in DSM-IV)

(ICD-10 code T88.7)

This optional category may be used to code other adverse medication effects that are a focus of clinical attention (e.g., hypotension, cardiac arrhythmia, priapism).

□ □ □ □

RELATIONAL PROBLEMS

ESSENTIAL FEATURES. These are difficulties of interaction between or among family members or, in the words of DSM-IV, members of other "relational units." Relational problems are not considered mental disorders, but they should be acknowledged when they cause clinically significant symptoms or impairment of the relationship. They may be listed on Axis I if they are the primary clinical focus, or on Axis IV if they are incidental to another disorder. They may aggravate mental disorders or their treatment.

(127)

(128)

V61.9 Relational Problem Related to a Mental Disorder or General Medical Condition
(new in DSM-IV)

(ICD-10 code Z63.7)

This diagnosis is used when the clinically significant relational problem is related to a mental disorder or general medical condition.

❑ ❑ ❑ ❑

V61.20 Parent-Child Relational Problem
(Parent-Child Problem in DSM-III-R)

(ICD-10 code Z63.8; Z63.1 if child focus)

This category may be used, for example, for a conflict between a healthy child or adolescent and his or her parents (including step- or foster parents) that results in clinically significant symptoms in child or parent.

❑ ❑ ❑ ❑

V61.1 Partner Relational Problem
(Marital Problem in DSM-III-R)

(ICD-10 code Z63.0)

This category should be used when the focus of attention or treatment is a clinically significant or impairing problem in a marriage or similarly intimate relationship.

❑ ❑ ❑ ❑

V61.8 Sibling Relational Problem
(new in DSM-IV)

(ICD-10 code F93.3)

This category should be used when the focus of attention or treatment is a problem between siblings (including half- or foster siblings), causing clinically significant symptoms or impairment.

❑ ❑ ❑ ❑

V62.81 Relational Problem Not Otherwise   *(ICD-10 code Z63.9)*
Specified (NOS)
(Other Interpersonal Problem, or Other Specified
Family Circumstances, formerly 61.80, in DSM-III-R)

This category is used for clinically significant problems in other important relationships (e.g., with a coworker).

❑ ❑ ❑ ❑

PROBLEMS RELATED TO ABUSE OR NEGLECT

This section was added, consistent with ICD-10, to address significant
symptoms or impairment caused by abuse or neglect of a vulnerable person by
one or more others.

CODING NOTE: Codes are used when the focus of attention is
the perpetrator; use 995.5 or 995.81 when the focus of clinical
attention is the victim. ICD-10 does not differentiate between
perpetrator and victim in this context, but additional codes
should be used for mental disorders or related medical conditions caused by the abuse or neglect.

V61.21 Physical Abuse of Child   *(ICD-10 code T74.1)*
(995.5 for victim)
(new in DSM-IV)

V61.21 Sexual Abuse of Child   *(ICD-10 code T74.2)*
(995.5 for victim)
(new in DSM-IV)

V61.21 Neglect of Child   *(ICD-10 code T74.0)*
(995.5 for victim)
(new in DSM-IV)

V61.1 Physical Abuse of Adult   *(ICD-10 code T74.1)*
(995.81 for victim)
(new in DSM-IV)

V61.1 Sexual Abuse of Adult   *(ICD-10 code T74.2)*
(995.81 for victim)
(new in DSM-IV)

❑ ❑ ❑ ❑

ADDITIONAL CONDITIONS THAT MAY BE A FOCUS OF CLINICAL ATTENTION

The following are not considered mental disorders, but they should be acknowledged when they cause clinically significant symptoms or functional impairment. They may aggravate mental disorders or their treatment. Except where noted, they are similar to the corresponding DSM-III-R V-code disorders.

> CODING NOTE: These conditions may be listed on Axis I if they are currently an important clinical focus, or on Axis IV if they are incidental to another disorder.

V15.81 Noncompliance With Treatment   (ICD-10 code Z91.1)

This category may be used when the focus of attention or treatment is noncompliance with, or refusal of, treatment for a mental disorder or general medical condition. The result of the noncompliance must be sufficient to warrant individual clinical attention. The source of the noncompliance is immaterial, and might, for example, be related to personal beliefs, denial, misunderstanding, cost, or side effects.

□ □ □ □

V65.2 Malingering   (ICD-10 code Z76.5)

ESSENTIAL FEATURES. Malingering implies intentional faking or gross exaggeration of physical and/or psychological symptoms, motivated by a clear expectation of personal gain (e.g., money, avoiding work, evading criminal prosecution, obtaining drugs). Malingering is a diagnosis of exclusion; this *Training Guide* suggests caution when diagnosing it. DSM-IV, like DSM-III-R, lists four items that should lead the clinician to suspect Malingering:

1. Medicolegal context of presentation (e.g., referral by an attorney)
2. Marked discrepancy between the person's claimed stress or disability and the objective findings
3. Lack of cooperation during the diagnostic evaluation and in complying with the prescribed treatment regimen
4. The presence of Antisocial Personality Disorder

DIFFERENTIAL DIAGNOSIS. Malingering is differentiated from Factitious Disorder by the presence of external incentives (rather than the intrapsychic ones of Factitious Disorder). It should also be differentiated from Dissociative and Somatoform Disorders.

□ □ □ □

V71.01 Adult Antisocial Behavior   (ICD-10 code Z72.8)

This code denotes antisocial (e.g., criminal) behavior not due to an Axis I or II mental disorder.

DIFFERENTIAL DIAGNOSIS. Conduct Disorder, Antisocial Personality Disorder, and Impulse Control Disorders are considered.

□ □ □ □

V71.02 Child or Adolescent   (ICD-10 code Z72.8)
Antisocial Behavior

This category is appropriate when antisocial behavior, including criminal behavior, in a child or adolescent is a focus of clinical attention and is not primarily a symptom of a mental disorder.

DIFFERENTIAL DIAGNOSIS. Conduct Disorder and Impulse Control Disorder are considered. *Patterns* of antisocial behavior are often better diagnosed elsewhere, especially in children or younger adolescents.

□ □ □ □

V62.89 Borderline Intellectual Functioning   (ICD-10 code R41.8)

CODING NOTE: Code on Axis II.

This category is appropriate for individuals whose intellectual functioning is between that of normal persons and those with Mental Retardation, and whose intellectual performance is a focus of clinical attention or causes significant impairment. The generally accepted Borderline range is a measured IQ of 71 to 84.

DIFFERENTIAL DIAGNOSIS. Differential diagnosis can be difficult, particularly when there are social, cultural, language, or clinical factors that make meaningful measurement of intelligence difficult. Mental Retardation requires an IQ of 70 or below. Many mental disorders may either divert the clinician's attention from intellectual assessment or, conversely, cause the clinician to assume poor intellectual functioning when the apparent impairment is actually caused by a mental disorder.

□ □ □ □

780.9 Age-Related Cognitive Decline   (ICD-10 code R41.8)
(new in DSM-IV)

This category may be used when there is clinically significant or functionally impairing decline in cognitive functioning which is caused by normal aging, and which is not better accounted for by a mental disorder or general medical condition.

DIFFERENTIAL DIAGNOSIS. Any Dementia, cognitive loss due to stroke or other neurological disease or event, and pseudodementia associated with depression are considered.

□ □ □ □

V62.82 Bereavement   (ICD-10 code Z63.4)
(Uncomplicated Bereavement in DSM-III-R)
(significantly modified from DSM-III-R)

> NOTE: DSM-IV considers bereavement to be limited to the death of a loved one. Many clinicians consider this category also appropriate for other significant losses, such as by divorce or geographic separation.

This category may be used when one's reaction to the loss or death of a loved one is clinically significant or functionally impairing. Depressive symptoms or syndromes are common in such circumstances, but appropriate handling of feelings and situations by the individual, over time, with adaptive resolution, should preclude diagnosis of a mental disorder. The patient usually knows that a depressed mood is typical of such a loss but may seek help for relief of symptoms (e.g., difficulty sleeping). The course of Bereavement is also affected by grief work done before actual death, such as in the case of a terminal illness. It should be noted that "normal" grief feelings and behaviors (and their duration) vary considerably among individuals and cultural groups.

DIFFERENTIAL DIAGNOSIS. Major Depressive Episode, which may be suggested by such symptoms as guilt about things unrelated to the death or lost person; thoughts of death other than those associated with the loss or with joining the deceased person; morbid preoccupation with worthlessness; marked psychomotor retardation; hallucinatory experiences other than culturally acceptable transient perceptions of the voice of (or, in some cultures, the image) of the deceased; and prolonged, marked functional impairment are considered in the differential diagnosis. Diagnosis of a Depressive Disorder is generally not made unless severe symptoms continue beyond 2 months. Adjustment Disorder is not coded when death of a loved one is the cause of the symptoms, although other serious losses (e.g., divorce) may suggest that diagnosis.

□ □ □ □

V62.3 Academic Problem   (ICD-10 code Z55.8)

This category may be used when the focus of attention or treatment is an academic problem, generally not due to a mental disorder (e.g., underachievement in the absence of a Learning Disorder or other clinical explanation). When related to a mental disorder, the academic problem must be severe enough to merit specific clinical attention.

□ □ □ □

V62.2 Occupational Problem   (ICD-10 code Z56.7)

This category may be used when the focus of attention or treatment is occupational, such as clinically significant or impairing job dissatisfaction, generally not due to a mental disorder. When related to a mental disorder, the occupational problem must be severe enough to merit specific clinical attention.

□ □ □ □

313.82 Identity Problem   (ICD-10 code F93.8)
(Identity Disorder in DSM-III-R, formerly under
"Disorders Usually First Evident in Infancy,
Childhood or Adolescence")

This category may be used to describe clinically significant or impairing distress related to, for example, uncertainty in one's life goals, career preferences, patterns of interpersonal relating, sexual orientation and behavior, values, or loyalties.

□ □ □ □

V62.89 Religious or Spiritual Problem   (ICD-10 code Z71.8)
(new in DSM-IV)

This category describes clinically significant or impairing religious or spiritual difficulty, such as that associated with lost or questioned faith. The spiritual issues may or may not be related to an organized religion.

□ □ □ □

V62.4 Acculturation Problem   (ICD-10 code Z60.3)
(new in DSM-IV)

This category may be used to describe clinically significant symptoms related to adjustment to a different culture (e.g., following immigration), but not meeting criteria for an Adjustment Disorder.

□ □ □ □

V62.89 Phase of Life Problem   *(ICD-10 code Z60.0)*
(Phase of Life or Other Life Circumstance Problem
in DSM-III-R)

These conditions include clinically significant or impairing problems associated with, for example, going to a new school, leaving the parental home, beginning a new career, experiencing a marriage or a divorce, or adjusting to retirement. The symptoms may be caused by a mental disorder; however, the Phase of Life Problem must be severe enough to merit specific clinical attention.

❑ ❑ ❑ ❑

DIFFERENCES BETWEEN DSM-III-R AND DSM-IV OTHER CONDITIONS THAT MAY BE A FOCUS OF CLINICAL ATTENTION

❑ The following are new in DSM-IV: **Neuroleptic-Induced Parkinsonism, Neuroleptic Malignant Syndrome, Neuroleptic-Induced Dystonia, Neuroleptic-Induced Acute Akathisia, Neuroleptic-Induced Tardive Dyskinesia, Medication-Induced Postural Tremor, Relational Problem Related to a Mental Disorder or General Medical Condition, Sibling Relational Problem, Religious or Spiritual Problem, Age-Related Cognitive Decline**, and **Acculturation Problem**.

❑ Clinical significance or impairment of functioning is emphasized as a requirement for coding **Noncompliance With Treatment, Malingering, Adult** or **Child/Adolescent Antisocial Behavior, Borderline Intellectual Functioning, Age-Related Cognitive Decline, Bereavement, Academic Problem, Occupational Problem, Identity Problem, Religious or Spiritual Problem, Acculturation Problem**, and **Phase of Life Problem**.

❑ **Psychological Factors Affecting Medical Condition** has been broadened, separated from the mental disorders, and given more specific subcategories.

❑ **Relational/Interpersonal/Family Problems** are now grouped together. Those that were found in DSM-III-R are similar in DSM-IV. Clinical significance or functional impairment is emphasized as a requirement for coding.

❑ **Abuse and/or Neglect** conditions are new in DSM-IV.

❑ **Partner Relational Problem** is the appropriate DSM-IV category for problems involving intimate but unmarried couples, not Relational Problem NOS as in DSM-III-R.

❑ **Bereavement** is no longer "uncomplicated" bereavement, and is better differentiated from Major Depressive Episode.

❑ **Identity Problem** is no longer listed under "Disorders Usually First Evident in Infancy, Childhood, or Adolescence."

....

CASE VIGNETTES: OTHER CONDITIONS THAT MAY BE A FOCUS OF CLINICAL ATTENTION

Case Vignette 1

M.T., a 40-year-old man, has been arrested for the fifteenth time since he finished high school, this time for armed robbery. He was on parole when he committed the alleged offense. M.T. has never held a job, other than criminal behavior, for more than 6 months. He has been married and divorced twice, and has often been cited for failure to pay child support. He gets into fights often, both when intoxicated and when sober. M.T. is impulsive and irresponsible, and at one time traveled with a partner from town to town robbing filling stations and convenience stores. Although a frequent drinker and suspected to be a former user of marijuana and amphetamines, M.T. denies alcohol or drug problems at present and no corroborating information is available. Further information about Substance Abuse is being sought.

As a child and adolescent, M.T. was considered intelligent, friendly, and prone to manipulate others. He was arrested once at age 16 (for possession of alcohol), but was not known to be particularly dishonest, irresponsible, or aggressive. He graduated from high school with good marks and attendance.

DIAGNOSIS AND DISCUSSION

Axis I—V71.01 Adult Antisocial Behavior (ICD-10 Z72.8)
Axis II—301.9 Personality Disorder Not Otherwise Specified (ICD-10 F60.9)

The lack of clear-cut childhood antisocial behavior or Conduct Disorder eliminates Antisocial Personality. Although no specific Personality Disorder appears likely, the pervasive, maladaptive quality of M.T.'s behavior and lifestyle, and his marked social impairment, suggest an "NOS" Axis II diagnosis. One should be cautious about equating a Personality Disorder diagnosis with "mental illness" in chronically antisocial people, especially when it may be used to excuse them from responsibility for their behavior. A Deferred (799.9) or No Diagnosis (V71.09) Axis II code could also be defended.

There is insufficient information for a clear Axis I diagnosis of a Substance-Related Disorder, but it is probable and further information is being sought. A presumptive diagnosis might be considered.

Case Vignette 2

V.K. is a 34-year-old woman who is seen for an unscheduled appointment in the mental health clinic for new and acute complaints of "I can't sit still; I've got ants in my pants." Staff observes V.K. shuffling her feet while seated and repeatedly getting up to pace about the room. Abnormal Involuntary Movement Scale (AIMS) testing is negative for orobuccal symptoms or other movements of her extremities. She has no significant tremors.

Her mental illness—Schizophrenia, Paranoid Type—was in poor remission at her last clinic visit, 3 days ago, prompting a change in medication to haloperidol and an increase in dose. Pacing has not been one of her schizophrenic symptoms; if anything, her illness appears to be in somewhat better remission. A psychiatrist prescribed benztropine several years ago, for unknown symptoms, but V.K. has not taken any recently. No other medications or physical abnormalities are apparent.

DIAGNOSIS AND DISCUSSION

Axis I—295.30 Schizophrenia, Paranoid Type, With Residual Symptoms but Unspecified Pattern (ICD-10 F20.08)
Axis I—333.99 Neuroleptic-Induced Acute Akathisia (ICD-10 G21.1) (ICD-9-CM substance code E939.2 [haloperidol])
Axis II—V71.09 No Diagnosis on Axis II (ICD-10 Z032) or 799.9 Diagnosis Deferred on Axis II (ICD-10 R46.8)
Axis III—Adverse effects from Psychotropic Agent (E939.2)

The Schizophrenia diagnosis is mentioned in the vignette, although it is not clear whether the course is episodic or continuous. The new symptoms meet both informal and suggested research criteria for Neuroleptic-Induced Akathisia. Other likely causes or related disorders have been ruled out. Although this syndrome is due to neurotoxicity, it is coded on Axis I rather than Axis III. The optional ICD-9-CM E code is noted on Axis I as well. There is no mention of Axis II symptoms or signs. If there were a history of Personality Disorder before the onset of Schizophrenia, the Personality Disorder diagnosis might be coded as "premorbid."

Case Vignette 3

J.D., a 16-year-old, outwardly normal male, is referred to the psychiatrist because of J.D.'s continuing reluctance to adhere to his diabetic treatment regimen. He has been insulin dependent for several years, yet regularly "forgets" his injections and glucometer testing. Ignoring his dietary restrictions has contributed to his being overweight and his blood sugar is often out of control.

J.D. tells the psychiatrist that he doesn't "feel sick" and sees no need to treat himself differently from his peers. Later in the interview, J.D. expresses doubts about his health, and even his virility, related to the diabetes: "My grandfather had it and all he ever did was take his insulin and eat what my grandma told him and sit around till he died. They had to cut off his toes."

J.D. describes some self-doubt and dysphoria and has occasional problems sleeping, but he does not meet criteria for a Mood or Anxiety Disorder. He is doing well in school.

DIAGNOSIS AND DISCUSSION

Axis I—316 Psychological Symptoms Affecting Diabetes (ICD-10 F54); V15.81 Noncompliance With Treatment (ICD-10 Z91.1)
Axis II—V71.09 No Diagnosis on Axis II (ICD-10 Z03.2)
Axis III—Diabetes Mellitus, Type I/Insulin Dependent (ICD-10 250.1)

Both the psychological factor and the noncompliance with treatment for diabetes are clinically significant and merit psychological treatment focus, although the noncompliance might be coded on Axis IV in some situations. There is no indication that the problem meets criteria for an Axis I mental disorder (e.g., a Mood or Adjustment Disorder). No Identity Problem or Phase of Life Problem is described, although one might consider them in light of J.D.'s apparent view of himself as infirmed and/or destined to be disabled.

CHAPTER 27

ADDITIONAL CODES

300.9 Unspecified Mental Disorder (Nonpsychotic)   *(ICD-10 code F99)*

This code is indicated for specific mental disorders not included in DSM-IV, when none of the available Not Otherwise Specified (NOS) categories is appropriate, and/or when a qualified clinician decides that a mental disorder is present but information is insufficient for diagnosis.

V71.09 No Diagnosis or Condition on Axis I   *(ICD-10 code Z03.2)*

There is no clear indication of an Axis I disorder or condition.

799.9 Diagnosis or Condition Deferred on Axis I   *(ICD-10 code R69)*

This code should be used when incomplete data preclude diagnostic judgment about an Axis I diagnosis or condition.

V71.09 No Diagnosis on Axis II   *(ICD-10 code Z03.2)*

There is no clear indication of an Axis II disorder.

799.9 Diagnosis Deferred on Axis II   *(ICD-10 code R46.8)*

This code should be used when incomplete data preclude diagnostic judgment about an Axis II diagnosis.

CHAPTER 28

DSM-IV APPENDICES

DSM-IV provides a number of appendices which are very useful for the student, clinician, researcher, or coding technician. Although this *Training Guide* does not reproduce all their content, it is important to know what they contain and when they may be important. The appendices also contribute to one's understanding of the place of DSM-IV codes and criteria in the context of unfamiliar cultures, the previous DSM-III-R, the worldwide standard tenth edition of the International Classification of Diseases (ICD-10), and the general medical codes of ICD-9-CM and ICD-10.

APPENDIX A: DECISION TREES FOR DIFFERENTIAL DIAGNOSIS

There are six decision trees for differential diagnosis in this appendix:

Mental Disorders Due to a General Medical Condition
Substance-Induced Disorders
Psychotic Disorders
Mood Disorders
Anxiety Disorders
Somatoform Disorders

They contain or imply brief questions one might ask at each "branch point," which reflect (but pointedly do not duplicate) important items from the DSM-IV diagnostic criteria.

> NOTE: Except for the psychotic disorders, these diagnoses are not mutually exclusive within a particular decision tree. Since more than one disorder may be present, within or outside each decision tree, diagnosis must be made in a context of all DSM-IV criteria sets and an overall diagnostic process.
> DSM-IV states that the purpose of the decision trees is to promote understanding of the DSM-IV classification system. We suspect that many students and clinicians will also use them for clinical diagnosis. This being the case, it is important that one be aware of the limitations of the decision trees as well as their usefulness. The DSM-IV decision trees present a very sim-

ple diagnostic scheme for a particular clinical problem (e.g., Differential Diagnosis of Psychotic Disorders). In addition, many individuals with mental disorders have several disorders on Axis I and/or Axis II. For these reasons, we *do not* recommend employing these decision trees as standards or stand-alone guides for clinical protocols in training programs, clinics, or health care systems.

(131)

....

APPENDIX B: CRITERIA SETS AND AXES PROVIDED FOR FURTHER STUDY

These are new categories and axes suggested by professionals and/or groups for inclusion in DSM-IV. Although each has some merit, the DSM-IV Task Force determined that there was insufficient information to either include or exclude them. The criteria listed here provide a standard foundation for their study.

(132)

....

PROPOSED NEW DISORDERS

....

We will briefly describe each proposed disorder but will not reproduce the research criteria here. None of these conditions is an official DSM-IV disorder.

NOTE: Except where noted, all disorders in this section require clinically significant distress or impairment, and are not due to the direct physiological effects of a substance or general medical condition.

Postconcussional Disorder

ESSENTIAL FEATURES. Impaired cognitive functioning due to a closed-head injury with concussion is the essential feature. There must be quantitatively documented impairment of attention or memory, as well as at least three symptoms or signs from a list of eight. Significant functional impairment must be present. The symptoms are not better accounted for by a DSM-IV mental disorder. This disorder is preempted if DSM-IV criteria for Dementia Due to Head Trauma are met.

Mild Neurocognitive Disorder

ESSENTIAL FEATURES. There is neurocognitive impairment due to a general medical condition, with significant distress or interference in social or occupational function but only mild impact on daily activities. (DSM-IV is not clear about this apparent inconsistency.) The deficits must be in two cognitive areas, such as language, memory, attention, "executive" functioning, perceptual-motor activities, or information processing. Delirium, Dementia, and Amnestic Disorders preempt this diagnosis.

Caffeine Withdrawal

ESSENTIAL FEATURES. Withdrawal symptoms, including headache, due to sudden decrease of caffeine intake are seen. Marked fatigue, anxiety, depression, or nausea accompanies the headache.

Alternative Dimensional Descriptors for Schizophrenia

Some studies indicate that schizophrenic symptoms occur in three distinct "dimensions"—psychotic, disorganized, and negative (or deficit)—each possibly related to different pathophysiology and treatment response. These alternative dimensional descriptors may represent a more accurate way of characterizing and understanding Schizophrenia, both in the present and over the course of the illness.

In this model, each of the three dimensions must be specified as absent, mild, moderate, or severe in the present and during the lifetime of the patient. The *psychotic* dimension refers to hallucinations and delusions; *disorganized* refers to inappropriate affect or disorganized speech or behavior, and the *negative* (deficit) dimension refers to negative symptoms such as flattened affect or suppressed volition. Symptoms due to medication, depression, or reactions to delusions or hallucinations are not considered part of the dimensions.

Postpsychotic Depressive Disorder of Schizophrenia

ESSENTIAL FEATURES. There is a major depressive episode whose occurrence is limited to the residual phase of Schizophrenia. Depressed mood is required (as contrasted with depressive episode characterized by loss of interest or pleasure). The symptoms are not caused by the negative or psychotic symptoms of the Schizophrenia itself, nor by medication side effects.

Simple Deteriorative Disorder (Simple Schizophrenia)

ESSENTIAL FEATURES. There are prominent negative symptoms, different from the patient's premorbid state, causing a distinct deterioration of social, occupational, or academic functioning. Alogia, avolition, and/or flattened affect develop gradually over at least a year. Social isolation or withdrawal and poor interpersonal relationships are usual.

The patient never meets Criterion A for Schizophrenia, and the symptoms are not better accounted for by another Axis I or II disorder.

Premenstrual Dysphoric Disorder

ESSENTIAL FEATURES. There are multiple dysphoric symptoms that occur regularly during the postluteal phase of the menstrual cycle, remit after onset of menses, and are absent during the week after menses. At least five symptoms from the

DSM-IV list of 11 must be present, one of which must be marked depression, marked anxiety, marked lability, or marked anger/irritability. The symptoms and other criteria must be confirmed by prospective daily ratings (e.g., from a journal kept by the patient).

Alternative Criterion B for Dysthymic Disorder

The DSM-IV Mood Disorders field trial suggested that the Criterion B currently used for dysthymia might better be replaced by the following:

B. Presence, while depressed, of three (or more) of the following:
   (1) low self-esteem, self-confidence, or feelings of inadequacy
   (2) feelings of pessimism, despair, or hopelessness
   (3) generalized loss of interest or pleasure
   (4) social withdrawal
   (5) chronic fatigue or tiredness
   (6) feelings of guilt or brooding about the past
   (7) subjective feelings of irritability or excessive anger
   (8) decreased activity, effectiveness, or productivity
   (9) difficulty thinking, reflected by poor concentration, poor memory, or indecisiveness

Minor Depressive Disorder

ESSENTIAL FEATURES. There are depressive periods that are similar in length to Major Depressive Episodes but lack their level of symptoms and impairment. Sadness, depression, loss of interest, or loss of pleasure is common to each episode, and two to five other criteria from those of Major Depressive Episode are met. Minor Depressive Disorder is not diagnosed if the patient has ever met criteria for Major Depressive, Manic, Mixed, or Hypomanic Episode; currently meets criteria for an Axis I mood disorder; or has symptoms only during a Psychotic Disorder.

Recurrent Brief Depressive Disorder

ESSENTIAL FEATURES. This disorder resembles recurrent Major Depressive Disorder except that (1) the depressive episodes meet only symptom number and severity criteria for Major Depressive Episode and not duration criteria (i.e., the episodes last less than 2 weeks), and (2) depressive episodes must occur at least monthly for 1 year. They are not associated with the menstrual cycle.

Mixed Anxiety-Depressive Disorder

ESSENTIAL FEATURES. There are persistent or recurrent dysphoric mood and symptoms of anxiety, both of which endure for at least 1 month. In addition to dysphoria, the symptoms must include at least 4 of 10 items listed, about half of which suggest anxiety (e.g., difficulty concentrating/mind going blank, worry, hypervigilance, anticipating the worst).

Factitious Disorder by Proxy

ESSENTIAL FEATURES. The fraudulent describing by one person of physical or psychological symptoms in another person, often a small child, who is being cared for by the first, is the essential feature of this disorder. As with conventional Factitious Disorder, there is no apparent source of external gain for the feigning person (such as money), but rather an internal, psychodynamic need to be in a patient role by proxy. The "perpetrator" is often the mother of the "victim."

Dissociative Trance Disorder

ESSENTIAL FEATURES. The individual enters an unintended trance state, outside cultural or religious norms, with altered consciousness or loss of feeling of identity. Two possible forms of trance are suggested by the research criteria: simple trance associated with a narrowing of awareness or focus on particular stimuli, or stereotyped movements that feel outside one's control or "possession trance," in which a new, perhaps spiritual identity appears to replace one's own.

Binge-Eating Disorder

ESSENTIAL FEATURES. There is recurrent binge eating that appears outside the control of the patient, without the compensatory behaviors seen in Bulimia Nervosa (vomiting, purging, intense exercise). The patient is distressed by the behavior, which includes rapid, driven eating of unusually large amounts of food, often without feeling hungry and in spite of feeling full. The symptoms are present for an average of 2 days a week over at least 6 months.

Depressive Personality Disorder

ESSENTIAL FEATURES. There is a pervasive pattern of depressive feelings and demeanor that starts in childhood or early adulthood, permeates one's experience, and includes at least five of seven depressive signs and symptoms listed in DSM-IV Appendix B. The characteristics do not occur exclusively during exacerbations of Axis I Mood Disorders and are not better accounted for by Dysthymic Disorder.

Passive-Aggressive Personality Disorder
(Negativistic Personality Disorder)

Persons with this disorder are chronically negativistic and passively resist others' calls for occupational or social performance. Passive criticism of authority, chronically finding excuses for lack of performance, and resentment of those who are more successful are common. The traits begin in adolescence or early adulthood and permeate one's behavior and experience. They are not limited to exacerbations of Mood Disorders and are not better explained by Dysthymic Disorder.

❑ ❑ ❑ ❑

....
MEDICATION-INDUCED MOVEMENT DISORDERS

NOTE: These conditions are listed in DSM-IV "Other Conditions That May Be a Focus of Clinical Attention." Appendix B contains suggested descriptions and research criteria.

Descriptions, criteria, and ICD-10 codes for these conditions are found on pages 298–304 of this book.

❑ ❑ ❑ ❑

....
PROPOSED NEW AXES AND SCALES
....

Defensive Functioning Scale

The Defensive Functioning Scale attempts to assess the patient's internal (largely unconscious) ability to cope with anxiety-producing impulses or events. It depends on the clinician's understanding the patient's current and recent psychological defense mechanisms and coping styles, then comparing them with categories of functioning provided by the scale (e.g., high adaptive level, major image-distorting level). A glossary of specific defense mechanisms and coping styles is provided in DSM-IV.

Global Assessment of Relational Functioning (GARF) Scale

The GARF is an effort to provide an overall judgment of family or other "relational unit" functioning. It does not assess specific persons but considers the clinician's descriptions of the group or couple. Those descriptions are compared with suggested criteria for various levels of relational functioning (e.g., satisfactory, clearly dysfunctional, obviously and seriously dysfunctional). The scale is analogous to the Global Assessment of Functioning (GAF, Axis V) for individuals.

Social and Occupational Functioning Assessment Scale (SOFAS)

The SOFAS is a new instrument which, although similar to the GAF in format, attempts to assess an individual's social and/or occupational functioning independent of the overall severity of his or her mental disorder. It focuses on specific limitations to social and/or occupational activities, including both mental and physical impairment. Like the GAF, it excludes external or environmental factors, such as minority prejudice or lack of opportunity.

□ □ □ □

APPENDIX C: GLOSSARY OF TECHNICAL TERMS

(133) DSM-IV provides a brief glossary of terms used in the text. The terms and definitions are similar to, but less comprehensive than, those in the *American Psychiatric Glossary* (7th ed., 1994, American Psychiatric Press, Inc., Washington, DC). See the glossary in this *Training Guide*, page 324.

APPENDIX D: ANNOTATED LISTING OF CHANGES IN DSM-IV

(134) Most of the major differences between DSM-III-R and DSM-IV are listed here, by disorder and section. Many of the minor changes have been omitted. See differences listed in each section of this *Training Guide*.

APPENDIX E: ALPHABETICAL LISTING OF DSM-IV DIAGNOSES AND CODES

(135) This listing is useful when one knows the exact name of a disorder and needs to code it, for example, for a medical records or reimbursement purpose.

APPENDIX F: NUMERICAL LISTING OF DSM-IV DIAGNOSES AND CODES

(136) This listing allows one to begin with only a code number and find the disorder to which it refers.

APPENDIX G: ICD-9-CM CODES FOR SELECTED GENERAL MEDICAL CONDITIONS AND MEDICATION-INDUCED DISORDERS

(137) These two sections provide selected *International Classification of Diseases, Ninth Edition, Clinical Modification* (ICD-9-CM) codes for use on Axis III (general medical conditions) and occasionally on Axis I (E codes for medications that may be involved in Medication-Induced Disorders). The list is not exhaustive but may be helpful in many cases. More complete information is available in the *ICD-9-CM Diseases: Tabular List*.

NOTE: In most parts of the world, ICD-9 was superseded by ICD-10; the transition to ICD-10 in the United States (including the mental and behavioral disorders chapter) is expected to be complete within the next several years.

APPENDIX H: DSM-IV CLASSIFICATION WITH ICD-10 CODES

ICD codes for mental and behavioral disorders are the standard for most of the world, and are used in several record and reimbursement systems in this country. DSM-IV diagnoses are consistent with ICD-10, and virtually all of the diagnoses and specifiers are represented in the ICD-10 list. See list on pages IX–XXIV of this *Training Guide,* and specific disorder sections for ICD-10 codes.

(138)

APPENDIX I: OUTLINE FOR CULTURAL FORMULATION AND GLOSSARY OF CULTURE-BOUND SYNDROMES

The first section of this appendix is a brief effort to help the clinician deal with issues that arise when the clinician, patient, and/or environment are from differing cultures. The second section lists about 25 regional syndromes found in various countries and cultures in which the syndromes are viewed as aberrant. They deserve clinical attention but are not necessarily associated with DSM-IV disorders.

(139)

APPENDIX J: DSM-IV CONTRIBUTORS

This last appendix is a list of the great many individual and organizational contributors to the creation and validation of DSM-IV.

(140)

GLOSSARY OF TERMS USED IN DSM-IV

NOTE: The names of specific disorders are defined in the text and are not listed in this glossary.

Abstracting, Abstracting Ability—Refers to one's ability to use abstract, symbolic thought, as differentiated from concrete or literal thought.

Acute—Current; currently visible; related to the present or recent past; not *chronic* (q.v.).

Affect—The outward, often facial, manifestation of subjective feelings or emotions.

Agnosia—An inability to recognize and name objects.

Agoraphobia—A morbid fear, and intolerance of, unfamiliar surroundings or open spaces.

Akinesia—Lack of movement.

Alogia—Lack of thought content, inferred from lack of verbal productions.

Ambivalence—Vacillation between or among two or more thoughts or feelings; indecision, perhaps to a pathological extent; also, coexistence of contradictory feelings or impulses toward something.

Amenorrhea—Absence of menses.

Anergia—Loss of strength or energy; feeling a loss of strength.

Anhedonia—An inability to experience pleasure.

Anorexia—Absence of appetite or eating; refusal to eat.

Anxiety—A feeling of apprehension or uneasiness, similar to fear, due to the anticipation of internal or external danger. The source of the danger, in some definitions, is unknown. In psychoanalytic theory, the danger stems from threats (usually unconscious) to the ego.

Anxiolytic—Refers to the amelioration of anxiety; as a noun, a class of medications that alleviate anxiety.

Apathy—Marked lack of interest or motivation.

Aphasia—An inability to understand or produce language, not related to sensory (e.g., deafness) or motor (e.g., dysarthria) deficit.

Aphonia—Inability to speak or produce normal speech sounds.

Apraxia—Loss of a motor skill not explained by simple weakness or previously existing incoordination.

Arylcyclohexylamine—Any of a class of psychoactive substances, which includes phencyclidine (PCP).

Associations—With repect to thought process, the relationship (normal or abnormal) between one idea or thought and the next (see also Tangential, Loose Circumstantial, Clang).

Asterixis—A neurological sign characterized by flapping of the hands, associated with toxic or metabolic encephalopathy.

Ataxia—Muscle incoordination, especially affecting gait.

Athetoid—Refers to slow, regular, twisting motion of limbs.

Autistic—Refers to autism (q.v., in text); refers to marked disturbances in relating to, and apparent unawareness of, others and one's environment.

Autonomic—Refers to normally involuntary innervation of cardiac and smooth muscle tissue (e.g., internal organs).

Avolition—Lack of initiative, especially for goal-directed activity.

Belle Indifférence—An apparent indifference to symptons that would be expected to elicit worry or distress (also La Belle Indifférence).

Benzodiazepine—A class of antianxiety and hypnotic medications.

Bereavement—Grief over a loss.

Bestiality—See Zoophilia; also, the practice of sexual activity with nonhuman animals.

Biopsychosocial—Refers to the multideterminate nature of psychiatric syndromes and disorders, and to multideterminate approaches to their understanding and treatment.

Blocking—An interruption of communication before a thought or idea has been completed, caused by psychological factors that are unconscious or unknown to the individual.

Blunting—With respect to affect, marked reduction in normal intensity.

Bulimia—Episodic, usually uncontrollable eating binges, sometimes accompanied by ingestion of large amounts of foods. Self-induced vomiting or diarrhea is characteristic.

Butyrophenone—A class of antipsychotic medications.

Cannabis—Marijuana.

Cardiac Neurosis—The fear or erroneous belief that one has heart disease; also a feeling of physical incapacity related to past heart disease, out of proportion to one's actual disability, or to fear of having a heart attack.

Catalepsy—Diminished responsiveness, often trancelike; may be related to organic or functional disorders or to hypnosis. Includes waxy flexibility (q.v.).

Cataplexy—Episodic loss of muscle tone, often to the extent of falling and often triggered by strong emotions.

Catatonic—Refers to any of several striking motor anomalies, generally described as related to a psychosis, including extreme excitement, stupor, negativism, rigidity, or posturing.

Cerea Flexibilitas—Waxy flexibility (q.v.).

Choreiform—Writhing.

Chronic—Long persisting; not acute or limited to the present.

Circadian—Refers to 24-hour biological rhythms.

Circumstantial—When referring to thought process, describes conversation or a train of thought that wanders from the point but eventually returns to it.

Clairvoyance—The experience or feeling of being able to sense others' thoughts (not usually considered psychotic).

Clang—With respect to associations or thought process, speech or train of thought largely governed by sound or rhyme rather than logic (e.g., "Turn on the light, tight, bright; bright enough to bite. Watch out for biting dogs.").

CNS Depressant—In pharmacology, refers generally to central nervous system sedation (does not refer to depression of the mood).

Complex Tics—Tics that involve more extensive behaviors than simple motor tics (e.g., grooming behaviors, coprolalia).

Compulsion—A powerful impulse toward a specific purposeful behavior which is often repetitive and unwanted, and often in response to an obsession.

Concordant—In genetics, refers to a characteristic or trait found in two genetically related (especially twin) animals or people.

Concrete—Refers to literal thought, as differentiated from abstract, symbolic thought.

Confabulation—Creation of inaccurate memories or fabrications, unconsciously, to substitute for unrecalled events.

Congenital—Present at birth, but not necessarily implying genetic or familial transmission.

Conjugal—Refers to marital, especially sexual, relationships.

Constricted—With respect to affect, a reduction or circumscribing of range and/or intensity.

Constructional Apraxia—Loss of the ability to produce or copy drawings, shapes, or designs.

Continence—The ability to control voluntarily one's urination or defecation.

Conversion—Refers to a physical symptom or dysfunction that unconsciously expresses an emotional conflict or need (cf., conversion reaction).

Coprolalia—Pathological use of obscene or unacceptable words.

Coprophilia—Reliance on feces as a primary source of sexual gratification.

Covert—Hidden.

Defense Mechanism—See Neurotic Defense Mechanism.

Delirium—An acute, organically caused brain disorder characterized by confusion and altered consciousness.

Delirium Tremens—A severe, life-threatening delirium caused by withdrawal from alcohol.

Delusion—A fixed, false belief not ordinarily accepted by other members of an individual's culture. In DSM-IV, a **bizarre** delusion is one that involves very unusual or completely implausible elements. A delusion **of reference** is one in which elements in the environment, such as comments from the news media, have particular significance and/or refer to oneself.

Dementia—An organically caused mental disorder characterized by loss of previously held mental abilities, including intellect, memory, and judgment.

Depersonalization—A strong feeling of not being oneself or of being detached from oneself or the environment.

Depression—A sad, despairing, or discouraged mood; such a mood or feeling sufficient to be a symptom or a mental disorder; a syndrome (e.g., Major Despression) characterized by depressed mood.

Derailment—A disorder of thought process in which one's thoughts unexpectedly and inappropriately leave the topic. Similar to loose associations (q.v.).

Derealization—A strong feeling of strangeness or detachment from the environment or from reality.

Dereistic—Refers to feelings or thoughts that are grossly illogical, not in accordance with reality.

Diplopia—Double vision.

Diurnal—Daily.

Dizygotic—Refers to multiple fetuses (e.g., fraternal twins) developed from more than one zygote.

Dysarthria—Difficulty in speech production related to anatomical or coordination deficit.

Dysfluency—A disturbance of language fluency.

Dyskinesia—A movement disorder involving involuntary muscle contractions; may be mild (e.g., benign orofacial dyskinesia) or severe (e.g., hemiballismus).

Dyslexia—Difficulty understanding or manipulating words (e.g., in reading) that is not related to education or intelligence.

Dysmenorrhea—Irregularity or other abnormality of menses.

Dysmorphophobia—Preoccupation with an imagined defect in appearance; Body Dysmorphic Disorder.

Dysphonia—An impaired ability to create or understand sounds.

Dysphoric—Uncomfortable, painful.

Dyssomnia—A disorder of sleep, whether organic or functional.

Dystonic—With respect to movement, refers to involuntary, often painful or disfiguring muscle contractions; also, not in agreement with (see also Ego-dystonic).

Echokinesis—Pathological imitation of another's movements.

Echolalia—Pathological imitation of a just-heard word or sound.

Ego—Literally, the self, refers to one's inner self or personality; in psychoanalytic theory, a major part of the (largely unconscious) psychic apparatus, which is primarily responsible for defense mechanisms.

Ego-alien—Foreign to one's view of oneself.

Ego Boundary—The conceptual delineation between oneself (especially one's perception of oneself) and the external world.

Ego-dystonic—Inconsistent with an acceptable view of oneself.

Ego-syntonic—Consistent with an acceptable view of oneself.

Empathy—Being aware of another's feelings as if through that person's eyes (e.g., putting oneself in another's shoes).

Encapsulated—Circumscribed, well delineated (e.g., referring to delusions; see also Fragmented).

Endogenous—Arising from intrapsychic causes (see also Reactive).

Erotomania—A delusion of idealized, secret romantic love, usually involving a famous or highly visible person.

Etiology—Cause.

Euphoria—A feeling of extraordinary happiness or well-being.

Exacerbate—Make worse.

Expressive—In language, refers to the construction, production, and expression of communication, largely words.

Factitious—Refers to symptoms or disorders voluntarily produced by the patient for unconscious reasons (separate from Malingering).

Familial—Transmitted within families, not necessarily genetically (see also Hereditary, Congenital).

Fetish—A body part or nonliving object not ordinarily associated with sexual excitement that nevertheless causes inordinate sexual arousal in an individual; the condition of being attracted to such an object.

First-degree Relative—In genetics, a parent, full sibling, daughter, or son.

Flagellation—Beating, usually whipping, with a sexual, religious (e.g., absolving), or self-punitive context; slang for masturbation.

Flashback—An intense, dissociative experiencing of a past event or feeling; may be reality based or substance induced.

Flight of Ideas—Rapid movement from topic to topic, out of proportion for ordinary conversation, usually verbal.

Florid—Highly visible, unmistakable; "in full bloom."

Folie à Deux—A condition in which two people, usually living together, affect each other's psychotic syndromes in such a way that when one is symptomatic, the other improves.

Fragmented—Not whole; poorly circumscribed (e.g., referring to delusions; see also Encapsulated).

Functional—Usable; able to function; with respect to psychiatric disorders, refers to those not associated with known or presumed anatomical, physiological, or other "organic" causes.

Gamma Alcoholism—An alcohol abuse syndrome characterized by the inability to stop drinking once one begins.

Ganser Syndrome—A dissociative syndrome occasionally seen under conditions of isolation or incarceration.

Gender Identity—One's personal assumption of, or identification with, his or her maleness or femaleness.

Globus Hystericus—Emotional feeling of a "lump in the throat."

Grandiose—Refers to size or importance greatly out of proportion to reality.

Gran Mal—A form of seizure including both loss of consciousness and generalized movements (also Grand Mal).

Hallucination—A sensory experience in the absence of external stimulation of the relevant sensory organ. Hallucinations are separate from thoughts, feelings, obsessions, and illusions (q.v.), and are experienced as if they were real.

Hallucinogen—A substance that induces hallucinations.

Hallucinosis—Hallucinations during clear consciousness.

Hebephrenic Schizophrenia—A non–DSM-IV term for Schizophrenia, Disorganized Type; *Hebephrenia* connotes inappropriate, shallow, silly affect and behavior.

Hemiballismic—Refers to gross, irregular movements of large parts of the body.

Hereditary—Having to do with genes and/or chromosomes; genetically transmitted (see also Familial, Congenital).

Homosexuality—Persistent adult sexual preference for members of one's own gender, whether or not accompanied by a homosexual lifestyle. Persistent homosexual preference should be differentiated from occasional homosexual or bisexual fantasies or behavior among adults, and from ordinary, transient sexual play or experimentation among children and adolescents.

Hostile-Dependent—A situation in which one's dependence on someone or something engenders guilt, irritation, or inconvenience in the dependent individual, leading to anger against the other person or the object. As a personality trait, refers to a person who is routinely dependent on others but also hostile toward them because of the feelings and conflicts associated with that dependency.

Hyperacusis—Overarousal; hypersensitivity to sensory stimulation, especially sounds.

Hypervigilance—A condition of emotional and physiological preparedness, to an unnecessary extent, in anticipation of an anxiety-producing stimulus.

Hypnagogic—Refers to the semiconscious state just before sleep.

Hynopompic—Refers to the state just as one awakens from sleep.

Hypnotic—In pharmacology, a medication to induce sleep.

Hypoxyphilia—The practice of strangling or suffocating oneself, almost to the point of unconsciousness, for sexual stimulation.

Hysterical—Histrionic; also, refers to a Conversion Disorder (Briquet's syndrome); having flamboyant, superficially stereotypic gender characteristics; frightened or panicked to the point of being out of control. (Note: The many meanings of this disorder in clinical and lay settings often make its understanding in any one context difficult.)

Ideas of Reference—Ideation, often short of a delusion, that occurrences or objects in the environment have particular, special meaning for oneself.

Identity—The sense of self, providing a unity of personality over time.

Idiosyncratic—Characteristic of one individual; limited to one person.

Illusion—The misperception or misinterpretation of an external stimulus, differentiated from hallucinations by the presence of some form of sensory stimulation.

Immediate Memory—In the mental status examination, the portion of memory that exists a few seconds after an event (e.g., repetition of words or numbers immediately after they are spoken by the examiner).

Incidence—In epidemiology, the number of new cases that occur over a given period of time (see also Prevalence).

Incontinence—Inability to control urination or defecation.

Infibulation—Piercing the skin, especially for sexual reasons.

Insufflation—"Snorting" or sniffing, as with powdered cocaine.

Involutional—Refers to the menopausal or postmenopausal period of life, especially depressive disorders arising at that time.

Jacksonian—In epilepsy, seizures with localized convulsive movements without loss of consciousness.

Kleine-Levin Syndrome—Episodic hypersomnia, beginning in adolescence and associated with bulimia.

Klismaphilia—Reliance on enemas as a primary source of sexual gratification.

Klüver-Bucy Syndrome—Primitive impulse-control symptoms associated with memory defect and other changes, caused by loss of both temporal lobes.

Korsakoff's Psychosis—A psychosis characterized by confabulation, often related to chronic alcoholism (see also Wernicke's Encephalopathy).

La Belle Indifférence—See Belle Indifférence.

Labile—Rapidly shifting; unstable.

Lacrimation—Tearing.

Lesch-Nyhan Syndrome—A metabolic defect associated with Mental Retardation.

Limited Symptom Attack—In Anxiety Disorders, a single or small number of symptoms of anxiety that do not meet DSM-IV criteria for Panic Attacks.

Loose; Loose Associations—With respect to associations or thought process, lack of logical connection between one's thoughts or ideas, usually expressed in confusing conversation. Similar to Derailment.

Macropsia—The illusion that objects appear larger than they actually are.

Magical Thinking—The belief that one's thoughts or behavior will affect the environment in some way separate from natural cause and effect.

Malingering—Symptoms or disorders that are voluntarily produced for conscious reasons of personal gain (separate from factitious).

Melancholia—Severe, anhedonic depression (implies an endogenous source).

Metaphorical Language—Idiosyncratic communication meaningful only to those familiar with the speaker's (e.g., a child's) past experience.

Micropsia—The illusion that objects are smaller than they actually are.

Milestones—The significant accomplishments of human growth and development (e.g., walking unassisted, speaking in sentences), especially the ages at which they occur.

Monoamine Oxidase Inhibitors (MAOI)—In psychopharmacology, a class of antidepressant medications.

Monozygotic—Refers to multiple fetuses (e.g., identical twins) developed from a single zygote.

Mood—Breadth of sustained emotion (e.g., sadness, euphoria); a pervasive and sustained emotion.

Mood Congruent—Apparently consistent with the mood being exhibited (e.g., mood-congruent behavior, mood-congruent delusion).

Mood Incongruent—Not consistent with the mood being exhibited.

Morbid—Occurs during or after an exacerbation of a disease; severe, predisposing to serious illness or other problems (e.g., morbid obesity).

Multiaxial—Refers to several classes of information used in psychiatric evaluation. DSM-IV uses five axes, the first three of which constitute the official diagnostic assessment.

Munchausen's Syndrome—A factitious (i.e., voluntary but unconsciously motivated) disorder or set of symptoms.

Myoclonic—Refers to irregular, brief, usually generalized muscle contractions.

Narcissism—Focus on and regard for oneself, to either a healthy or abnormal extent.

Narcotic Antagonist—A drug that counteracts the physiological effect of a narcotic.

Necrophilia—Reliance on dead sexual objects (in reality or fantasy) as a primary source of sexual stimulation.

Negative Symptoms—With repect to Schizophrenia, often subtle but pervasive absence of normal thought or behavior, as differentiated from presence of abnormal symptoms. Negative symptoms include absence of normal affect or social interaction, as differentiated from presence of hallucinations or delusions.

Negativism—Active or passive resistance, for example, to movement (as in catatonia) or to verbal responsiveness (as in autism).

Neologism—A "word" invented by an individual, often having an idiosyncratic meaning.

Neuroleptic—In common usage, refers to antipsychotic medication; also, a neuroleptic medication.

Neurotic—Refers to internal, unconscious conflict; also refers to a neurosis (e.g., a neurotic disorder or conflict characterized by unconscious defense mechanisms).

Neurotic Defense Mechanism—An unconscious pattern of feelings, thoughts, or behaviors designed to prevent or alleviate anxiety that stems from internal conflict. The presence of this pattern—in combinations called defensive systems—is generally normal and adaptive, but in many people it reaches maladaptive proportions. Examples include denial, displacement, intellectualization, projection, rationalization, reaction formation, and undoing. All defense mechanisms involve repression, which is the mechanism by which the person prevents unconscious material from reaching awareness. Some writers describe some defense mechanisms as voluntary. Lists of defense mechanisms vary from text to text.

Nihilistic—Refers to nonexistence or lack of existence (e.g., of oneself).

Nonrestorative Sleep—Sleep that does not satisfy one's need for sleep.

Nystagmus—A specific, rhythmic motion of the eyeballs, sometimes in response to certain neurological tests.

Obsession—A persistent, intrusive thought.

Opioid—In pharmacology, any class of drugs or other substances with actions similar to opium (e.g., heroin, meperidine).

Overt—Open, easily seen.

Palilalia—Pathological repeating of one's own sounds or words.

Parallel Play—In young children, play with another child, but not involving interpersonal interaction.

Paranoia—A condition of oversuspiciousness, sometimes to a grossly unrealistic, even psychotic extent; old term (usually *paranoia vera*) for Delusional Disorder.

Paraphilia—Any of a class of recurrent, intense, pervasive sexual urges or fantasies that are associated with psychosocial dysfunction and/or are not socially acceptable; commonly synonymous with sexual deviation.

Paresthesia—Numbness or tingling, usually of the extremities.

Partialism—In paraphilias, focus on specific nonsexual parts of the body as a primary source of sexual stimulation.

Passive-Aggressive—Unconscious aggressive impulses manifested in passive ways (e.g., by obstructing progress or purposeful inefficiency).

Pathognomonic—Refers to a symptom or sign that is found in only one disease or disorder, and in no other.

Pathological Intoxication—Intoxication, generally from alcohol, in response to only a small amount of intoxicant, and out of proportion to that amount.

Pathophysiology—Organic abnormality related to disease.

Pavor Nocturnus—Sleep terrors (q.v.).

Perseveration—Persistent, often rhythmic repetition of words or ideas, not generally controllable by the individual.

Personality Trait—Enduring patterns of perceiving, relating to, and thinking about the environment and oneself, exhibited in a wide range of social and personal contexts.

Pervasive—Broadly and comprehensively found; involving all or almost all things.

Petit Mal—A form of seizure that involves loss of consciousness with impulsive movements (also Petite Mal).

Phenomenologic—Refers to descriptions or descriptive characteristics. DSM-IV descriptions of disorders are often phenomenological (i.e., based on observations) rather than etiological (based on cause).

Phenothiazine—In psychopharmacology, a class of antipsychotic medications.

Phobia—A persistent, irrational, morbid fear of an object or an activity, recognized by the individual as unreasonable but nevertheless leading to significant avoidance of the phobic object.

Piloerection—Stiffening or raising of the hair on one's body.

Postpartum—After delivery of one's child.

Poverty of Speech—Restricted quantity of speech. Differentiated from poverty of speech content, which implies adequate quantity but little information.

Premorbid—Before the onset of illness.

Preoccupation—A repetitive, often continuous thought or focus of one's thoughts (see also Obsessive).

Presenium—The period just before old age.

Pressure of Speech/Pressured Speech—Accelerated, often loud and emphatic speech which is difficult to stop and may continue even in the absence of a listener.

Prevalence—In epidemiology, the number of cases present in a population at or during a particular time (see also Incidence).

Primary Gain—The unconscious gratification, from alleviation of neurotic conflict, that motivates neurotic behaviors (e.g., somatoform symptoms) (see also Secondary Gain).

Prodromal—Premonitory; preparatory.

Prognosis—A prediction of the outcome of an illness or disorder, based on clinical experience with similar cases.

Pseudodementia—A dementia-like syndrome not actually related to organic illness.

Pseudologia Fantastica—Telling of elaborate, intriguing lies.

Psychoactive—In pharmacology, having some effect on the psyche, emotions, or psychiatric/psychological symptoms.

Psychogenic—Caused by the emotions or psyche.

Psychomotor—A combination of physical and mental functions.

Psychomotor Agitation—Continuous activity (often with pacing, wringing of the hands, or inability to sit still) related to emotional distress.

Psychomotor Retardation—General slowing of emotional and physical responses.

Psychosocial—Refers to a combination of psychological and social factors or interventions.

Psychosomatic—Refers to the interaction between the mind and body, especially illnesses in which emotional disorder or conflict gives rise to, or significantly affects, physical signs or symptoms. Closely related or identical to psychophysiological, in which physiological mechanisms are affected by emotional factors.

Psychotic—Refers to serious impairment in reality testing, with inaccurate perceptions and/or thoughts about external reality (implying the creation of a new, internal reality).

Querulous Paranoia—A delusion of injustice that one feels must be remedied by legal action.

Reactive—Refers to symptoms associated with, or exacerbated by, one's external environment (as opposed to the intrapsychic environment); more specifically, emotional symptoms that change (e.g., get better or worse) with changes in the external environment (see also Endogenous).

Recent Memory—In the mental status examination, memory for items or names 3 to 5 minutes after hearing them.

Receptive—In language, refers to the taking in, processing, and interpretation of sensory input, generally words.

Reciprocal Play—In children, play that involves interacting with another child (see also Parallel Play).

Reflex Memory—See Immediate Memory.

Remission—Abatement of symptoms, commonly to the point at which no indication of disease is present (but it is not considered cured).

Remote Memory—In the mental status examination, memory for items or events that occurred in the distant past.

Residual Phase—When referring to psychiatric illness, the part of the course in which acute or florid symptoms are no longer present.

Rhinorrhea—Nasal discharge.

Ritualistic—Refers to an activity, usually repetitive, employed for a magical or anxiety-relieving, often idiosyncratic purpose.

"Rum Fits"—Seizures precipitated by alcohol withdrawal.

Rumination—Obsessive repeating of a thought or idea; in infants, regurgitation and reswallowing of food.

Scanning—A condition, often associated with hypervigilance, in which a person tries intensively to be aware of his or her environment, in fear or anticipation of an anxiety-producing event.

Scapegoating—In families or groups, the involuntary appointing of one member to represent the pathological characteristics of the group.

Scatologia—Lewd or obscene speech.

Seasonal Depression—Depression whose symptoms are regularly associated with a particular time of year, usually winter (cf., Seasonal Affective Disorder).

Secondary Gain—Indirect gratification or reward, not consciously sought, from illness or symptoms. Easily confused with Primary Gain (q.v.) and with direct rewards for malingered symptoms.

Seizure Equivalent—Motor, sensory, autonomic, or emotional feelings or behavior that are ictal in nature. Also called Epileptic Equivalent.

Self-esteem—Regard for oneself.

Self-image—One's mental picture of oneself, particularly with regard to strengths, weaknesses, expectations, and ethics.

Senium—Old age.

Sensory—Related to the senses (e.g., sight, smell, touch); differentiated from motor.

Sign—A manifestation of a pathological condition observed (directly or indirectly) by an examiner rather than subjectively experienced by the individual. Separate from symptoms (q.v.).

Simple Schizophrenia—A non–DSM-IV classification that refers to a form of schizophrenia without florid symptoms.

Simple Tic—Reasonably delimited tics, such as eye blinking, grimacing (see also Complex Tic).

Sleep Apnea—Any of several physiologically based conditions in which one stops breathing while asleep.

Sleep Paralysis—Inability to move just before falling asleep, or just after awakening.

Sleep-related Myoclonus—Myoclonus that occurs exclusively during, or is related to, sleep.

Sleeptalking—A non-REM parasomnia similar to, and probably related to, sleepwalking.

Somatic—Refers to the body or human biology.

Somatopsychic—Refers to psychological symptoms caused or exacerbated by somatic illness or injury.

Speech Melody—The intonation or inflection of one's speech.

"Speedball"—Any of several combinations of abusable drugs, especially cocaine and heroin mixed in a syringe.

Stammering—An impairment in speech fluency similar to stuttering.

Startle Response—A condition, often related to hypervigilance (q.v.), in which an individual reacts abruptly, and out of proportion, to a minor physical stimulus.

Stereotyped/Stereotypic—Refers to movements or verbalizations repeated mechanically, without apparent purpose (see also Ritualistic).

Stressor—An object or situation, real or symbolic, that gives rise to stress.

Stuporous—Physically and verbally unresponsive, especially because of an illness, intoxication, injury, or altered state of consciousness.

Subacute—Having the potential to become acute; likely to become acute.

Superego—In common usage, the *conscience*; in psychoanalytic theory, that portion of the psyche formed by identification with and introjection of parental characteristics that foster ethics, empathy, and self-criticism.

Surrogate—Substitute.

Symbolic—Substituting for a real feeling, memory, object, or event. In a psychodynamic context, the thing symbolized is unconscious, and the symbol may bear only an indirect relationship to it.

Sympathomimetic—Refers to a substance whose action mimics that of the sympathetic nervous system.

Symptom—An outward manifestation of pathological condition, perceived by the patient, especially subjective complaint.

Syndrome—A group of symptoms and/or signs associated with each other (but not necessarily occurring at the same time), sometimes suggesting a particular disorder or diagnosis.

Tangential—Refers to thoughts or words that depart from the current train of thought in an oblique or irrelevant way.

Terminal Insomnia—Awakening significantly earlier than planned, with an inability to return to sleep.

Thought Broadcasting—The delusion that one's thoughts can be heard by others.

Thought Insertion—The delusion that others have placed thoughts in one's mind.

Thought Withdrawal—The delusion that thoughts have been removed from one's mind.

Tic—An involuntary, rapid, recurrent, nonrhythmic, stereotyped motor movement or vocalization.

Tolerance—In pharmacology, physical habituation to a drug (prescribed or not), leading to loss of its effect unless the dose is increased (not synonymous with addiction); generally, loss of effectiveness of a particular treatment or stimulus at its current level.

Toucherism—Frotteurism, but sometimes distinguished from Frotteurism by its fondling characteristics.

"Trailing"—The auditory illusion that sounds echo or persist.

Trance—A nonorganic alteration of consciousness, produced voluntarily (e.g., during hypnosis) or involuntarily (e.g., during a dissociative disorder).

Transsexualism—One's deep and persistent belief that one's physical gender is inappropriate, and that he (or, more rarely, she) should be of the opposite sex. It is accompanied by marked gender dysphoria and a near-constant wish to change one's gender. Transsexualism should be differentiated from transvestism and ordinary homosexuality.

Transvestic Fetishism (Transvestism)—A paraphilia in which cross-dressing (e.g., a male wearing typically female clothing) is prominent; should be differentiated from transsexualism and homosexuality.

Trichophagy—The mouthing or eating of one's hair.

Tricyclic—In psychopharmacology, a class of antidepressant medications.

Unconscious—Out of awareness; not under voluntary control; that part of the psyche not available to voluntary control or awareness.

Urophilia—Reliance on urine as a primary source of sexual gratification.

Vertigo—A feeling of dizziness, usually including the sensation that one's environment or oneself is spinning.

Visual Tracking—Following objects with one's eyes.

Voluntary—Under conscious control.

Vorbeireden—A psychological symptom involving giving approximate answers or talking past the point, done consciously in Factitious Disorder and unconsciously in Ganser's syndrome.

Waxy Flexibility—A symptom of catatonia characterized by the ability of an examiner to move the patient's body or limbs into different positions, which are then held indefinitely by the patient (also Cerea Flexibilitas).

Wernicke's Encephalopathy—Central nervous system dysfunction due to thiamine deficiency, as in chronic alcoholism (part of the Wernicke-Korsakoff syndrome).

Zoophilia—Reliance on sexual activity with nonhuman animals (in reality or fantasy) as one's primary source of sexual stimulation.

INDEX

**The Complete DSM-IV TRAINING PROGRAM
for use with the
DSM-IV Training Guide
by
William H. Reid, M.D., M.P.H.,
and
Michael G. Wise, M.D., F.A.C.P.**

The *Complete DSM-IV Training Program* consists of a hard-cover edition of the *DSM-IV Training Guide*, the two-volume *Video-taped Clinical Vignettes,* and either a set of 35 mm slides, or a set of overhead transparencies. The copy that appears on either the *Overhead Transparencies* or the *Instructional Slides* is identical, and is keyed by circled numbers (3) in the margins of this book. To order, contact the publisher:

**Brunner/Mazel, Inc.
19 Union Square West
New York, NY 10003**

(800) 825-3089; (212) 924-3344; Fax: (212) 242-6339

NOTES

NOTES

NOTES

NOTES